MW01200792

An Introduction to

HEALTHCARE
and
MEDICAL TEXTILES

Wen Zhong, Ph.D.
University of Manitoba

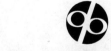

DES*tech* Publications, Inc.

An Introduction to Healthcare and Medical Textiles

DEStech Publications, Inc.
439 North Duke Street
Lancaster, Pennsylvania 17602 U.S.A.

Copyright © 2013 by DEStech Publications, Inc.
All rights reserved

No part of this publication may be reproduced, stored in a
retrieval system, or transmitted, in any form or by any means,
electronic, mechanical, photocopying, recording, or otherwise,
without the prior written permission of the publisher.

Printed in the United States of America
10   9   8   7   6   5   4   3   2   1

Main entry under title:
    An Introduction to Healthcare and Medical Textiles

A DEStech Publications book
Bibliography: p.
Includes index p. 285

ISBN No. 978-1-60595-020-4

HOW TO ORDER THIS BOOK

BY PHONE: 877-500-4337 or 717-290-1660, 9AM–5PM Eastern Time

BY FAX: 717-509-6100

BY MAIL: Order Department
DEStech Publications, Inc.
439 North Duke Street
Lancaster, PA 17602, U.S.A.

BY CREDIT CARD: American Express, VISA, MasterCard, Discover

BY WWW SITE: http://www.destechpub.com

To
my father (Liangming Zhong)
my mother (Feifei Yin)
my husband (Malcolm Xing)
and my children (Harvey and Max)

Table of Contents

Preface

FOR eight years at University of Manitoba I've been teaching two courses related to what I am writing about: *Textiles for the Healthcare Sectors* and *Advanced Textiles for the Healthcare Sectors*. All these years, I've tried in vain to find for my students a textbook that is commercially available. Dealing with an interdisciplinary topic, I've been trying to accommodate the needs of students for such varied areas as materials (including textiles) science and engineering, biomedical engineering, and health studies. On the one hand, students with a background in materials science and engineering may have difficulties understanding the basic mechanisms of the interaction between biotextiles and host cells/tissues; on the other hand, students without the background in textiles may get confused with the various textile structures, including wovens, knits and different types of nonwovens. Similarly, when I am approached by graduate students or professionals in the areas of Materials Science or Biomedicine for a book that will give them some background knowledge about fibers and textiles and how their structures and properties influence their biomedical applications, I've had similar difficulties recommending sources that are tailored to their needs. Such experience has caused me to believe that it is a good idea to write a book of this nature.

The text of this book is organized into two parts besides the first introductory chapter. Four chapters dealing with the basics of what is involved in the area of healthcare textiles comprise Part I. The six-chapter Part II addresses the various applications of healthcare/medical textiles.

Introductory in nature, this is a textbook for students but, since it also includes the latest developments in the related areas, it also suits

the needs of professionals who happen to want to learn the basics of
fibers and textile structures that can be used in the healthcare sectors,
as well as information on design and product development in medical
and healthcare textiles. To that end, I have tried to connect the basics
of textile engineering and related concepts to the design and development of textile materials and structures for medical end uses. The text
of the book is prepared in such a way as to accommodate readers with
different backgrounds and intentions, and those who wish to get deeper
into a related subject discussed in the book can refer themselves to the
abundant literature at the end of each chapter. Specifically, this book is
intended to benefit:

1. Senior undergraduate students or graduate students in the disci-
   plines of Textile Sciences, Materials Science and Engineering, or
   Biomedical Engineering who need a textbook or reference book;
2. Professionals in medical/healthcare textile product development
   who may find a handbook of this nature useful; and
3. Other professionals (in Materials Science and Engineering, Biomedical Engineering, or Biomedicine) who now and again need to
   know something about textiles.

At the close of my endeavor, I wish to extend my appreciation to the
individuals and parties that have made this book possible. The book
would never have been written or be like what it is now had it not been
for the opportunity provided by Faculty of Human Ecology, University
of Manitoba, an opportunity that has involved me in an interdisciplinary field, provided me valuable interactions and collaborations with researchers in the many related areas, and thus had me well prepared. I
also wish to extend thanks to undergraduate and graduate students that
I have been working with in the past seven years in my courses about
medical textiles. They have had to deal with a situation where the essential *textbook* is so miserably lacking that they have had to learn their
lessons depending on handouts and copies of reading materials from
various sources, never making a complaint. Instead, their inputs and
suggestions have been valuable for the improvement of the courses,
and have certainly functioned as a pat on my back during my efforts to
teach and write. I also wish to say a word of thanks to faculty colleagues
who have reviewed my book in such a way as to be in a position to help
eliminate errors and suggest improvement; they are, especially, Drs. &
Professors Lena Horne and Michael Eskin.

Special thanks are due to my family—people who have provided any type of support I need. Among them, my father, Professor Liangming Zhong, has been the first reader of my draft book and has tried to make sure that this book can be understood by those who are totally outside of the field; my husband and collaborator, Dr. Mengqiu (Malcolm) Xing, a professional of Biomaterials and Regenerative Medicine, has provided insights as such.

Finally I wish to express my appreciation to *you,* readers of the book, who are the ones most likely and able to offer comments and suggestions essential for improvement to be made in the future, which will benefit all who will use the book, including my students and me as a teacher. So let me know such comments and suggestions, please. Please contact me at zhong@cc.umanitoba.ca.

It is proper to make known that any reference within this book to any specific commercial or non-commercial product or process by trade name, trade mark, manufacturer or otherwise does not constitute or imply an endorsement, recommendation, or favoring by the author.

WEN ZHONG

CHAPTER 1

Introduction

W^HAT are healthcare and medical textiles? It is the first question that must be answered in this book. The Textile Institute (UK) defines *medical textiles* as "a general term which describes a textile structure which has been designed and produced for use in any of a variety of medical applications, including implantable applications" (Denton, 2002). Following the same line of thinking, we can define *healthcare textiles* as textile structures designed and produced for use in the various healthcare sectors. Although there are slightly different implications between the practices of medicine and healthcare, the two terms, medical textiles and healthcare textiles, are often used together or interchangeably, and will be treated as such in this textbook.

Healthcare and medical textiles are a major growth area within the scope of *technical textiles,* which is defined as "textile materials and products manufactured primarily for their technical performance and functional properties rather than their aesthetic or decoration characteristics" (Denton, 2002). Technical textiles include, in addition to healthcare and medical textiles, aerospace, industrial, marine, military, safety and transport textiles and geotextiles (Horrocks and Anand, 2000; Denton, 2002). Over the last few decades, there have been significant changes in the textile market, where traditional textile products, or the textile products produced primarily for their aesthetic or decoration properties (e.g., *apparel*), account for an increasingly smaller portion, while technical textile products constitute an increasingly larger portion.

According to the end use survey reports on the use of fiber quantities (manufactured and natural fibers) released by the U.S. Fiber Economics Bureau, the market share of apparel dropped dramatically from 35% to 15% between 1999 and 2010. Home textiles also showed sizable shrinkage in the market, from 16% to 8%. On the contrary, floor cover-

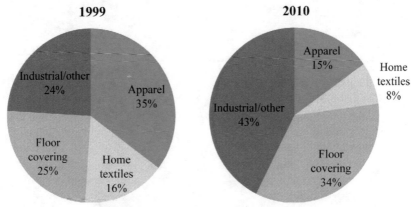

FIGURE 1.1. *Market shares of end use categories.*

ing increased its share from 25% to 34%, and industrial and other consumer-type textile products demonstrated the largest increase in market share, from 24% to 43%, as shown in Figure 1.1 (Horn, 2011). According to U.S. Fiber Economics Bureau, the category of industrial and other consumer-type textile products overlap a major portion of technical textile products, including narrow fabrics, medical, surgical and sanitary products (excluding sutures), transportation fabrics, tires, hose, belting, electrical applications and reinforced plastics, felts, filtration, sewing thread (including medical sutures), rope, cordage and fishline, bags and bagging, coated and protective fabrics, paper and tape reinforcing, fiberfill, stuffing and flock, and unallocated nonwovens. Figure

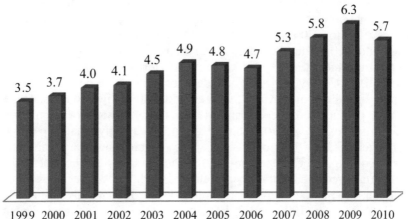

FIGURE 1.2. *Market share of medical, surgical and sanitary products (sutures not included).*

1.2 also shows a steady increase of market share of medical, surgical and sanitary products (excluding sutures) in the last decade.

1.1. MATERIALS FOR HEALTHCARE AND MEDICAL TEXTILES

Traditionally, a textile product starts from such raw materials as natural or synthetic fibers. Fibers are spun into yarns and then woven or knitted into fabrics. After the dyeing and/or finishing processes, the fabrics can be further turned into a product like apparel, bed sheets or curtains.

The last century witnessed the creation and commercialization of a number of synthetic fibers, which helped bring about the mass production of textile fibers with better performances and specific functional attributes, including better mechanical strength, thermal/chemical resistance, and UV/microorganism resistance. These advantages expanded the end uses of textile materials, especially of technical textile products.

With the progress of materials science and related research work in the last few decades, new fibrous materials (created or as a result of modifications on existing fiber materials) are now available and are being applied in a vast variety of end uses. A striking example is the application of new biocompatible and biodegradable polymer and fiber materials in surgical implants. Modifications on existing fiber materials, both physical and chemical, allow end products to perform such important functions as absorption or cause them to be antibacterial, flame retardant or antistatic.

New fabrication methods have also been developed to create fibrous structures other than woven and knit. For example, nonwoven technology has enabled the manufacturing of fabrics without the yarn spinning process, which not only substantially reduces production cost but also causes the end products to have porous and highly absorbent structures to meet the requirement of hygiene products. The technology of electrospinning allows the production of ultrafine fibers in the size of nanometers, which is way beyond the capacity of traditional fiber spinning technology. Combination of a fibrous material and another material such as polymer, metal or ceramic helps produce various kinds of composite materials that will bring about a synergy between two dissimilar materials.

Due to these new technologies, a much wider range of textile materials, structures and processing techniques are now available for the design and development of advanced products for many purposes, including healthcare and medical applications. As a result, readers of this book will be exposed to a vast variety of materials and structures that are not used for traditional textile products, or for other technical textile products, but are especially suitable for medical and healthcare purposes. Readers will also learn that design principles and evaluation criteria for these special-purpose textile materials differ significantly from those for other applications. To facilitate such understanding, Part I of the book will be devoted to the discussion of such basics for the healthcare and medical textiles: Chapter 2 briefly introduces the fundamentals of textile materials and structures, and how these textile components may be used in the design and development of healthcare and medical products; Chapter 3 discusses medical and healthcare nanofibers, which are not produced via traditional textile processing methods but are of importance in the development of a variety of biomedical textile products. The following two chapters focus on important design criteria for healthcare and medical textiles. Chapter 4 emphasizes textile-related comfort issues and healthcare problems, which are essential for the design and development of medical and healthcare textiles for external end uses; Chapter 5, on the other hand, concentrates on biocompatibility, biostability, and bioresorbability, which are critical criteria for the design of any medical textile product for internal applications.

1.2. APPLICATIONS OF HEALTHCARE AND MEDICAL TEXTILES

Healthcare and medical textiles are found in a wide variety of applications. A non-exhaustive list of these is given here and is discussed in greater detail in Part II of the book.

Hygiene is critical in the practices of healthcare and medicine to prevent diseases and infections and to preserve health. Various textile products are available to facilitate hygiene in both personal life and in healthcare facilities. Highly absorbent products, mostly disposables, have been used to retain body fluids/waste to keep skin surfaces clean and dry. Depending on their end users, they are referred to as *diapers, sanitary napkins* or *incontinent pads.* The development of these products has gone through a long journey; improvements of product performance in terms of absorbency and comfort continue to be made. Since use of these products often has environmental consequences, the discussion will naturally encompass related issues, especially those associated with the so-called *disposables.* For more details about *hygiene textiles,* see Chapter 6.

Since we have extremely tender *skin* as opposed to our audaciously hard surroundings, for many hundred years, we humans have dreamed of having it assisted by something that is as light as cloth but as strong as iron, able to keep us warm and *protect* us as well! Nowadays such wonder clothes/devices are no longer miracles. The last few decades witnessed the development of high performance fibers/fabrics, which, due to their specially-engineered structures or finishes, have rendered a clothing system "protective". Also, depending on the nature of external hazards, different types of protective clothes have been developed to keep us safe from extremely high/low temperatures, mechanical impact, harmful chemicals, microorganisms, insects, UV radiation, and so on, as a result of our having rendered them *fireproof, bulletproof, waterproof, dust-impermeable,* etc. More detailed information on *protective textiles,* especially those used in the medical/healthcare sectors, will be given in Chapter 7.

A large part of the practice of medicine is to aid healing. The treatment of an open wound to facilitate its healing usually involves the use of wound care products like wound dressings. Numerous wound care products are now available on the market to treat wounds of different types and with diverse severity. Many of these are in textile structures. More details about *wound care textiles* can be found in Chapter 8.

Replacement, reparation or regeneration of injured or diseased human tissues or organs has long been a challenge in the practice of medicine. Tremendous progress has been made in the area of tissue or organ transplantations, which save or improve the life of millions of people every year. However, the severe shortage of donors for tissue/ organ transplantation makes it critical to develop alternative means. As a result, implantable biomaterials, including *biotextiles* (see Chapter 9), have been developed to be used in a biological environment to replace or repair the damaged human tissues/organs or to assist such repairing processes: sutures are used to close surgical wounds, and vascular grafts, ligament prostheses and hernia repair mesh grafts are also used clinically. However, for most of the grafts made of biotextiles (or other biomaterials)—especially those for permanent implants—their performances are still far from being satisfactory in terms of biocompatibility and biostability. As a promising effort to overcome the drawbacks of current grafts made from biomaterials, tissue engineering approaches aim at developing biological substitutes for the repair or replacement of damaged human tissues or organs. In such a process, appropriate living cells are seeded on a matrix or scaffold and then guided to develop into a new and functional living tissue for implantation. A number of such products, known as *bioengineered grafts,* are already used in clinics. More details about these *tissue engineered grafts* are provided in Chapter 10.

Recent advances in nanotechnology, electronics, materials science and the collaboration among scientists in these fields have resulted in the development of *smart* or *intelligent* textiles that can sense and/or respond to mechanical, light, thermal, chemical, electrical and magnetic stimuli. This is possible because, since these stimuli are able to change the appearances (e.g., color) and/or structures of the smart materials incorporated into the textiles during their fabrication, these changes will emit a warning signal (e.g., a flashing light). Smart textiles may have applications in such end uses as sports/recreation or special work wear for first responders or for use in extreme environments (e.g., space exploration), where early signals of distress would enable timely interventions. More commonly and to the benefit of still more people, they can be used by people whose heartbeat, respiration, blood oxygen saturation, temperature or body motion needs monitoring. Chapter 11 provides a detailed discussion about medical/healthcare *smart textiles*.

1.3. SUMMARY

To a large degree, progress of textile science and technology comes hand in hand with the expanding application of textile materials and structures. Traditional textile products, or those manufactured primarily for their aesthetic or decorative properties, have been shrinking greatly in their market share of fiber usage. On the other hand, interdisciplinary collaboration between textile science and technology and other fields (e.g., engineering, architecture, biology and medicine) have resulted in the creation of technical textiles, covering such sectors as transportation, architecture, sports and medicine.

The future of the textile science and industry lies in the development of new advanced textile materials and structures to meet the demanding needs in the various fields. Among them, medical/healthcare textiles have been one of the most rapidly-growing sectors for a number of years. Born from the marriage of textile science and medicine, these new textiles help prevent and cure diseases or injuries. Aimed at the promotion of human health, the research and development of medical/ healthcare textiles have attracted enormous attention and effort. This book will give a description, as comprehensive as possible, of the wide variety of textiles for medical and healthcare end uses.

1.4. REFERENCES

Denton, M.J. (2002). Textile terms and definitions, 11th Ed. Manchester, UK: Textile Institute.

Horn, F. (2011). Market share of end use categories. *In:* Fiber Organon. Arlington, VA: Fiber Economics Bureau.

Horrocks, A.R. and S. Anand. (2000). Handbook of technical textiles. Boca Raton, FL: CRC Press/Woodhead Pub.

Part I
Basics

CHAPTER 2

Textile Materials and Structures

THIS chapter contains the basics of textile materials and structures, especially those used in healthcare and medical textiles. They are reinforced by discussions of the contribution of the characteristics of these textile materials and structures to the functionality of the products and their special end uses.

2.1. MATERIALS AND STRUCTURES USED FOR HEALTHCARE AND MEDICAL TEXTILE PRODUCTS

Textile is defined as "a general term for fibers, yarn intermediates, yarns, fabrics, and products that retain all the strength, flexibility, and other typical properties of the original fiber or filaments" (ASTM, 2008). In other words, textiles are made from the basic elements of fibers. However, to develop healthcare and medical textiles, materials other than textiles have to be included. This makes it necessary, at the very beginning, to list related materials and structures that comprise healthcare and medical textiles. In Figure 2.1, they are shown in such a way that each lower-level constituent component (i.e., *raw material*) is related by an arrow to a higher-level component (i.e., *transformation,* or *product*) that is composed of the lower one. If a component, whatever its rank, is related by several arrows to several higher components, they are each and all composed of that lower one as a constituent component.

Shown also in Figure 2.1 is a chain of traditional textile transformation processes (highlighted in bold text): *fibers* composed of natural or synthetic *polymers* are spun into *yarns,* followed by being woven or knitted into *fabrics* and further fabricated into specific *products,* including *apparel.*

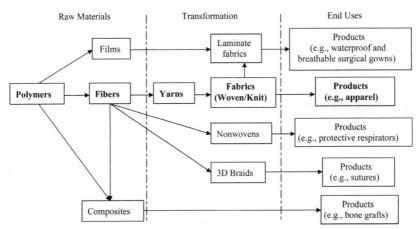

FIGURE 2.1. *Materials and structures used for healthcare and medical textile products.*

Beyond that, there is a variety of structures that are more often used in technical end uses: laminated fabrics can be made by bonding a fabric(s) with a polymeric film(s)/foam(s) by using an adhesive or by the adhesive properties of one of the layers. By controlling the pore sizes in micro-porous films, waterproof but breathable (i.e., water vapor permeable) fabrics can be obtained. Such fabrics are desirable in applications like surgical gowns, where both protection (e.g., against body fluid through which diseases may be transmitted) and comfort are essential. Fibers can also be directly processed into nonwoven fabrics, in which fibers are bonded together via mechanical, thermal or chemical means. Skipping the yarn-spinning procedures, nonwoven fabrics are known for their low cost, making them desirable for applications in disposable hygiene and protective products. Filaments can be braided into 3-dimensional (3D) braids for specific products that require exceptional mechanical properties in the longitudinal direction. Sutures and ligament prostheses are two examples of medical textile products made of braids. Fiber-reinforced composites are another form of structure that can be used for products that require both excellent tensile and compression strength, which can be realized through the synergy effects of the two components that constitute the composite material. Periodontal and bone grafts, for example, can be made of such composite materials.

Although processed through different routes, as listed in Figure 2.1, textile products are entirely or partially composed of fiber materials. In this book, ANY product, device, material or structure that is for medical and healthcare use and is made of fiber materials will be included in the discussion.

The following sections constitute a discussion of the various components of textiles as listed above, and of their proven or potential applications in the medical and healthcare sectors.

2.2. POLYMERS

All fibers are made of macromolecules or *polymers* (in which *poly* means "many" while *mer* refers to "repeating units"). A polymer is formed when hundreds or thousands of small molecules (units) are covalently bonded, usually into a linear chain. A repeating unit of a polymer is known as *monomer*. The number of repeating units in a polymer chain is called the *degree of polymerization*.

2.2.1. Types of Polymers

Polymers can be categorized in different ways according to their structures. They can be divided into homopolymers, copolymers or block polymers, as shown in Figure 2.2. A *homopolymer* is composed of one monomer [as represented by the symbol A in Figure 2.2(a)] that repeats itself throughout the polymer chain. Most of the general-use fibers, including cotton, rayon, wool, silk, polyester, nylon, and polypropylene fibers, are composed of homopolymers. A *copolymer* usually contains two or more monomers [e.g., symbols A and B represent two different monomers in Figure 2.2(b)] that appear alternatively along the polymer chain. Acrylic fibers are composed of copolymers. A *block polymer* has two or more repeating blocks or segments along the polymer chain, each of which is a homopolymer, as shown in Figure 2.2(c). Spandex fibers are made of block polymers.

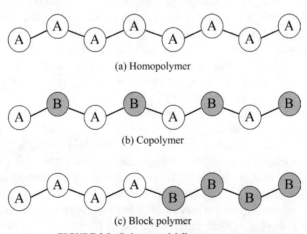

(a) Homopolymer

(b) Copolymer

(c) Block polymer

FIGURE 2.2. *Polymers of different structures.*

Polymers can be either thermoplastic or non-thermoplastic polymers. *Thermoplastic polymers* will soften and melt when heated and harden when allowed to cool down, with their polymeric structure remaining intact if the temperature is below that for their decomposition. Polyester, nylon and polypropylene fibers are composed of thermoplastic polymers. Cellulosic, acrylic and aramid fibers, on the other hand, are made of *non-thermoplastic polymers,* and will not soften or melt before irreversible decomposition occurs. These thermal properties may determine the way in which the manufactured fibers can be produced. Thermoplastic polymers can be spun into fibers via *melt spinning,* whereby a molten polymer is extruded through the holes in a spinneret, and then solidifies while traveling in the cool air to form fibers. Non-thermoplastic polymers cannot be processed by melt spinning. They are usually dissolved in appropriate solvents. The polymer solution will be extruded through the spinneret into a hot air or liquid bath, so that the solvents will be evaporated in the hot air (in the case of *dry spinning*) or extracted by the liquid bath (*wet spinning*) to yield fibers.

2.2.2. Structures and Properties of Fiber Polymers

The performance of fibrous materials originates from the structures and properties of their constituent polymers. The backbone of most polymers for textile fibers contains covalently bonded carbon atoms (C). Other atoms such as oxygen (O) and nitrogen (N) may also appear in the polymer backbone and be covalently bonded to carbon atoms. The atoms in the backbone can be covalently bonded to hydrogen atoms (H) and other side groups.

Polymer chains are arranged in certain ways to form a fiber. In a linear polymer structure, the degree of parallelism of the chain molecules to the fiber axis is referred to as *degree of orientation.* On the other hand, a polymer chain may run through different regions in a fiber with different packing density (Figure 2.3). Polymer chains pack tightly in an orderly fashion in the so-called *crystalline regions,* while distributing loosely in a disordered pattern in the *amorphous regions.* The highly packed crystalline regions contribute to the mechanical strength of the fiber, while the loosely packed amorphous regions allow the uptake of water molecules or other chemicals that may be incorporated into the textile products (e.g., dyes, finishing agents). As a result, a high degree of orientation and crystallinity usually contribute to high mechanical strength, low elasticity, and low absorbency.

Various interactions are involved within a polymer chain and between the polymer chains that constitute a fiber. The atoms within a polymer chain are mostly linked by the *covalent bond,* in which the

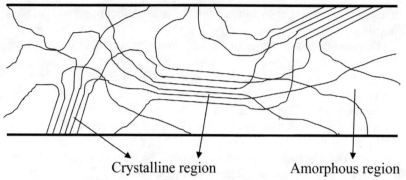

Crystalline region   Amorphous region

FIGURE 2.3. Crystalline and amorphous regions within a fiber.

electrons that are shared by two atoms shift away from the center or stay unchanged due to the difference between the capacities of the two atoms to attract electrons. The tendency for an atom to attract electrons is known as *electronegativity*. The more one atom attracts electrons, the more electronegative it is. O and N are atoms that are very electronegative; O has even higher electronegativity than N. These atoms can pull electrons from atoms with less electronegativity (e.g., C and H) when forming covalent bonds. A covalent bond formed between two atoms with similar electronegativity is referred to as *non-polar covalent bonds*, such as those between two carbon atoms (including single C–C bond in which one pair of electrons are shared between the two atoms, double C=C bond in which two pairs of electrons are shared, and triple C≡C bond in which three pairs of electrons are shared) and between carbon and a hydrogen atoms (C–H). On the other hand, a covalent bond formed between two atoms with different electronegativity is called a polar covalent bond, like C–O, C=O, C–N, O–H.

A molecule or a chemical group (i.e., two or more atoms that are bonded together as a single unit to appear as a part of a molecule) is usually composed of one of more covalent bonds; it may be regarded as a polar or non-polar molecule (or group) as a result of the arrangement of the bonds. In the simplest case, the polarity of a molecule or group containing only one covalent bond can be determined by the polarity of the bond; for example, carbon monoxide (CO), hydroxyl (–OH) and nitrile (–C≡N) groups are known as polar molecule/groups. For a molecule or group with more than one covalent bond, its polarity depends on the distribution of the bonds: Non-polar molecules or groups may be composed of exclusively non-polar bonds. Examples are polypropylene (Figure 2.10) and methyl groups (–CH$_3$). On the other hand, a molecule or group containing polar bonds is most likely a polar molecule/group (e.g., –COOH carboxyl group), unless the polar bonds are arranged in an asymmetric manner to balance out the polar effect (e.g., CO_2 carbon dioxide).

The polarity of a polymer or its side groups can affect the properties of the polymer. Non-polar groups are usually less reactive than polar groups. Polar groups, such as hydroxyl (–OH), have better affinity to water molecules via the *hydrogen bonds,* which occur between a hydrogen attached to an electronegative atom (e.g., oxygen, nitrogen) of the molecule and an electronegative atom of a different molecule. Hydrogen bonds are the strongest intermolecular forces. Figure 2.4 shows a hydrogen bond between a water molecule (H_2O) and a hydroxyl group in a polymer (e.g., cotton). The high electronegativity of the oxygen renders the oxygen atoms (in both the water molecule and hydroxyl group) slightly negatively charged ($\delta-$) and the hydrogen atoms slightly positively charged ($\delta+$). The oxygen in the water molecule, which has two additional lone electron pairs, may utilize one pair to attract the hydrogen in the hydroxyl group to form a hydrogen bond, and may use the other pair to attract the hydrogen in a second water molecule to form another hydrogen bond. This explains why fibers with polar groups tend to attract water molecules and adhere to them tightly.

Neutral or non-polar molecules attract each other via very weak electrostatic forces, known as *Van der Waals forces,* which is one of the most important long-range forces between macroscopic particles and surfaces. They are general forces that always operate in all materi-

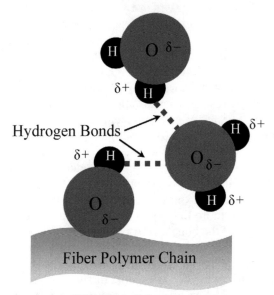

FIGURE 2.4. *Hydrogen bonds.*

als and across interfaces. Van der Waals forces are much weaker than chemical bonds. Random thermal agitation, even at around room temperature, can usually overcome or disrupt them. However, they play an important role in all phenomena involving intermolecular forces, especially those interactions between electrically neutral molecules. Nonpolar polymers, such as polypropylene, attract water to their surfaces via the Van der Waals forces.

2.3. FIBERS

A fiber is the basic, smallest element of a textile material. It is usually long, flexible and extremely thin. Traditionally, a minimum length of 0.5 inch (15 mm) and a length-to-diameter ratio of at least 100 are required for fibers that will be used in spinning and weaving.

The development and introduction of new structures of textiles have made revolutions first in our mind and then in the market, so that nowadays we have, in relation to their origin, *natural* and *man-made* fibers. Natural fibers are derived from plants, animals, or minerals, to be respectively referred to as *cellulosic* fibers, *protein* fibers, and *inorganic* fibers. Man-made fibers are regenerated from natural resources (regenerated fibers) or synthesized from small, organic molecules (synthesized fibers).

2.3.1. Natural Fibers

Natural fiber is defined as "any fiber that exists as such in the natural state" by the Federal Trade Commission (FTC, 1958). Natural fibers include cellulosic fibers and protein fibers. They vary in macroscopic size, length and shape.

2.3.1.1. Cellulosic Fibers

Cellulosic fibers are characteristic of a polymeric structure of linear cellulose, which is composed of β-D-glucose (Figure 2.5). Plenty of hydroxyl groups (–OH) are present in the molecular structure of cellulose. As a result, cellulose fibers are known to be hydrophilic, meaning they are "water-loving", making them absorbent.

Cotton is the most common cellulosic fiber with a white or off-white color. It is a hair of the seed taken from the boll of the cotton plant. Cotton fibers are short or staple fibers with a length in the range of 1/8 to 2.5 inches (0.32–6.35 cm) and a diameter in the range of 16–20 μm (Hatch 1993). Multiple layers exist at a cross section of a cotton fiber, including the outer skin (i.e., the cuticle, which is a thin waxy layer), the

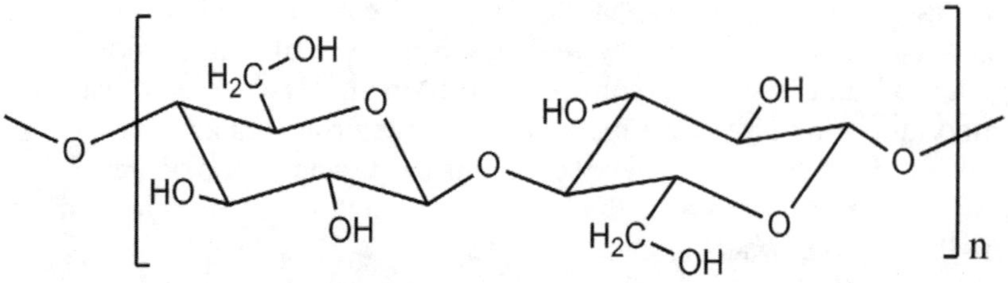

FIGURE 2.5. *The cellulose polymer.*

primary and the secondary cell walls (composed of spiral fibrils, which are natural ultra-fine fibers in nanoscale sizes), and a hollow canal (i.e., lumen). The lumen contains cell sap when the fiber is on a plant. When the sap evaporates, the lumen collapses to render a twisted longitudinal ribbon and kidney-shaped cross section. Mature cotton fibers have smaller lumens than immature cotton fibers.

With its medium stiffness (i.e., resistance of a material to be deformed by an applied force) among all types of fibers, the cotton fabric has a relatively soft touch. The cotton fiber is low in elasticity, which is the ability of a material to stretch under a tensile force and return to its original dimension when the force is removed. The hydrophilic cotton fiber contributes to a reduction of static accumulation in the end products, even at a low humidity. Since cotton is a plant fiber, it is also safe for sensitive skin when no finishes have been applied. For these reasons, cotton has been a desirable choice for products that have contact with the human skin. In the medical textile context, it has been used for ages in products for wound care due to its absorption and comfort.

2.3.1.2. Protein Fibers

Protein fibers are composed of polymers of amino acids (i.e., a group of molecules containing both amine groups [$-NH_2$] and carboxyl groups [$-COOH$]), and are usually derived from animals.

Wool fibers are usually taken from the fleece of the sheep or lamb. They may also refer to fibers taken from the hair of the Angora or Cashmere goat, camel, alpaca, llama and vicuna. By far the most widely used, wool fibers from the sheep vary in color (off-white to brown), length (1.5–15 inches) and fineness (14–70 μm) (Hatch, 1993). They usually have three-dimensional (3D) crimp (i.e., waves, bends, twists or curls along the fiber length). Wool fibers are composed of numerous long and spindle-shaped cells, each of which is composed of countless fibrils. These fibrils are further composed of α-helix keratin (polypeptide) polymers, consisting of a long chain of amino acids arranged in a right-coiled, or spiral, conformation (Figure 2.6), which makes it difficult for the polymer chains to pack closely. The wool fibers are therefore highly amorphous (70–75%) and to a lesser degree crystalline (20–25%).

Wool fibers have the highest capacity of water absorption among commonly-used textile fibers, and are therefore referred to as hygroscopic, owing to the presence of hydrophilic groups (i.e., both amine and carboxyl groups) in the polymer and the high percentage of amorphous regions. On the other hand, wool fibers are low in mechanical strength because of the low percentage of crystalline regions. The three dimensional crimp and α-helix polymer structure give wool its high elasticity and elastic recovery. They consequently are prime candidates for apparel end uses, including sportswear, in cold weather.

A most distinguishing feature of wool fibers is that their surfaces are covered with a layer of scales, which are overlapping surface cells. There are undesirable effects of scaly surfaces. These scales interlock with each other during laundry, leading to considerable shrinkage. They may also cause itchy sensations when placed next to the human skin. There have even been reports on allergic reactions caused by wool fibers (see Chapter 4 for more details); hence their limited applications in the medical or healthcare sectors.

Silk is produced by the larva of cultivated or wild silkworms for the construction of their cocoons. Silk is the only natural filament or continuous fiber, with a length up to 600 m and a fine diameter between 12 and 30 μm (Hatch, 1993). The silk fiber is composed of a protein polymer called fibroin, which consists of amino acids arranged in a pleated β-sheet structure (Figure 2.7). Such a structure allows the poly-

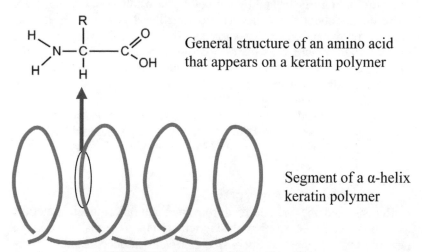

General structure of an amino acid that appears on a keratin polymer

Segment of a α-helix keratin polymer

FIGURE 2.6. *α-helix keratin (polypeptide) polymer.*

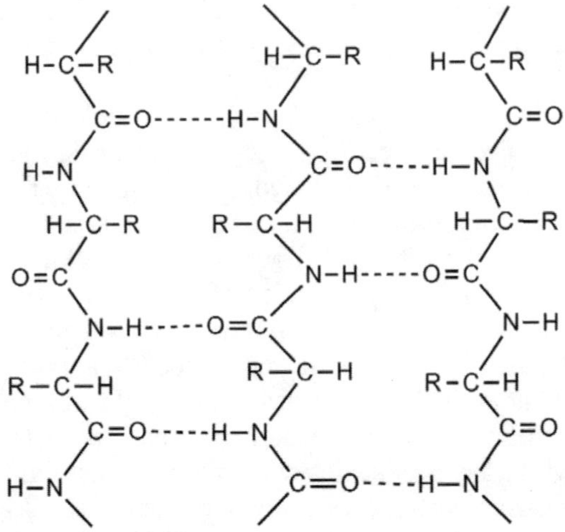

-------- hydrogen bonding

FIGURE 2.7. The pleated β-sheet structure.

mer chains to pack so tightly that the silk fiber is high in terms of its crystalline regions (70–75%), and low in amorphous regions (25–30%).

The surface of silk fibers is covered with a layer of sericin, also referred to as silk gum. Most of the gum on the fiber surface is removed to allow further textile processing procedures. Silk is a hydrophilic fiber. It is very tough (i.e., hard to rupture), has a smooth surface, and has good biocompatibility (i.e., acceptance of an artificial implant by the surrounding tissues and by the body as a whole. See Chapter 5 for more details about this concept). Reasonably, it began to be used as sutures for wound closure as early as 5000–3000 B.C. But silk fibers are no longer regarded as the best choices for sutures because of the undesirable tissue reactions they may induce. More recently, however, studies on silk-based biomaterials suggested that the residual sericin on the silk fibers was the likely cause of these reaction problems. Studies have also revealed that the core silk fibroin fibers exhibit as good biocompatibility as some of the commonly used biomaterials (Altman, Diaz *et al.,* 2003).

2.3.2. Regenerated Fibers

Regenerated fibers are derived from such natural cellulosic materials as wood or bamboo. Along with synthetic fibers (to be discussed in the next section), regenerated fibers are *manufactured* fibers, namely, fibers "derived by a process of manufacture from any substance which, at any point in the manufacturing process, is not a fiber" (FTC, 1958). Regenerated fibers are therefore known also as manufactured cellulosic fibers.

Rayon, or the so-called viscose, artificial silk, is the first manufactured fiber in history, introduced in the 1910s. A manufactured fiber, rayon fibers vary in both diameter and length. The rayon fiber shares the polymer structure with other cellulosic fibers, as shown in Figure 2.1. However, its degree of polymerization (i.e., the number of repeating units in a polymer, as indicated by n in Figure 2.1) is around 400, much lower than that of cotton (6,000–10,000). The short polymer chains make it difficult for them to pack closely with each other. As a result, the rayon fibers have a 60–65% crystalline region, somewhat lower than the cotton fibers (with a 65–70% crystalline region) (Hatch, 1993). On the other hand, rayon fibers have a 35–40% amorphous region, higher than that of the cotton fibers (30–35% amorphous region). As the crystalline region contributes to mechanical strength/stiffness and amorphous region affects the absorbing capacity of a fiber, rayon fibers have lower mechanical strength, lower stiffness and higher water absorption than cotton fibers. In fact, the moisture absorbing capacity of rayon fibers is only second to wool fibers among the regularly used textile fibers. As a result, rayon fibers are softer and more absorbent than cotton fibers, providing a higher level of comfort when used in medical and healthcare textile products. In addition, they do not have any static buildup to cause discomfort or allergic reactions to the skin. They have therefore been used frequently in next-to-skin products, including apparel, bed-sheets, wipes and wound dressings.

Several modifications, or derivatives, of regenerated cellulosic fibers have been developed. For example, cuprammonium rayon fibers are produced by dissolving cellulose in an aqueous cuprammonium hydroxide solvent to form the spinning solution. Acetate fibers are obtained by partially acetylating the hydroxyl groups (i.e., the hydroxyl groups [–OH] are substituted by the acetyl groups [–OCOCH$_3$]) in the cellulose fibers. Triacetate fibers refer to cellulose fibers in which almost all the three hydroxyl groups in the six-membered rings are acetylated. Since the hydroxyl groups in these modified/derived cellulosic fibers are partially or mostly removed, they are less absorbent than other cellulose fibers. In addition to their applications in apparel, these modified cellulose fibers have a special application in the medical/healthcare sectors: hollow fibers for hemodialyzers (known also as artificial kidney; see Chapter 9).

2.3.3. Synthetic Fibers

A synthetic fiber is composed of a polymer originating from small organic molecules via the process of polymerization to form long linear chains.

The *nylon fiber* is the first in this class, commercialized in the 1930s. Nylon is defined by the Textile Fiber Products Identification Act as "a manufactured fiber in which the fiber forming substance is any long chain synthetic polyamide in which less than 85% of the amide linkages are attached to two aromatic rings" (FTC, 1958). According to the number(s) of carbon atoms in the monomer(s) that form the nylon polymer, the variety of nylon fibers are named nylon 3, nylon 4, nylon 5, nylon 6, nylon 6,6 (i.e., two six-carbon atom monomers are involved in the polymerization), etc. Among them, nylon 6 and nylon 6,6 (Figure 2.8) are the most frequently used for textile end uses. They contain zigzag soft chains that are highly aligned and packed closely together, and bonded together by strong intermolecular forces. Nylon fibers are therefore highly crystalline (65–85%) and low in amorphous percentage (15–35%) (Hatch 1993), which account for their high mechanical strength, abrasion resistance and toughness. The presence of the zigzag polymer chains also renders such merits as good elasticity and elastic recovery. Nylon is hydrophobic, although it has the highest moisture absorption capacity among synthetic fibers due to its polar amide group, as shown in Figure 2.8.

Nylon fibers have been used widely in the medical and healthcare sectors, including external (e.g., pressure garment, dental floss) and internal (e.g., sutures) applications. Due to the combination of high mechanical strength and good elasticity, nylon fibers are an appropriate material for applications such as apparel, home furnishing, sports

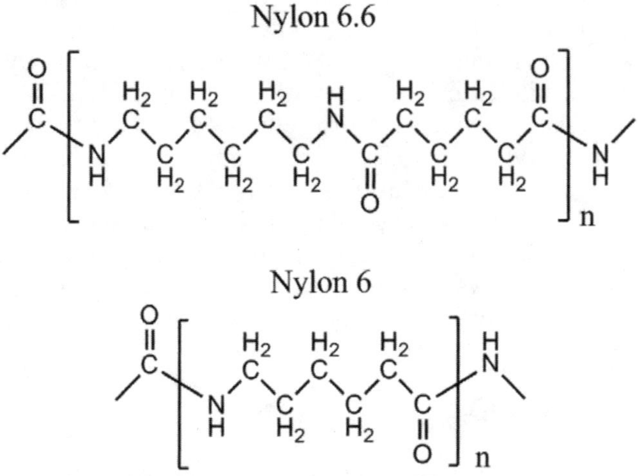

Nylon 6.6

Nylon 6

FIGURE 2.8. *Nylon 6 and Nylon 6,6.*

PET

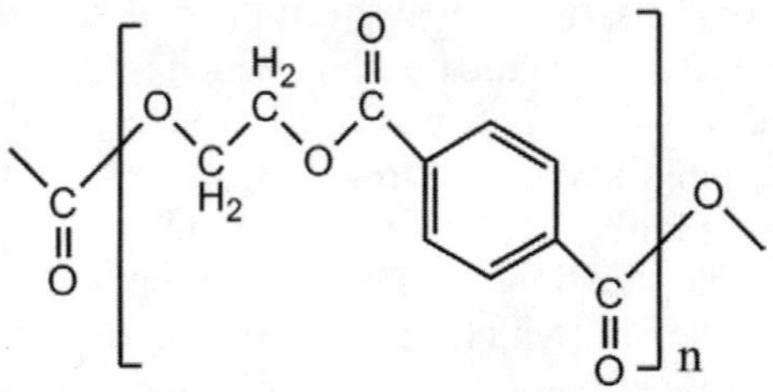

FIGURE 2.9. *Polyethylene terephthalate (PET).*

and recreational devices (e.g., sportswear, tents, parachutes, sleeping bags) and industrial instruments (e.g., tire cord, hoses, conveyer and seat belts, ropes and nets).

Polyester fibers consist of "long-chain polymers composed of at least 85% by weight of an ester of a substituted aromatic carboxylic acid" (FTC, 1958). Polyethylene terephthalate (PET) (Figure 2.9) accounts for 95% of the polyester fibers produced, and is also the most widely used synthetic fiber in the world. Polyester fibers are 35% crystalline and 65% amorphous (Hatch 1993). However, the polymer chains are highly aligned along the fiber axis, even in the amorphous region. The polymers are also bonded together by strong intermolecular forces. As a result, polyester fibers have high mechanical strength, toughness and abrasion resistance, as well as high elongation and elastic recovery. However, polyester fibers require higher forces to elongate as compared to nylon fibers. They also have higher resistance to heat and chemicals (including acids and oxidizing agents) than nylon fibers. Its hydrophobic nature and low moisture absorption can cause static buildup.

An inert material, polyester fibers have found applications in medical and healthcare products for internal uses, such as nonabsorbable suture, vascular grafts and ligament prostheses. They are also used in apparel (usually blended with cotton and other natural or regenerated fibers), home furnishings, sports and recreational devices (e.g., sportswear, tents) and industrial uses (e.g., hoses, power belts, ropes and nets, thread, tire cord, auto upholstery, and sails).

The *polypropylene fiber* (PP) (Figure 2.10) contains a polymer obtained from the monomer of propylene. PP fibers are highly aligned along the fiber axis and packed closely together (50–65% crystalline) (Hatch, 1993), and are therefore known for their high strength, toughness and abrasion resistance. They have medium elasticity but high elastic recovery. PP fibers have the lowest capacity of water absorption among the commonly used fibers, and are thus called the zero absorbent fibers. Despite its hydrophobicity, the PP fiber is known for two distinguishing features. First, it has a high capacity for wicking, whereby water can be quickly transported away from the skin to the outer environment. Second, it has a low static buildup, which is usually a problem for hydrophobic fibers. The latter feature is due to the fact that the nonpolar polymer structure inhibits the electrons' escaping from the atoms to the fiber surface. The PP fiber is also the lightest in its class.

PP fibers have applications in medical and healthcare products that require zero absorbency (which means inert and low adherence to tissues) and/or a high wicking capacity, such as the top sheets for diapers and other disposable hygiene products, such as nonabsorbable sutures that can be easily pulled out from the flesh. They are also used in carpets and rugs (because of their low static buildup), next-to-skin sportswear (due to their high wicking capacity and light weight) and industrial instruments (e.g., geotextiles, filters).

Acrylic fibers are composed of polymers with characteristic acrylonitrile units, as shown in Figure 2.11. Acrylonitrile polymers have been developed for a variety of uses. Their properties also vary. Acrylic fibers for general use have a moderate mechanical strength and a low capacity of water absorbency. They are mostly used for apparel and furnishings.

Acrylic fibers can be modified into a series of variants with enhanced functions for specific end uses in the medical and healthcare sectors. These modacrylic (i.e., modified acrylic) fibers possess low levels of acrylonitrile units (35–85%). Among them, the most well-known are modacrylic fibers that serve as a flame retardant (FR) or are antibacterial. FR modacrylic fibers consist of polymers that are usually produced by copolymerization of an acrylonitrile monomer and a halogen-based monomer, as shown in Figure 2.11. Details about the mechanism of the flame-retardant, halogen-based compounds will be discussed in Chapter 7. An antibacterial modacrylic fiber can be obtained by the incorporation of cationic amines onto the backbone (i.e., via copolymerization) or side chain (i.e., via grafting) of an acrylonitrile polymer, as discussed in detail in Chapter 7.

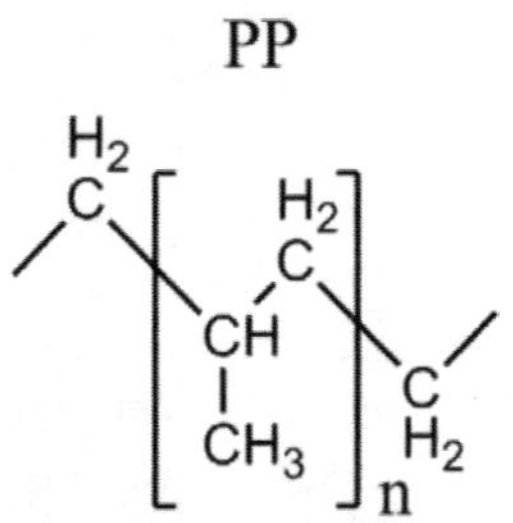

PP

FIGURE 2.10. *Polypropylene (PP).*

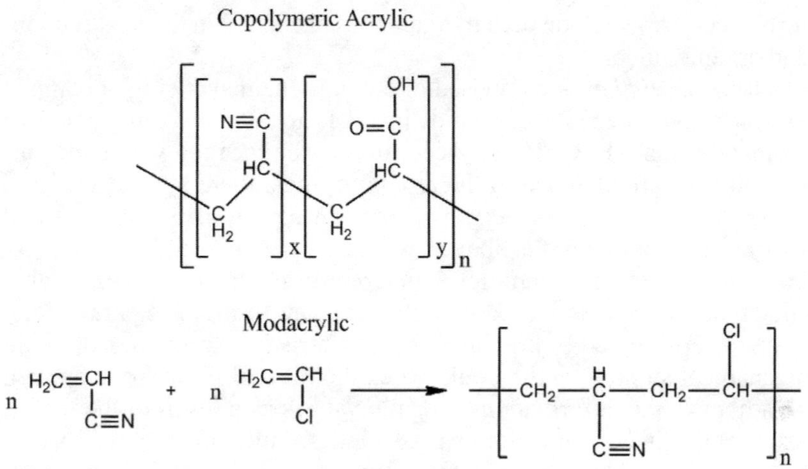

Copolymeric Acrylic

Modacrylic

FIGURE 2.11. *Acrylic and modacrylic.*

Elastomeric fibers have superior elasticity. At room temperature, an elastomeric fiber can be stretched repeatedly to at least twice its original length, and still return to its original length upon release of the force. Spandex fiber is the most widely used elastomeric fiber. It contains a block polymer composed of a hard and crystalline segment (usually polyurethane) and a soft and pliable segment (e.g., polyether, polyester), as shown in Figure 2.12. The soft segments in the polymer structure usually coil in a relaxed manner. They can be uncoiled to accommodate the stretch and recoiled to restore their original state upon the release of force. When the soft segments are extended, they become more aligned along the fiber axis to produce more crystalline regions, so that the mechanical strength of the spandex fiber is preserved.

Uses of spandex fibers can be found in such medical and health care products as pressure garments and elastic tubular bandages. Wider uses are found where it is desirable for the product to have a high elasticity and elastic recovery, as instanced by hosiery, swimsuits, exercise wear, waist bands, bra straps, side panels and cups.

High performance fibers are developed for special end uses, where such performances as exceptional flame resistance, heat resistance, chemical resistance, and/or mechanical strength are required. High per-

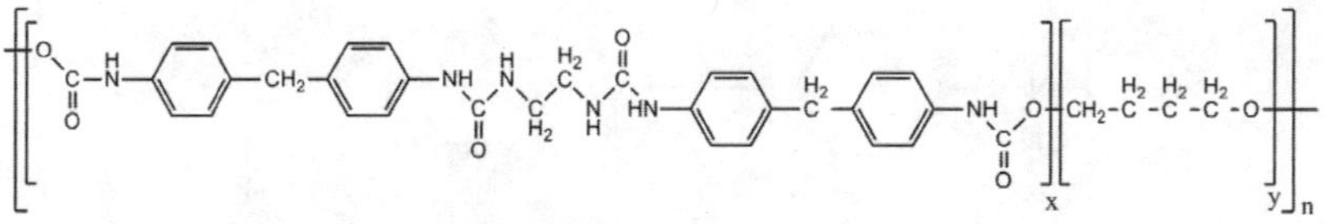

FIGURE 2.12. *Spandex fiber.*

formance fibers include both inorganic (as discussed in the next section) and organic fibers.

The *aramid fiber* is composed of a "long-chain synthetic polyamide in which at least 85% of the amide linkages are attached directly to two aromatic rings" (FTC, 1958). According to the location where the amide linkages are attached to the aromatic rings, there are meta-aramid fibers and para-aramid fibers, as shown in Figure 2.13. The first and best-known meta-aramid fiber is Nomex®. It has a high decomposition temperature, high ignition temperature, is almost non-flammable and is therefore widely used in firefighter's uniforms. The para-aramid fiber, as represented by Kevlar®, is characteristic of exceptionally high mechanical strength and modulus (i.e., the ratio of force/strain applied on a fiber to the deformation/elongation/stress as a result of the force). It therefore finds applications in parachutes, bullet-proof vests, ballistic fabrics, etc. These aramid fibers are also known for their excellent chemical resistance, even at elevated temperatures.

Other high performance organic fibers include, but are not limited to, PBI (flame, heat and chemical resistant), sulfar (flame, heat and chemical resistant), and ultra-high molecular weight polyethylene fibers (exceptionally high mechanical strength and modulus).

Because of their special performance, the above mentioned fibers are usually used in uniforms or devices for certain high-risk professionals (e.g., firefighters, policemen, soldiers), or in industrial products. They have not been used in the medical or healthcare sectors, however.

Fiber materials to be used for medical purposes, especially those to be used internally, should be both biocompatible and/or bioresorbable (i.e., can be broken down by the body so that no surgical procedure is required to have them removed). A more detailed discussion on bio-

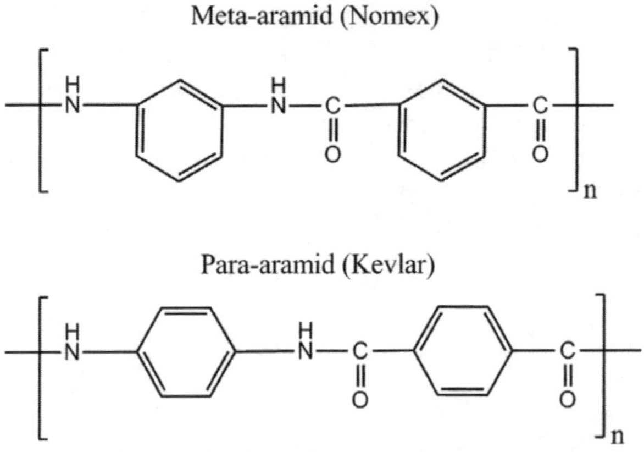

Meta-aramid (Nomex)

Para-aramid (Kevlar)

FIGURE 2.13. *Aramid fibers.*

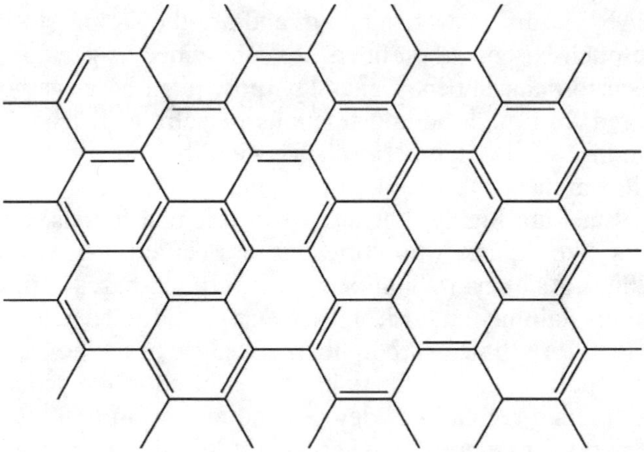

FIGURE 2.14.   *A small section of a graphite sheet.*

compatibility and bioresorbability of materials can be found in Chapter 5. Since most of the general-purpose textile materials cannot meet one or both of these requirements, a wide range of biomedical fibers or polymers have been developed. As most of these *biomedical polymers* can be processed into nanofibers, they will be delineated in Chapter 3.

2.3.4. Inorganic Fibers

Inorganic fibers have their applications mostly in technical end uses. Among them, the *glass fiber* (or *fiberglass*) is the oldest and most familiar performance fiber. It was invented in 1938, and soon became known for its high mechanical strength—higher than most commonly used synthetic fibers (e.g., polyester) and even steel. In addition to this is its low cost. For these reasons it soon found applications in architecture and the transportation industries (e.g., as glass fiber-reinforced composite materials for parts of vehicles or boats). Its good insulation properties account for its use in staple glass fiber mats for soundproofing or heat insulation. However, there have been health concerns about glass fibers, including skin irritation and toxicity upon inhalation, indicating that they are unlikely to function as medical and healthcare materials.

The *carbon fiber* is another high performance inorganic fiber under continuous development in the last 50 years. It is composed of long, thin graphite sheets (shown in Figure 2.14) stacking together in bundles to form fibers. Currently, there are a rich variety of carbon fibers available for different end uses, among which two are the most frequently used: the polyacrylonitrile (PAN)-based and pitch-based carbon fibers (Hearle, 2001). The PAN-based are processed from high molecular weight PAN via dry or wet spinning, and are the strongest carbon fibers. The pitch-based carbon fibers are subdivided as general purpose and high performance fibers. General purpose pitch-based carbon fibers are prepared from high boiling fractions of petroleum feedstocks via melt spinning, while high-performance pitch-based carbon fibers are produced from mesophase (or known as the liquid crystal phase) pitch. Liquid crystals are highly structured and oriented liquids: their molecules flow like liquids, while oriented in a certain way, like crystals (Khoo, 2007). As a result, high-performance pitch-based carbon fibers have high crystallinity and orientation, and therefore have even higher modulus than PAN-based carbon fibers. Because of their excellent mechanical properties, carbon fibers have been used in the aerospace industry, sports and recreational devices and architecture in the form of reinforcements for composite materials. Carbon fibers are also used in such implantable devices as ligament prostheses and reinforcements for bond grafts.

2.4. YARNS

A yarn is a continuous strand of textile fibers that can be used for the fabrication of fabrics or other textile structures. Staple fibers or short fibers are assembled together to form *spun yarns,* while filaments or continuous fibers are processed into *filament yarns.* There are also *compound yarns* in which two strands form a core and a sheath respectively.

All staple yarns and some filament yarns are twisted to hold the fiber together. Twist is defined as "the helical or spiral configurations induced by turning a strand about its longitudinal axis" (ASTM, 2008). Degree of twist is expressed as the number of turns about its axis per unit length, and is an important parameter that can affect the properties of yarns and fabrics. A yarn with 1–10 twists per centimeter (tpc) is referred to as a *negligible-twist* yarn. *Low-twist* yarns usually have 15–30 tpc, *moderate-twist* yarns 50–65 tpc, while *high-twist* yarns have 100–200 tpc. The degree of twist can affect mechanical strength: for spun yarns, an increase in the degree of twist can increase its strength at first, as increased friction among fibers causes the yarn strength to increase; however, if the degree of twist goes beyond a certain value, the fibers in the yarn will start to crush on each other and bring down its strength. For filament yarns, the yarn strength remains constant until the degree of twist reaches a critical value, at which point the strength starts to decrease. The amount of water taken up by a yarn decreases with the increase of the degree of twist, as a result of decreased interstices between fibers. Similarly, thermal insulation of a fabric may decrease due to a larger degree of twist, as a result of the smaller space for still air to

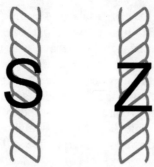

FIGURE 2.15.   *Direction of twist.*

get entrapped in the yarn structure. However, increased twist does make the surface of the yarn more impact and smooth, so as to make the yarn or its fabric more comfortable to the touch.

The direction of twist in a yarn is indicated as either *S* or *Z*, as shown in Figure 2.15. The direction and degree of twist can be utilized in the design and development of textile products expected to provide special performances. A good example of such product development is the self-adhesive elastic retention bandage for wound care, as detailed in Chapter 8.

2.5. FABRICS AND 3D STRUCTURES

"Fabric" usually refers to the two-dimensional (2D) structures formed by the interlacing or binding of fibers and/or yarns, including woven, knit, nonwoven and compound fabrics. There are also three-dimensional (3D) structures that are made from fibers and/or yarns and used for special applications. These structures will be briefly introduced in this section.

2.5.1. Woven Fabrics

Woven fabrics are composed of two or more sets of yarns that are interlaced usually at right angles, as shown in Figure 2.16. Some of the terms useful for the description of a woven fabric are listed below.

Warp, or *end,* indicates the lengthwise direction of a fabric, or the direction in which the fabric is taken off from the loom (i.e., the weaving machine). *Weft* (also called *filling* or *pick*), on the other hand, refers to the crosswise direction of a woven fabric. Any direction other than the lengthwise and crosswise is named as the *bias* direction. An *interlacing pattern* is a description of how the warp and weft yarns are interlaced with each other (i.e., the way one set of yarns moves over and under the other set of yarns) to form a fabric. A *weave repeat* is the smallest number of warp or weft yarns on which an interlacing pattern can be represented. A weave repeat for the weave pattern as shown in Figure 2.16 is indicated as enclosed in the dashed frame. A *float* is the length of a yarn (in terms of the number of intersecting yarns it passes over) that floats on the surface of a fabric between adjacent intersections. The weave shown in Figure 2.16 has a float number of 4, as its weft floats on the *fabric face* (i.e., the side of the fabric which usually has the more attractive appearance and is viewed during use and wear) and warp floats on the fabric back. The *progression of interlacing* is the number of filling yarns by which the interlacing of a warp yarn in a weave moves upwards relative to the warp yarn on its immediate left. The progression of interlacing of the fabric shown in Figure 2.16 is 3. There are three basic woven structures, as shown in Figure 2.17.

Plain weave is the most commonly used, in which each weft yarn passes alternatively over and under each warp yarn, and each warp yarn passes alternatively over and under each weft yarn, as shown in Figure 2.17(a). This is the simplest weave with the smallest weave repeat (2 × 2), smallest float (i.e., only 1) and highest frequency of yarn interlacing. Variations of plain weave include *basket weave,* in which two (or more) warp yarns interlace with two (or more) filling yarns, as shown in Figure 2.17(b). A similar weave with two warp yarns float over one filling yarn is called *half-basket weave.* Plain weave or its variations can usually be used in products that require a tight and dense structure to avoid penetration by liquid. In the healthcare sectors, for example, such

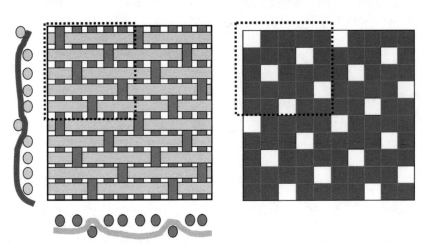

(a) Weave pattern: surface view
and cross-sectional views

(b) Weave diagram

FIGURE 2.16. *Structure of a woven fabric (satin).*

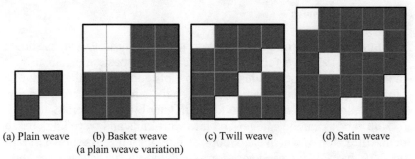

(a) Plain weave   (b) Basket weave   (c) Twill weave   (d) Satin weave
(a plain weave variation)

FIGURE 2.17.   *Basic weave structures.*

applications include waterproof and breathable fabrics for protection purposes (see Chapter 7) and vascular grafts (Chapter 9).

Twill weave repeats on three or more warp yarns and diagonal lines (i.e., twill lines) are produced on the fabric face [Figure 2.17(c)]. Denims are well-known twill fabrics. Twill fabrics have a smaller frequency of yarn interlacing, and may therefore have a greater yarn packing density than plain-woven fabrics.

Satin weave is characterized by its long floats, arranging from 4 to 12, which contributes to its smooth and lustrous fabric surface. Figure 2.17(d) shows a satin weave with its warp yarns floating on the fabric face, with a float number of 4. Satin fabrics with their weft yarns floating on the fabric face are also known as *sateens*.

More complex structures are available for woven fabrics to provide special patterns or designs. For example, leno fabrics are open and light fabrics that can be used as surgical gauze and cheesecloth, as shown in Figure 2.18. Since the truly complex woven structures are less likely to be applied in the healthcare and medical textile products, they will not be discussed in this book.

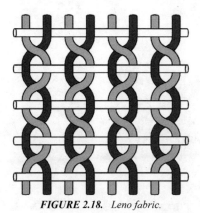

FIGURE 2.18.   *Leno fabric.*

2.5.2. Knit Fabrics

Knit fabrics are composed of intermeshing loops of yarn, as shown in Figure 2.19. *Loop* (also called *stitch*) is the basic element in knit fabrics. *Course* is used to describe a row of loops across the width of a fabric in the crosswise direction. *Wale,* on the other hand, refers to a row of loops along the length of the fabric in lengthwise direction.

Knit fabrics can be categorized into weft knits and warp knits based on the direction in which each loop-forming yarn lies. As shown in Figure 2.19, in *weft knit,* each yarn forming the loops runs across the fabric in the crosswise direction; in *warp knit,* the yarn runs in the lengthwise direction. Figure 2.19(a) shows the simplest form of weft knit fabrics, single jersey (or known as plain stockinette) knit, in which only one yarn system is used to form one layer of loops, and all of the knitted loops are of the same type and meshed in the same manner. Figure 2.19(b) demonstrates the structure of a single-bar tricot knit (a warp knit), which also contains only one yarn system and one type of loops.

Fabricated from yarns in an entirely different manner, knit and woven fabrics are quite different in performance. The loops in knit fabrics endow them with a much higher flexibility than woven fabrics in general. As a result, knit fabrics are noted for their elasticity and elastic recovery, and are thus suitable for form-fitting garments to allow freedom of body movement, or other products that require close fit (e.g., pressure garment for patients with burn wounds, see Chapter 8). Warp knits usually have lower elasticity than weft knits. Woven fabrics, on the other hand, have higher dimensional stability (i.e., are better able to retain their original dimensions) than knit fabrics, and are therefore used in applications where it is necessary to guard against deformation. Other features of knit fabrics, in comparison with the woven, are ease of

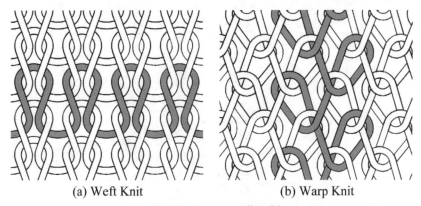

(a) Weft Knit   (b) Warp Knit

FIGURE 2.19.   *Structures of knit fabrics.*

care, soft draping quality, and greater warmth in still air. However, knit fabrics have very high relaxation shrinkage (i.e., shrinkage due to the relief of tension) as a result of the distortion and extension of the loops during manufacturing processes. Knit fabrics also have the tendency to snag (i.e., for part of the yarn to be pulled out from the surface of a fabric). Broken snags may cause the knit fabrics (mostly the weft knit type) to run or ladder to form holes or vertical flaws across the entire product. Such structural instability of the knit fabrics (especially weft knits) may cause problems with, or even failure of, implantable products (e.g., vascular grafts, see Chapter 9) in their end uses.

2.5.3. Nonwoven Fabrics

Different from woven or knit fabrics, nonwoven fabrics are fabricated directly from fibers instead of yarns. In nonwoven fabrics, staple fibers or filaments are usually randomly laid and bonded together by mechanical (e.g., needle-punching, fluid jet entangling, stitching), thermal (e.g., thermal bonding) or chemical (e.g., adhesive bonding) means. Most of the general purpose fibers can be used in the production of nonwoven fabrics.

Nonwoven fabrics have several advantages over woven or knit fabrics. Firstly, the production of nonwovens skips the yarn-forming procedures, considerably reducing the cost of production. Secondly, the nonwovens are highly porous, and allow air and water permeability. Furthermore, the random distribution of the fabric-forming fibers makes the fabric isotropic (i.e., exhibiting the same or similar properties in all directions). These advantages justify the wide application of nonwovens in disposable hygiene products, such as the coverstock for diapers, feminine hygiene products, wipes and towels (see Chapter 6). A summarized list of nonwoven fabrics, along with their forming mechanisms, properties and applications, are shown in Table 2.1.

2.5.4. Compound Fabrics and 3D Textile Structures

Compound fabrics are multi-layered structures containing at least one layer of fabric. The other component layers may comprise yarns, fibers, films and/or foams. Different layers are usually held together by mechanical (e.g., stitching), thermal (e.g., fusing) or chemical (e.g., adhesives) means.

A good example of compound fabrics is the *coated fabric,* in which a base fabric is covered on one or both surfaces, with a layer (or layers) of substantially continuous polymeric coating materials. The base can be the woven, knit or nonwoven fabric, and the coating material is usually

TABLE 2.1. A Summary of Nonwoven Fabrics.

	Bonding Method	Properties	Application
Needle-punched nonwovens	Mechanical bonding by needle punching	Coarse, low cost	Filter media, apparel interlinings, road underlay, and auto trunk liners
Spun-laced nonwovens	Entangled by high pressure water jet	Soft drape, low strength, dimensional stability	Draperies and bedspreads, tablecloths, and apparel
Wet-laid nonwovens	Paper-making techniques followed by adhesive bonding	Paper-like	Wipes, towels, surgical gowns, and diaper cover stocks
Dry-laid nonwovens	Deposition fiber layers from an air stream/carding, followed by adhesive bonding	Soft hand and excellent drape	Diaper cover stocks, wipes and sanitary napkins
Melt-blown nonwovens	Microfibers extruded, entangled by air stream, and bonded at cross-over points before solidification	Uniformity, lower to moderate strength	Surgical mask, drape and gown, and sanitary products
Spun-bonded nonwovens	Filament extruded, laid down, bonded at cross-over points before solidification	High tensile and tear strength	Filtration, geotextiles, and protective apparel

natural or synthetic rubber, PVC (polyvinyl chloride), or PU (polyurethanes) (Horrocks and Anand, 2000).

The *laminated fabric* is another type of compound fabric composed of at least one layer of fabric and another component like film(s), fabric(s) or foam(s). The different layers are bonded together by adhesives or the adhesive properties of one or more of the components.

Depending on the properties of coating/laminating polymeric materials, the coated and laminated fabrics can be rendered UV resistant or waterproof. They have been developed into waterproof and breathable (i.e., permeable to water vapor) products and used in sports and recreational devices (e.g., tents), as well as protective apparel or devices against waterborne pathogens (i.e., any infectious or disease-producing agent, including bacteria, viruses or other microorganisms), as discussed in Chapter 7. They can also be used in a variety of end uses, from automotive (e.g., seat covers, headliners, airbags, covering for convertibles, etc.), to marine (e.g., inflatable boats, life jacket, sails, etc.) to household products (e.g., furniture upholstery, shower curtains, man-made leather, etc.).

Other compound fabrics less likely to be used in the healthcare and medical textiles and will not be discussed in this book.

3D (three-dimensional) textile structures are mostly used for specific advanced applications. Currently, 3D textile structures can be fabricated by 3D braiding or weaving techniques.

The *braiding* technique is used to bring about a textile structure by diagonal intersection of yarns or filaments. 2D braiding produces flat strip or tape, while 3D braiding provides tubular- or rod-shaped textile structures. 3D braids have been used in the reinforcement structure of composite materials to be applied in high-end products, such as those employed in the military or aerospace sectors. Braided structures are also found in healthcare and medical textile products, such as sutures and ligament prostheses (see Chapter 9).

Conventional or modified weaving looms can be used to construct multilayered woven fabrics, with extra set(s) of weft yarns that interlace through the thickness of the fabric. Such multilayered woven fabrics usually have lower delaminating strength, but can be produced with relatively low cost. As a rule, 3D wovens are produced in some special equipment, where 3 sets of yarns interlace with each other in the 3D space, with each set of yarns being perpendicular with the other two sets of yarns. Such 3D fabrics are costly, and their uses are reasonably limited to the reinforcement of advanced composite materials applied in high-end industries, including those related to the medical and healthcare sectors.

2.6. FIBER-REINFORCED COMPOSITES

Composite materials are composed of two or more physical distinct components, one of which (i.e., the reinforcement) can be dispersed into the other(s) to achieve optimum properties. The final material may have superior properties to those of the individual components (Hull, 1981; Swanson, 1997). Fiber materials are common reinforcements in composite materials; such composite materials are called *fiber-reinforced composites.* Fiber-reinforced composites usually contain two components: fiber as the reinforcement, and the matrix, which is usually a polymer.

Reinforcement fibers for composites are mostly high-performance fibers, including glass fibers, carbon fibers, and aramid fibers. Recently, bast fibers such as hemp and flax have also been used in composite reinforcements because of their high mechanical strength and environmentally benign features. These fibrous reinforcements can be in the form of discrete short fibers, continuous filaments, fabrics (e.g., woven, knit or nonwoven), 3D braids and 3D woven structures, depending on the end uses.

The polymeric matrices of composites can be classified into two general groups: thermosets and thermoplastics. Thermosets, also known as thermoset resins (e.g., epoxy), are converted into hard and brittle solids during the composite fabrication processes via chemical cross-linking (i.e., curing). Such processes, however, are not reversible. Thermoplastics, or thermoplastic resins (e.g., polyester, nylon and polypropylene), on the other hand, can be repeatedly heated to melt, and cooled down to consolidate. As a result, thermoplastics make it possible for the composite materials or parts to be repaired or reformed. Other matrices, like metals and ceramics, are also available to construct composite materials for high-temperature end uses.

Compared with conventional materials, composite materials usually have higher specific strength (i.e., strength per unit weight) and/or specific modulus (i.e., modulus per unit weight). This feature is very important for transportation vehicles and/or devices, since a reduction in weight leads to greater efficiency and energy savings. As a result, composite materials have been widely used in the automotive and aerospace industries. Other application areas include sporting and recreational devices, and in infrastructures, like bridges and buildings. Carbon fiber reinforced composites have found applications in medical implants, such as dental and bone grafts.

2.7. FINISHING FOR TEXTILE PRODUCTS

A wide range of finishing methods are known for textiles to provide or enhance specific properties or functions of the end products. They can be achieved via chemical, mechanical or thermal means. Among them, the most relevant for medical and healthcare textiles are comfort and protective finishes, as explained briefly in the following:

A variety of finishing methods can be used to change the surface appearance/smoothness of fabrics, and subsequently affect their sensorial comfort (see Chapter 4) when being applied in products that are in direct contact with the human skin. *Glazing* or *polishing,* for example, refer to a finishing method in which a fabric is impregnated with a solution of starch, wax or resin, and then passed through a friction calender (i.e., a set of hard pressure rollers that can be used to smooth a sheet material) to obtain a smooth and even layer of the applied chemicals. *Schreinerizing* is another approach to enhance the surface smoothness of a fabric. In this process, a fabric is passed through a Schreiner calendar (which usually includes a heated roller) to flatten the yarns and smooth out the fabric surface.

Water-repellent finishes aim at minimizing the spreading, wetting and the penetration of water. Such effects can usually be achieved by application of water repellents, but the use of such chemicals is not preferred in medical and healthcare applications. Laminated fabrics containing waterproof and breathable film(s) are mostly used in products that require water repellency. Alternatively, physical modification of material surface is another approach to change the hydrophilicity of the textile materials without incurring chemical compounds in the procedures. More detailed information about waterproof products can be found in Chapter 7.

Flame-retardant finishes are used to ensure that fabrics meet established standards for ease of ignition, rate of flame spreading, and capacity of self-extinguishing after the removal of fire source. Different flame-retardant finishing agents have been developed for such purposes. See Chapter 7 for more details.

Antimicrobial finishes are important for healthcare and medical textiles. The treated fabrics will usually have reduced rate of growth and spread of microorganisms due to the presence of antimicrobial agents that have been incorporated into the fibers or fabrics via different approaches. A more detailed explanation is given in Chapter 7.

Antistatic finishes are applied to provide textile products with increased electrical conductivity and, consequently, decreased static buildup that may lead to discomfort or even injury. Antistatic agents or conductive materials can be used to achieve these objectives, as will be further discussed in Chapter 7.

2.8. SUMMARY

Textiles are highly versatile. This versatility is attributed to the multiplicity of textile materials and structures, each with some special features, which are combined to give end products a great variety of special properties and performances, which are determined in the course of product design and development.

Fibers can be composed of natural or synthetic polymers, and organic or inorganic compounds, which provides a spectrum of properties and performance. For example, they can range from highly hydrophilic (e.g., wool) to zero absorbent (e.g., polypropylene), from exceptionally elastic (e.g., spandex) to very stiff (e.g., carbon). Fibers of natural polymers (both natural fibers and regenerated fibers) have higher absorbency, but lower mechanical strength as compared to synthetic fibers, and some items are well known for some special performance (e.g., carbon fiber for its great mechanical strength).

Fibers are *assembled* into yarns, fabrics or even 3D structures. Thus, the end products can be either stable in dimension, low in elasticity (like the wovens), or have high elasticity and elastic recovery (e.g., knit fabrics). In contrast, nonwoven fabrics are capable of skipping some of the composition processes as needed in the production of woven and knit fabrics, to result in a very desirable product property: low cost, a merit admired by, say, those who produce disposables. Design and production of compound fabrics and composite materials with fiber reinforcement give the various "high-performance" products: coated or laminated fabrics used in protective clothing or devices, and composite materials for industrial or medical applications.

The medical and healthcare application of textiles depends solely on the textiles' versatility. That is to say, textiles, when property designed and fabricated, provide not only such properties as needed in keeping the human body warm and comfortable, but also can be rendered antibacterial, antistatic, waterproof, or capable of assisting in healing.

2.9. REFERENCES

Altman, G.H., F. Diaz, *et al.* (2003). Silk-based biomaterials. *Biomaterials* **24**(3): 401–416.

ASTM. (2008). D123-07 Standard terminology relating to textiles. West Conshohocken, PA: American Society for Testing and Materials.

FTC. (1958). The Textile Fiber Products Identification Act: 15 U.S.C. § 70, Federal Trade Commission

Hatch, K.L. (1993). Textile science. Minneapolis/Saint Paul: West Pub.

Hearle, J.W.S. (2001). High-performance fibres. Boca Raton, FL: CRC Press/Woodhead Pub.

Horrocks, A.R. and S. Anand. (2000). Handbook of technical textiles. Boca Raton, FL: CRC Press/Woodhead Pub.

Hull, D. (1981). An Introduction to composite materials. Cambridge: Cambridge University Press.

Khoo, I.-C. (2007). Liquid crystals. Hoboken, N.J.: Wiley-Interscience.

Swanson, S.R. (1997). Introduction to design and analysis with advanced composite materials. Upper Saddle River, N.J.: Prentice Hall.

CHAPTER 3

Medical and Healthcare Nanofibers

CONVENTIONAL fibers for apparel or industrial applications are relatively coarse, ranging from millimeters to micrometers. However, there are fibers that are much, much finer than the conventional, the making of which requires different production techniques than those used for conventional fiber production. They are "ultrafine" fibers, technically called *nanofibers*.

Nanofibers are valued for their ultra-high specific surface areas (i.e., surface-to-volume or surface-to-mass values), and have been found potentially useful in many applications, such as wound dressing, selective separation, immobilization of biologically or pharmacologically active agents and molecules, and as scaffolds for tissue engineering. The versatile performance of nanofiber materials is the result of the choice, control and optimization of nanofiber properties in the course of production, and they characterize the various means of fabrication, as discussed in the following.

3.1. FABRICATION OF NANOFIBERS

Nanofibers can be produced by a number of methods. They can be extracted from natural materials (e.g., cellulose or protein fibers) via physical separation and/or chemical extraction. They can also be produced by means of drawing, template synthesis, phase separation, self-assembly and electrospinning.

3.1.1. Extraction of Nanofibrils From Natural Resources

Many cellulosic fibers, such as those from cotton, hemp, flax, bamboo and wood, or protein fibers such as wool and silk from silkworms

37

or spiders, have hierarchical structures composed of fibrils in nano-scale sizes. These nanofibrils are bonded to each other via relatively weak forces like the Van der Waals forces. There have been trial efforts to break down such microsized natural fibers into nanosized fibrils by mechanical, or a combination of mechanical and chemical, means.

Mechanical separation of cellulose fibrils from natural fiber resources (e.g., wood pulp, cotton, chitosan and silk) may involve the process of grinding to apply shear stress to the longitudinal axis of the fibers, so that the fibrillated fibers will have diameters ranging 20–90 nm (Taniguchi and Okamura, 1998). Ultrasonic extraction is another approach to disrupt the adhesions among the fibrils so as to extract nanofibrils from both cellulosic and protein fiber sources (Zhao, Cao et al., 2007). High frequency ultrasound is capable of creating, growing and collapsing micro-bubbles in an aqueous suspension containing natural fibers. The violent collapse produces microjets and shock waves to impact the surface of the fibers, forcing them to split along the fiber axis. Different fiber resources may need different ultrasonic frequencies and treating times to individualize the nanofibrils. Although the mechanical approaches are more environmentally friendly because no chemicals are involved, the nanofibrils may be broken during the process. Furthermore, with mechanical separation one cannot ensure that the fibrils will be completely "clean", as residuals of non-fibril substances (e.g., lignin and pectin in cellulosic fibers) may get attached to and remain on the fibril surface. Interestingly, this is not necessarily a disadvantage: it has been reported that the lignin in hemp fibers may function as a UV blocker and an anti-bacterial agent (Zimniewska, Kozlowski et al., 2008).

Chemical/mechanical approaches are typically applied to the treatment of cellulosic fibers, especially bast fibers from hemp and flax. They provide long and strong fibers consisting of bundles of individual cells held together by polysaccharide, pectin and lignin. The wall of such a cell is composed of nanosized cellulosic fibrils embedded in an interpenetrating matrix of hemicelluloses and pectins (Bhatnagar and Sain, 2005). In order to remove the non-cellulosic components, the bast fibers are subjected to pre-treatment with alkali to loosen the fiber structure, followed by acid hydrolysis and a second alkali treatment to remove part of the non-cellulose components. After the chemical treatment, which functions to weaken or break up the association between the nanofibrils and plant cells, the materials are cryo-crushed, that is, frozen in liquid nitrogen, and crushed by mechanical forces to isolate the cellulose nanofibrils (Bhatnagar and Sain, 2005; Wang and Sain, 2007). The mechanism of such a process is to form ice crystals within the wall of the fiber cell and to wait for these high pressure ice crystals to crush the cell wall into individualized fibrils.

The choice of production approaches can influence properties of the products. For example, use can be made of a solvent to swell the cellulose, followed by ultrasonication to isolate the nanofibrils (Oksman, Mathew *et al.*, 2006). This combination of chemical and mechanical approaches may bring about cleaner fibrils than the mere mechanical ones, but may cause damage to the fibers.

"Cellulose" used to be a term for the fibrillar cell wall of various plants. Then it was found that some species of bacteria (generally called *Acetobacter xylinum*) can also produce pure cellulose containing no lignin or other foreign substances (Iguchi, Yamanaka *et al.*, 2000). Studies have been performed to explore the optimum physical (e.g., temperature and pressure), chemical and biological conditions that allow cultured bacteria to produce considerable quantities of high quality cellulose fibrils (Hult, Yamanaka *et al.*, 2003). This product can be a useful material for biomedical applications because of its high purity and crystallinity, and its relatively low production cost, as well.

These extraction methods were developed to liberate natural nanofibrils in their original forms from the specific matrices in which they grow. Most of the other fabrication methods involve the assembling of polymers—either extracted from natural resources or synthesized from monomers—into nanofibers. These regenerated or synthetic nanofibers will be explained in the next few sections.

3.1.2. Electrospun Nanofibers

Electrospinning is a method to produce ultra-fine (in nanometers) fibers by charging and ejecting a polymer melt or solution through a spinneret under a high-voltage electric field and to solidify or coagulate it to form a filament. Introduced in 1934 (Formhals, 1934), the technology has recently recaptured attention due to its capacity to produce nano-size fibers from both natural and synthetic polymers.

A typical electrospinning apparatus is shown in Figure 3.1. The process of electrospinning is as follows. Solution ready for the spinning is delivered to a stainless spinneret via a syringe pump. A high voltage power supply applies voltage up to 30 kV between the spinneret and a grounded fiber collector, where the pendant drop of polymer solution at the nozzle of the spinneret becomes highly electrified and the repulsive electrostatic forces overcome the surface tension, causing a charged jet of fluid to be ejected. Charges on the polymer jets lead to "splaying" or splitting of the jet into finer filaments, which are deposited on the collector after solvent evaporation. The collector varies in its design. In its simplest form, it can be a metal board for collecting a nanofibrous membrane with fibers randomly distributed. Or it can be

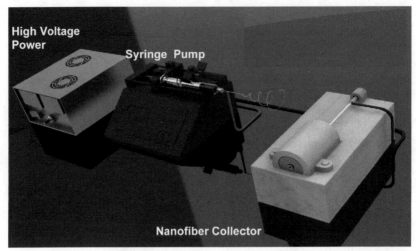

FIGURE 3.1. *The electrospinning apparatus.*

a rotating mandrel (as shown in Figure 3.1) for collecting a tubular-shaped nanofibrous substance that can be a material for vascular grafts to be used in tissue engineering. As compared to nanofibers electrospun from polymer solutions, nanofibers electrospun from molten polymers, although possible, are rarely used and therefore will not be discussed in this book.

Quite a few factors influence the morphology and properties of nanofibers:

Polymer solutions suitable for electrospinning cannot be beyond a certain range of *viscosity,* which is affected by the *molecular weight* and *concentration* of the polymer in the solution. An increased molecular weight means a longer polymer chain and a higher viscosity of the polymer solution due to the greater polymer chain entanglement in the solution. Similarly, an increased concentration leads to a higher viscosity. It follows that a well balanced consideration of the two factors is essential for the fabrication of electrospun nanofibers. A minimum molecular weight or concentration of the polymer is necessary for the formation of fibers; however, if the polymer chains are too short, or if there is too small a number of polymer chains in the flow field, they will be less likely to assemble into a continuous strand upon the high-speed stretching under the high electric field. Instead, they may form polymer particles or beads rather than filaments. On the other hand, if the molecular weight or concentration is too high, it will be difficult for the highly viscose polymer solution to be injected through the small orifice of the syringe needle (Ramakrishna, 2005), causing it to be blocked altogether.

Surface tension (a measure of the amount of energy required to increase the surface area of a liquid by one unit) of the polymer solution is another important parameter for electrospinning. It is caused by the attractive forces (cohesive forces) between the liquid molecules. The higher the surface tension, the more difficult it is for the liquid to expand its surface area. As a result, the high surface tension of the polymer solution is inversely related to the formation of fine and smooth nanofibers, because it makes it difficult to: (1) initiate the electrospinning process, as the repulsive electrostatic forces have to overcome the surface tension to shoot the fluid jet from the syringe needle tip; and (2) split the fluid jet into multiple finer filaments before it hits the collector. In order to bring down the surface tension of a polymer solution, a solvent with low surface tension (i.e., ethanol) can be used or mixed with another solvent for the electrospinning process. The surface tension of the polymer solution can also be reduced by the use of a surfactant (Ramakrishna, 2005).

Solution conductivity affects the amount of charges that the solution jet carries. The higher the conductivity, the more charges the electrospinning jet will carry, and the greater stretching force will be applied on the jet to yield finer and smoother fibers, although there is a limit to the decrease of the fiber diameter. The conductivity of a polymer solution can be raised by using a solvent with high conductivity or adding ionic compounds like salts (Choi, Lee *et al.*, 2004).

Processing parameters are also influential. *Voltage,* for example, is the critical factor to cause the polymer jet to be ejected from the syringe. An appropriate voltage between the needle tip and the grounded

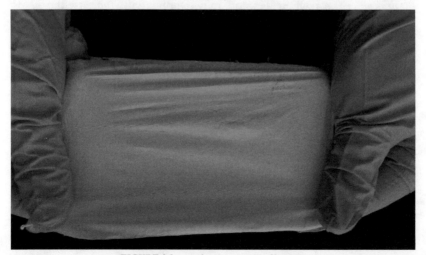

FIGURE 3.2. *An electrospun nanofiber mat.*

collector is important: too low a voltage will not initiate the ejection of the polymer jet; too high a voltage may overdraw the solution from the tip of the needle and lead to an unstable electrospinning process and uneven fibers. Within the working range of voltage, it is usually believed that the diameter of the nanofibers decrease with the increase of the voltage, which leads to a greater stretching on the polymer jet (Buchko, Chen *et al.*, 1999; Deitzel, Kleinmeyer *et al.*, 2001).

The distance between the needle tip and collector affect the flight time of the polymer jet as well as the strength of the electric field. A shorter distance means less travel time of the polymer jet before it hits the collector. On the other hand, the strength of the electric field increases with the decrease of the distance, and the increase of such strength may cause the polymer jet to accelerate to further shorten the trip. As a result, there will not be enough time for the solvent to completely evaporate during the trip, and the resulting fibers may get fused with each other (Buchko, Chen *et al.*, 1999), or it may lead to an unstable electrospining process and result in uneven fibers (Megelski, Stephens *et al.*, 2002). When the distance is too long, however, no fibers will be deposited on the collector.

Other processing parameters that affect the morphology and properties of nanofibers include *feed rate* (which influences the amount of solution available for electrospinning), *orifice size* of the needle (which affects the possibility of clogging at the orifice during electrospinning), and the *conductivity of the collector* (which affects the stability of potential difference between the needle tip and the collector).

Ambient conditions may also affect the electrospinning process. *Ambient temperature,* when elevated, may exponentially increase the evaporation rate of the solvents and reduce (also exponentially) the viscosity of the polymer solution during electrospinning. The resulting morphology of the nanofibers is dependent upon the evaporation rate or viscosity that dominates the process (De Vrieze, Van Camp *et al.*, 2009). Within the range of relatively low temperatures, it is the evaporation rate that will dominate the process. When the temperature is brought down in this range, it will take more time for the polymer jet to become solidified, i.e., the polymer jet will undergo a prolonged, thorough stretching to result in much finer fibers. Otherwise, the solution viscosity dominates the process within a range of relatively high temperatures where, when the temperature is increased within the range, there will be a smaller viscosity to allow better stretching on the polymer jet to produce finer fibers. The more flexible polymer chains may even contribute to better orientations of the resulting fibers (Wang, Chien *et al.* 2007).

Humidity, another important ambient condition, has variant effects on the electrospun nanofibers depending on their chemical natures. One observation is that a high ambient humidity may lead to water condensation on the fiber surface to cause a porous surface on the resulting nanofibers (Casper, Stephens, *et al.*, 2004).

It is worth noting that the above factors that affect the morphology and properties of electrospun nanofibers are not independent. They play synergistic roles in determining the performance of the final nanofibers. It is therefore essential that ALL these factors be taken into consideration before the electrospinning process for any ONE specific polymer.

3.1.3. Other Nanofiber Fabrication Methods

Other nanofiber fabrication methods are not used as frequently as electrospinning, largely because they are not likely to lead to worthwhile production.

Drawing is a process similar to dry-spinning, with which nanofibers are *drawn* slowly from the droplet of a polymer solution by a micropipetter. The polymer solution is made from a viscoelastic material (i.e., one exhibiting both viscous and elastic characteristics upon deformation) that can both accommodate the extensive deformation caused by drawing and also retain the integrated form of an ultra-fine fiber (Ondarcuhu and Joachim, 1998).

The approach of *phase separation* starts with the dissolution of a polymer into a solution, followed by the gelation of the polymer solution. One phase of the mixture, the solvent, is then extracted in distilled water to leave behind the other phase—polymer—in a highly porous nanofibrous structure, which is further freeze-dried to remove excessive water to give a dry fibrous structure (Ma and Zhang, 1999).

Self-assembly is an intricate technique to build nanofibers from small molecules or polymers into bricks. There are different patterns in which molecules are assembled into nanofibers. For example, a designed amphiphile (i.e., a molecule with both hydrophilic and hydrophobic blocks and properties) can be induced to self-assemble into a cylindrical nanosized fiber, as shown in Figure 3.3. It can be seen that, at any cross section, the amphiphiles have self-assembled in such a way that their hydrophobic tails pack in the center of the structure, while their hydrophilic heads appear on the surface and expose themselves to the aqueous environment. These amphiphiles can be further bonded to adjacent molecules via reactions to compose the integrity of the nanofiber structure (Hartgerink, Beniash, *et al.*, 2001).

A comparison of the various methods for fabricating nanofibers explains why electrospinning has dominated our research interests: as a process, it is convenient to perform, can be applied in industrial mass production, and allows proper control on morphology and properties of

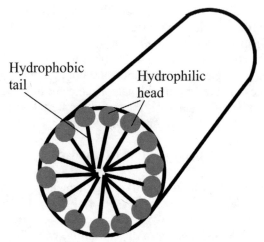

FIGURE 3.3. *Self-assembled nanofibers.*

the products. More importantly, it is the only approach capable of producing filaments from a large variety of natural and synthetic polymers. For this reason, electrospun nanofibers will be the focus of the rest of this chapter.

3.2. BIOPOLYMERS USED FOR NANOFIBERS

A wide range of biopolymers, both natural and synthetic, have successfully been electrospun into nanofibers. They are different in terms of chemical nature, mechanical property, biocompatibility (i.e., the ability of a material to provoke an acceptable cellular and biological response from the host environment; see Chapter 5) and bioresorbability (the ability of an implantable material to break down in the body, i.e., without having to be mechanically removed; see Chapter 5). Some of the widely used biopolymers will be discussed in this section.

3.2.1. Natural Biopolymers

Biopolymers electrospun from natural materials usually fall into two categories: proteins (e.g., collagen, gelatin, and silk fibroin) and polysaccharides (e.g., cellulose and its derivatives, chitin/chitosan, and hyaluronic acid).

Collagen is a biocompatible and bioresorbable natural polymer abundantly found in the connective tissue of animals. It accounts for about 20–30% of the total body proteins in vertebrates, existing in tissues of primarily mechanical functions (half of the total body collagen is found in the skin). It accounts for some 70% of the dry weight of dermis and tendon (Lee, Singla, *et al.*, 2001). Over twenty different types of collagen are known. Among them, type I and type III collagen are the principal structural elements of the extracellular matrix in most native tissues, while type II is mostly found in cartilages (Matthews, Wnek, *et al.*, 2002). Collagen exists naturally in the form of fiber; in structure, one collagen fibril is composed of three polymer chains in a triple helix, and thousands of overlapped fibrils form one collagen fiber (Figure 3.4).

Quite a few types of collagen (e.g., types I, II and III) have been electrospun into nanofibers, and found to be able to serve as a substitute for the extracellular matrix in tissue repair or regeneration. Collagen does not dissolve in water, but can be dissolved in acid solutions. It is usually electrospun from its solution in 1,1,1,3,3,3 hexafluoro-2-propanol (HFP) (Sell, McClure, *et al.*, 2009).

Collagen is one of the most frequently used biomaterials for such medical applications as wound care and tissue regeneration because of its many advantages: it is non-toxic, biocompatible, and can easily be absorbed in the body with very low immunogenicity (i.e., the ability of a substance to provoke an immune response; for greater details see Chapter 5). However, it is very costly to obtain highly purified collagen, and traces of foreign substances in it may negatively affect its biocompatibility. Also, since collagen has relatively low mechanical strength as compared to synthetic polymers, it is usually crosslinked to enhance its stability during the end uses.

Gelatin, a denatured collagen, is another frequently used biomaterial for electrospun nanofiber mats for medical applications because of its biocompatibility, bioresorbability and low cost. Two types of gelatin can be derived from collagen: type A is obtained from collagen through an acidic pretreatment, and type B through an alkaline pretreatment. The latter has a higher content of carboxyl groups than the former (Sell, McClure, *et al.*, 2009). Gelatin is similar to collagen in mechanical properties, biocompatibility and bioresorbability, but is much less costly, and is therefore related to many biomedical applications. It has, however, the demerit that that it dissolves in water at a temperature of no lower than 37°C, and would turn into a gel around room temperature

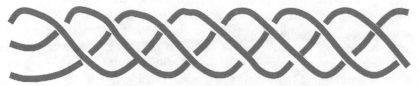

FIGURE 3.4. *The triple helix structure of collagen.*

(Barnes, Sell, *et al.*, 2007). Gelatin nanofibers, usually electrospun from the gelatin solution in organic solvents (e.g., HFP and trifluoroethanol (TFE)), acids (e.g., formic acid, acetic acid) or water, must be cross-linked so as to be stable enough in an aqueous environment.

Silk processed from cocoons of silkworms (Bombyx mori) has been used as a protein-based biomaterial (like sutures) for thousands of years. In the last few decades, its biocompatibility became somewhat problematic as an implantable material. It was suggested that the contained sericin may be to blame (Altman, Diaz, *et al.*, 2003). With all sericin removed, silk fibroin is processed from cocoons and applied in various biomedical uses. Silk nanofibers regenerated from *silk fibroin* have been developed in the last decade. A frequently used solvent for silk fibroin is formic acid (Min, Lee, *et al.*, 2004). Silk polymers obtained from other species of moth other than silkworm (Ohgo, Zhao, *et al.*, 2003), spiders (Oroudjev, Soares, *et al.*, 2002), and weaver ants (Siri and Maensiri, 2010) have also been used for the development of biomedical nanofibers. These silk nanofibers have been known for their biocompatibility, slow degradability and good mechanical properties (Wang, Kim, *et al.*, 2006).

Cellulose is the most abundant natural polysaccharide that has long been used for wound dressings in clinical applications (Lawrence, 1994; Foster and Moore, 1997). Cellulose or its derivatives have also been used in the development of nanofiber materials for biomedical applications because its ultrafine fibers provide maximum comfort with low costs. It is difficult to fabricate cellulose nanofibers directly from the cellulose polymer (non-derived), because cellulose can hardly be dissolved in common solvents or melted due to its high crystallinity and extensively hydrogen-bonded network (Xu, Zhang, *et al.*, 2008). Some commonly used cellulose solvents, such as N-methyl-morpholine N-oxide/water (nNMMO/H_2O, which is commercially used in the production of regenerated cellulose fibers known as Lyocell), are known for their low volatility—a reason why it is so difficult for them to be completely evaporated during electrospinning. Other solvent systems may contain non-volatile salts that have to be removed after electrospinning (Frey 2008). Due to these difficulties, most efforts have been devoted to the fabrication of nanofibers from cellulose derivatives, mostly cellulose acetate, followed by alkaline hydrolysis to remove the acetyl groups to restore the cellulose nanofibers (Frey, 2008). As a matter of fact, cellulose acetate was one of the first reported electrospun nanofibers. Nowadays, it is the most popular cellulosic material for electrospinning because of its good solubility in such solvents as acetone and DMAc (Dimethylacetamide) (Liu and Hsieh, 2002). In addition to cellulose acetate, cellulose derivatives used for the development of electrospun nanofibers include ethyl cellulose (Park, Han, *et al.*, 2007), hydroxypropyl cellulose (Shukla, Brinley, *et al.*, 2005) and bioresorbable oxidized cellulose (Son, Youk, *et al.*, 2004; Khil, Kim, *et al.*, 2005).

Chitin is the second most abundant natural polysaccharide, next only to cellulose. It can be derived from crab and shrimp shells. *Chitosan,* a N-deacetylated derivative of chitin (Figure 3.5), is a natural polysaccharide that has been extensively used in biomedical applications because of its biocompatibility, bioresorbability and antibacterial functions (Schiffman and Schauer, 2007). In terms of molecular structure, chitosan is quite similar to cellulose (Figure 2.5), except for an amino group (–NH$_2$) that replaces one of the three hydroxyl groups (–OH) attached to the six-membered ring. It is due to such amino groups that chitosan is a positive-charged (i.e., cationic) polymer in an acidic environment. The cationic nature of chitosan was believed to contribute to its capacity of bacterial inhibition, via the adhesion between the cationic polymer and the negatively-charged bacterial surface and the further disruption of the cell membrane of the bacteria (Kim, Choi, *et al.*,

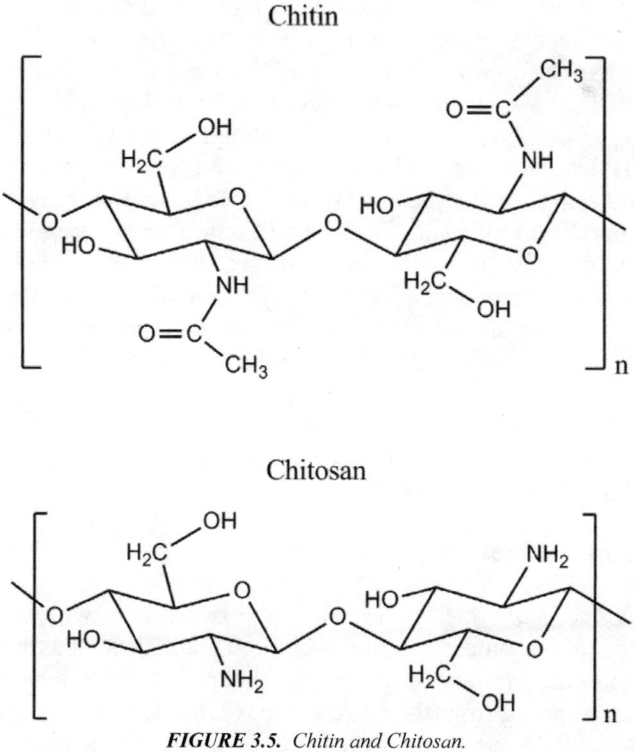

FIGURE 3.5. *Chitin and Chitosan.*

1997; Franklin, Snow, *et al.*, 2005). Chitosan does not dissolve in water, alkali, and most organic solvents. It is soluble in organic acids such as acetic and trifluoroacetic acids. However, viscosity of these solutions is high due to the strong hydrogen bonds between polymer chains, making their electrospinning processes difficult. As a result, chitosan is more often used in combination with other polymers, such as collagen (Chen, Chang, *et al.*, 2008; Chen, Mo, *et al.*, 2008), poly(ethyleneoxide) (PEO) (Desai, Kit, *et al.*, 2008) and Poly(lactide) (PLA) (Ignatova, Manolova, *et al.*, 2009) in electrospinning. Modified chitosan or chitosan derivatives have also been used in the development of biomedical nanofibers. For example, a water soluble N-carboxyethyl chitosan was developed to avoid the usage of organic solvents in electrospining so as to eliminate the toxic residue of the solvents, which can adversely affect the biomedical application of the fiber mats. Hybrid nanofibers containing carboxyethyl chitosan and poly(vinyl alcohol) can be prepared from their aqueous solutions. Such fiber mats were found able to promote cell attachment and proliferation, and are therefore useful for wound care (Zhou, Yang, *et al.*, 2008).

Other natural polymers that have been utilized in the design and development of biomedical nanofibers include Hyaluronic acid (HA) (Schiffman and Schauer, 2007), Poly-N-Acetylglucosamine (Muise-Helmericks, Buff, *et al.*, 2009), alginate-based materials (Park, Park, *et al.*, 2008), fibrinogen (Wnek, Carr, *et al.*, 2003), elastin (Miyamoto, Atarashi, *et al.*, 2009), poly(3-hydroxybutyrate-co-3-hydroxyvalerate (PHBV) (Han, Shim, *et al.*, 2007), wheat gluten (Woerdeman, Ye, *et al.*, 2005) and zein (a protein derived from corn) (Jiang, Reddy, *et al.*, 2010; Suwantong, Pavasant, *et al.*, 2011). The passion for the usage of natural polymers is partly due to the fact that they are usually obtained from such renewable resources as animals, agricultural crops or plants. One of the most important advantages of these natural polymers is that they are usually highly biocompatible and able to promote cell adhesion and proliferation. However, most natural polymers exhibit such drawbacks as relatively low stiffness and low mechanical strength, which can be alleviated by either having the nanofibers crosslinked, or by using synthetic polymers in combination.

3.2.2. Synthetic Polymers

Poly(vinyl alcohol) (PVA, the chemical structure of which is shown in Figure 3.6) is a biocompatible, non-biodegradable synthetic polymer traditionally used in wound dressings. PVA nanofibers can be obtained via electrospinning from the PVA/water solutions. However, the water solubility of PVA can be a problem that limits its application. As a re-

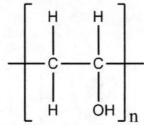

FIGURE 3.6. *The chemical structure of PVA.*

sult, various crosslinking treatments have been used to reduce its solubility in water. The fabricated PVC nanofibers can be crosslinked using such chemicals as glutaraldehyde. A crosslink can be obtained from the reaction between a hydroxyl group in the PVA and an aldehyde group (–CHO) in the glutaraldehyde in the presence of a strong acid (Yeom and Lee, 1996). Heat treatment is a chemical-free alternative method for the crosslinking of PVA, where the crosslinks are formed between two hydroxyl groups by losing H_2O molecules at a high temperature. Heat treatment also improves crystallinity of the electrospun PVA nanofibers (Hong, 2007).

Poly(lactide) (PLA) is another group of biodegradable and biocompatible polymers extensively used in biomedicine. PLA is hydrophobic, but it will undergo a slow degradation in an aqueous environment via hydrolysis at its ester bonds (see Figure 3.7), which causes random chain scission in the polymer chains to yield lactic acid. PLA usually becomes degraded in 30–50 weeks (Barnes, Sell, *et al.*, 2007). PLA can be electrospun into nanofibers from its solution in quite a few organic solvents, including HFP (He, Liao, *et al.*, 2010), dichloromethane (Schofer, Boudriot, *et al.*, 2009) and chloroform (Corey, Gertz, *et al.*, 2008). PLA is also frequently used in combination with other polymers, which represents the effort to take advantage of the different materials in biomedical applications. Thus, natural polymers, such as silk fibroin

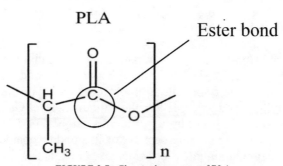

FIGURE 3.7. *Chemical structure of PLA.*

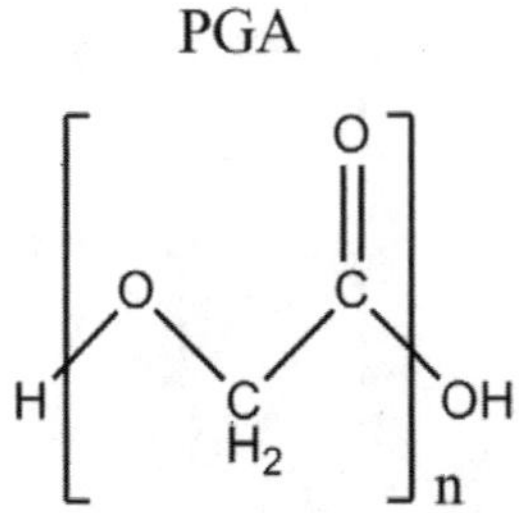

PGA

FIGURE 3.8. *Chemical structure of PGA.*

(Gui-Bo, You-Zhu, *et al.*, 2010), chitosan (Xu, Zhang, *et al.*, 2009) and gelatin (Su, Li, *et al.*, 2010), can be blended with PLA to form hybrid or composite nanofibrous structures, and PLA can be used as a block in co-polymers such as PEG-PLA (Xu, Zhong, *et al.*, 2010) and PLGA (Luu, Kim, *et al.*, 2003) in the fabrication of nanofibers.

Poly(glycolic acid) (PGA) is a biodegradable and bioresorbable polyester widely used in biomedical applications. It was first introduced as a material for bioresorbable sutures in the 1970s. PGA has good mechanical strength and a predictable bioresorbability (i.e., PGA monofilament sutures can be absorbed in the body in about 2 to 4 weeks depending on their hydrophilic nature), which is a desirable property for implants. As a result, it is also suitable for other end uses in which initial strength and fast degradation is needed, such as scaffolds for tissue repair and regenerations. For such purposes, PGA has been electrospun into nanofibers from its solution in HFP. However, the rapid degradation of PGA via hydrolysis may dramatically decrease the local pH value in the tissue and cause tissue responses if the local area does not have a high buffering capacity or effective mechanisms to remove the metabolic waste (Barnes, Sell, *et al.*, 2007). To date, PGA is usually used in combination with other polymers, such as PLA, in the form of co-polymers or blends, to provide desirable properties for biomedical applications.

Poly(caprolactone) (PCL) is a bioresorbable, biocompatible polyester frequently used in biomedical applications, including wound care and scaffolding for tissue repair and regeneration. PCL is hydrophobic and highly crystalline, thus capable of providing prolonged mechanical stability with a low rate of degradation (i.e., degrading in 1–2 years (Barnes, Sell, *et al.*, 2007)). PCL nanofibers can be produced from its solution in such organic solvents as chloroform, tetrahydrofuran (THF), N,N-dimethylformamide (DMF) or their mixtures (Del Gaudio, Bianco, *et al.*, 2009). PCL nanofibrous structures can be a good scaffolding material for tissue engineering because of its good mechanical properties and low degradation rate. Performance of PCL is usually enhanced with the use of natural polymers (e.g., gelatin (Alvarez-Perez, Guarino,

PCL

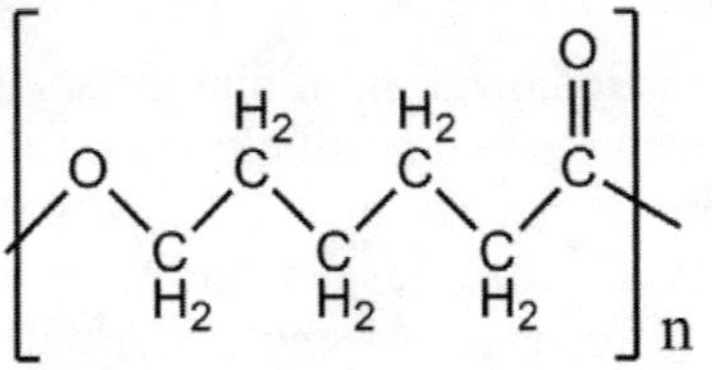

FIGURE 3.9. *Chemical structure of PCL.*

et al., 2010) and collagen (Powell and Boyce, 2009)) via blending or coating to improve its biocompatibility in biomedical applications.

Poly(ethylene glycol) (PEG), also known as *poly(ethylene oxide)* (PEO), is a hydrophilic, biocompatible polyether. PEG usually refers to a material with relatively low molecular weight (e.g., several thousand), while PEO refers to a material with high molecular weight (e.g., over tens or hundreds of thousands). PEO is water soluble, and therefore can be electrospun into nanofibers from its water solution (Deitzel, Kleinmeyer, *et al.*, 2001b). However, water solubility makes the material unstable in biological environments. Consequently, PEO or PEG is usually used in combination with other natural (e.g., collagen, chitosan) or synthetic polymers (e.g., PLA) in blends or copolymers (Subramanian, Vu, *et al.*, 2005; Szentivanyi, Assmann, *et al.*, 2009).

Other synthetic polymers that have been utilized in the development of biomedical nanofibrous structures include the nonbiodegradable polyurethane (Khil, Cha, *et al.*, 2003; Verreck, Chun, *et al.*, 2003; Kim, Heo, *et al.*, 2009) and biodegradable polydioxanone (Kalfa, Bel, *et al.*, 2010).

Generally speaking, synthetic polymers have better mechanical strength than natural polymers. They allow researchers more flexibility in the design and development of new products, but challenge them with the difficult task of minimizing cytotoxicity in such products. As a result, they are usually used in combination with natural polymers, or are modified or functionalized to improve their biocompatibility, as discussed in the next section.

PEG

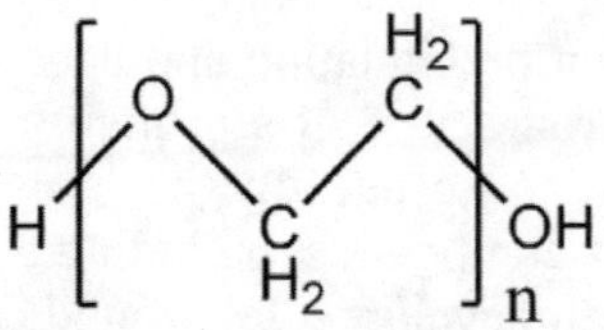

FIGURE 3.10. *Chemical structure of PEG.*

3.3. MODIFICATION OF NANOFIBERS

Modification or functionalization of nanofibers is necessary in order to engineer specific features that will help maximize their end-use performance. A spectrum of bioactive molecules, including antibacterial agents, anti-cancer drugs, enzymes, and proteins, can be incorporated into nanofibers via different approaches. The nanofibrous assemblies can be designed to have patterned orientations (e.g., uniaxial alignment), and fibers with a core/sheath structure can be obtained.

3.3.1. Modification for Drug-Loaded Nanofibers

Oral administration and venous injection are the most frequently used methods for drug delivery, but may not be the most efficient methods in some situations. Patients with locally damaged or diseased tissues or organs would benefit from localized delivery of drugs or other therapeutic agents. For example, patients with severe burn wounds or skin ulcers usually require antibiotics for infection control. However, with systemic administration of the antibiotics, the patient may run the risk of renal or liver toxicity, or only an insufficient portion of the prescribed drug may reach the wounded tissues (Stadelmann, Digenis, *et al.*, 1998). Furthermore, the ischemic wounds with little granulation tissues (i.e., newly formed vascular tissue normally produced during healing of wounds) can hardly be penetrated by the drug. In these situations, *topical administration* may function as a remedy (Jacob, Cierny, *et al.*, 1993; Stadelmann, Digenis, *et al.*, 1998; Fallon, Shafer, *et al.*, 1999), where the antibiotics are applied in minimal amounts at the site of infection and make sure that they function efficiently there. Accordingly, nanofibers with incorporated antibiotics have been studied as potential potent materials for wound care (Xu, Zhong, *et al.*, 2010; Chen, Zhou, *et al.*, 2011). Similarly, a lot of work has been concentrated on the development of nanofibers loaded with anti-cancer drugs, which, when topically administered, may help constitute a remedy for the many side effects (e.g., toxicity to healthy cells) and low efficiency that go with current chemotherapy.

Silver ions have long been known for their antimicrobial capacity. These positively-charged ions are readily bound to the negatively-charged proteins to favor precipitation and denaturation (i.e., a disruption of macromolecular structure of a protein, resulting in changes in its original characteristics—especially its biological activity). Products with various silver compounds, including silver nitrate and silver sulphadiazine, have been developed for wound care (Atiyeh, Costagliola, *et al.*, 2007). However, there have been concerns about the toxicity caused by the large excess amounts of silver released from the dressing becoming harmful to the wound (Poon and Burd, 2004). Reasonably, efforts have been made to develop dressing products capable of sustained release of silver ions so that wound dressings can be less frequently changed and the efficacy of infection control enhanced. Among those efforts, nanofibers have been frequently adopted as a potential efficient drug carrier for the silver (usually in the form of nanoparticles).

Two approaches have been used to prepare a silver-polymer nanofibrous structure: the *in situ* and *ex situ* methods. With the *ex situ* approach, nanoparticles are produced first and then dispersed into the polymer matrix to form a composite structure. However, this process may make it difficult for the silver nanoparticles to distribute into the polymer matrix in such a way that they can be the most effective, as the nanoparticles may easily be aggregated with each other to form clusters (Wang, Li, *et al.*, 2006). Alternatively, the *in situ* approach consists of electrospinning of the mixed solution of a silver salt (or compound) and a polymer, followed by a reductive reaction to yield silver nanoparticles within the nanofiber structure (Jin, Lee, *et al.*, 2005).

Generally speaking, if both the drug(s) and the polymer can be dissolved in a single solvent, they can be co-electrospun into nanofibers from a mixed solution of the drug(s) and the polymer (Ranganath and Wang, 2008). Otherwise, for drugs that are not soluble in any of the solvents for the polymer, or that can be destroyed by organic solvents, there are two options: emulsion electrospinning and coaxial electrospinning.

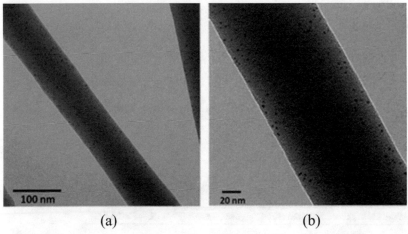

(a)   (b)

FIGURE 3.11. *TEM images of silver nanoparticle-filled nylon 6 nanofibers electrospun from 1.25% AgNO₃/nylon 6 solution. (a) 50,000×, and (b) 100,000×. (Shi, Vitchuli, et al., 2011)—Reproduced by permission of The Royal Society of Chemistry.*

1. For *emulsion electrospinning,* an aqueous solution of the drug is emulsified in a polymer solution to form a water-in-oil (w/o) *emulsion* (a mixture of two immiscible liquids, one of which is an aqueous solution and dispersed as microscopic or ultramicroscopic droplets throughout the other oily solution), and the emulsion is electrospun. During the electrospinning process, the water phase droplets (i.e., water solution of the drug) in the polymer jet are stretched into an elliptical shape in the fiber axial direction. In most circumstances, since the oil phase solvent evaporates faster than water, viscosity of the polymer/oily solvent phase increases more rapidly than that of the drug/water droplets. Also, the viscosity of the outer layer of the fiber increases more rapidly than that of the deeper layer. This difference in viscosity between the water and oil phases during the de-emulsification and the viscosity gradient from the outer layer to the inner layer lead to the inward movement of the water phase droplets (containing the drug), as well as their mergence during evaporation of the water, thus giving the electrospun nanofibers a core/sheath composition: the drug is encapsulated in the core and the polymer serves as the sheath (Figure 3.12) (Xu, Yang, *et al.,* 2005).

2. In *coaxial electrospinning,* use is made of a special coaxial spinneret (Li and Xia, 2004). Two coaxial capillaries allow the electrospinning of two components simultaneously: solution (either in water or organic solvents) of the medication in the core capillary, and the polymer solution in the outer capillary; hence, the fabrication of nanofibers of a core/sheath structure: the medication in the core and the polymer on the surface (He, Huang, *et al.,* 2006), as shown in Figure 3.13.

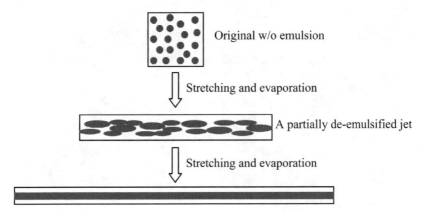

Original w/o emulsion

Stretching and evaporation

A partially de-emulsified jet

Stretching and evaporation

A final fiber with a core/sheath structure

FIGURE 3.12. *Fabrication of nanofibers with a core/sheath structure via emulsion electrospinning.*

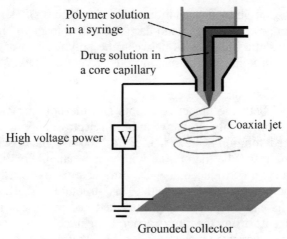

Polymer solution
in a syringe

Drug solution in
a core capillary

High voltage power   V   Coaxial jet

Grounded collector

FIGURE 3.13.   *The co-axial electrospinning setting.*

Nanofibers prepared via emulsion or coaxial electrospinning usually have a core/sheath structure—the fiber-forming polymer comprising the sheath, and the drug(s) encapsulated in the core. Such a structure provides sustained release of drugs from the nanofiber drug carrier.

3.3.2. Nanofibers Incorporated With Bioactive Agents

Nanofibrous structures have been identified as an excellent choice for scaffolds in tissue repair and regeneration (see Chapter 10). In these applications, there must be a favorable environment for the cells to attach to the scaffold, to migrate, to proliferate and to differentiate into the target tissues. To that end, the scaffolds should have appropriate physical properties, including high porosity, structural stability, controllable degradability (see Chapter 5), and, if necessary, desirably-tailored orientations (see the next section). Furthermore, the scaffolds are expected to provide an optimum biochemical environment for the growth of the cells/tissues. Most of the bioactive agents able to guide or stimulate the cellular activities (e.g., the growth factors) are proteins that have larger molecular weight (i.e., over tens of thousands) than the drugs (usually hundreds to thousands), as discussed in the previous section. Hence the extensive studies on the incorporation of such bioactive agents into/ onto the nanofibrous structures.

Proteins contain both acidic (e.g., carboxyl/–COOH) and basic (e.g., amine/–NH$_2$) functional groups, which combine to decide the overall charge of a protein molecule (e.g., positively or negatively charged). It follows that a polyelectrolyte (i.e., a charged macromolecule formed in an aqueous solution by dissociation of its charged units), like chitosan, may have an advantage as a nano-carrier for the bioactive protein, because electrostatic interactions between the polymer and protein help to entrap the protein into the nanofibrous structure (Liao, Wan, *et al.*, 2005).

Different methods have been adopted to incorporate proteins into nanofibers. If both the bioactive agents and the polymer can be dissolved into a single solvent, they can be co-electrospun into nanofibers from a mixed solution (Chew, Mi, *et al.*, 2007). Otherwise, co-axial electrospinning will be the option, with which nanofibers of the core/sheath structure are produced, usually with the bioactive agent(s) in the core and the polymer as the sheath. This structure has become well-known for its capacity to provide sustained and prolonged release of bioactive agents from the drug-carrier than nanofibers incorporated with randomly dispersed bioactive agents (Zhang, Wang, *et al.*, 2006).

Another alternative method is to immobilize bioactive proteins onto the fiber-forming polymer via the zero-length cross-linking agents, EDAC (1-ethyl-3-(3-dimethylaminopropyl) carbodiimide hydrochloride) and NHS (N-hydroxysulfosuccinimide), which may be removed completely after the reaction (Patel, Kurpinski, *et al.*, 2007). Figure 3.14 shows a PLA nanofiber with its surface immobilized with a fluorescein-labeled model protein, FITC (fluorescein isothiocyanate)-BSA (Bovine serum albumin) conjugation. Such functionalized nanofibers with bioactive agents immobilized on their surface have been demonstrated to

FIGURE 3.14. *Confocal image of a PLA nanofiber immobilized with FITC-BSA conjugation on its surface.*

be effective in promoting cell adhesion, proliferation, differentiation and/or wound healing (Choi, Leong, *et al.*, 2008; Paletta, Bockelmann, *et al.*, 2010; Chen, Zhou, *et al.*, 2011).

3.3.3. Modification for Specifically Oriented Nanofibers

The electrospinning processes usually provide nanofiber mats made up of randomly oriented fibers. Some applications, however, require materials in which the fibers are oriented as desired (e.g., in uniaxial alignment).

Since electrospun nanofibers are deposited from charged polymer jets, an extra electrical field can be applied to direct the alignment of the fibers. For example, a pair of parallel conductive electrodes separated by a gap can be used as a collector facing the ejected polymer jets. This dual-collector setting differs from the conventional electrospinning settings with a single collector in that it guides the electrical field lines in the vicinity of the collectors to split into two streams towards the opposite edges of the gap, so that the charged nanofibers can be stretched across and uni-axially aligned over the gap (Figure 3.15) (Li, Wang, *et al.*, 2003). Similarly, nanofibers with orthogonal and tri-axial orientations can be obtained by using two or three pairs of conductive electrodes that are arranged in different patterns as the collector, respectively; that is, each pair can be grounded alternatively for a certain period of time, allowing one layer of uni-axially aligned nanofibers to form at a time. With this layer-by-layer stacking approach, the nanofibrous mesh can be given a multi-axial alignment (Li, Wang, *et al.*, 2004).

Continuous aligned nanofibers can be produced by using a rotating mandrel as the collector, as shown in Figure 3.16. A high rotating speed of thousands of rpm (revolutions per minute) is needed to obtain aligned fibers around the mandrel. Different types of fiber-forming polymers may require different rotating speed of the collecting mandrel, and inadequate speed may be responsible for fibers randomly deposited (Boland, Wnek, *et al.*, 2001; Matthews, Wnek, *et al.*, 2002). Also, with the increase of the amount of fibers being collected on the mandrel, the accumulated electrostatic charges may apply a repulsive force to the incoming fibers to cause them to be less orderly oriented.

These aligned nanofiber meshes have been demonstrated to be capable of guiding and/or promoting the proliferation and/or differentiation of certain cells (e.g., neural stem cells (Yang, Murugan, *et al.*, 2005) and fibroblasts (Zhong, Teo, *et al.*, 2006), and are therefore useful as scaffold materials for tissue repair and regeneration. Figure 3.17, for example, shows a SEM (scanning electron microscope) image of mouse pre-osteoblasts (i.e., mesenchymal cells that can differentiate into osteoblasts) adhering to aligned PCL/gelatin nanofibers.

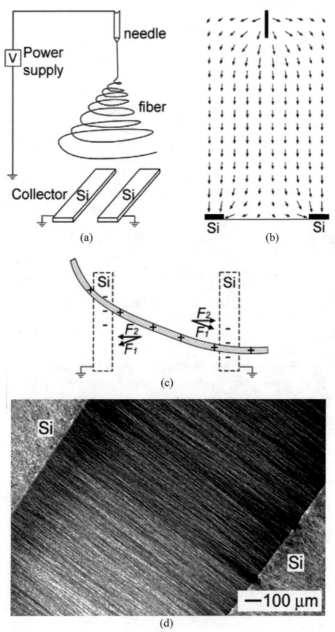

FIGURE 3.15. *(a) The electrospinning setup for generating uniaxially aligned nanofibers; (b) Electric field strength vectors in the region between the needle and the collector, with arrows denoting the direction of the electrostatic field lines; (c) Electrostatic force analysis of a charged nanofiber spanning across the gap. The electrostatic force (F_1) resulted from the electric field and the Coulomb interactions (F_2) between the positive charges on the nanofiber and the negative image charges on the two grounded electrodes. (d) dark-field optical micrograph of PVP nanofibers collected on top of a gap formed between two silicon stripes. [Reprinted with permission from (Li, Wang, et al., 2003). Copyright (2003) American Chemical Society].*

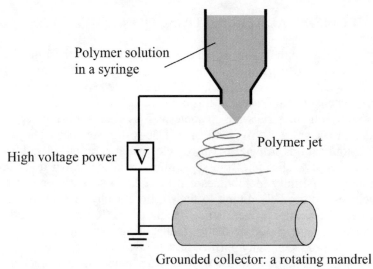

FIGURE 3.16. *Rotating mandrel as collector for the production of continuous aligned nanofibers.*

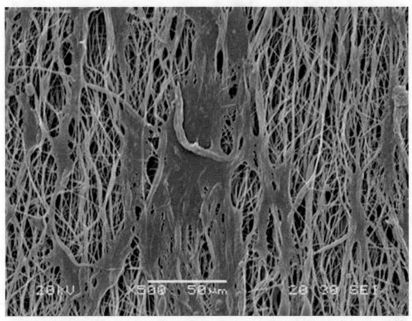

FIGURE 3.17. *A SEM image of pre-osteoblasts on aligned PCL/gelatin nanofibrous scaffold.*

59

3.4. BIOMEDICAL APPLICATIONS OF NANOFIBERS

Biomedical applications of nanofibers generally fall into three categories: selected separation, wound dressing and tissue engineering. They will be introduced in this section, and delineated in greater details in related chapters in Part II of this book.

Nanofibrous materials are characterized by their ultra-high specific surface areas (surface-to-volume or surface-to-mass values). They have found applications in what is called selective separation. Nanofibrous membranes used for selective separation are also known as affinity membranes. Affinity membranes can be used to separate one type of molecules from others owing to their different physical, chemical or biological properties, rather than molecular sizes (Ramakrishna, 2005). As such, they are important materials that allow the biopharmaceutical industry to produce highly purified therapeutic agents (e.g., antibodies). Purification is attained via use of a specific ligand (i.e., a molecule or molecular group that binds, or has specific affinity to, a target biomolecule known as a "receptor") that has been immobilized onto the surface of a fiber-forming polymer. For example, a regenerated cellulose nanofibrous membrane that is surface functionalized with protein A/G can be used as affinity membrane for the purification of the antibody immunoglobulin (IgG), as proteins A and G are known to be ligands for IgG (Ma and Ramakrishna, 2008).

A wound is "a disruption in the normal continuity of a body structure" (Shai and Maibach, 2005). Nowadays we have a variety of functionalized *wound dressings* that are capable of releasing antimicrobial agents and/or providing tissue regeneration agents (growth factors), and are therefore able to accelerate wound healing. Among these, electrospun nanofiber dressings are the most significant because of their high porosity, ultra softness, large surface-to-volume ratio, and great flexibility; these qualities have accounted for the development of a wide variety of natural and synthetic polymers. In addition, they exhibit higher drug encapsulation efficiency and better structural stability than other drug carriers. Different therapeutic agents, such as antibacterial agents and growth factors, can be incorporated into the nanofibrous dressings to enhance their functions in wound care.

The severely limited supply of donors for transplantation leads to thousands of deaths each year, and immune repression and disease transmission between patients and donors make things worse. An adequate solution to these problems should consist of two aspects: (1) stable supply of substitutes for tissues and/or organs, and (2) creation of a new environment as a substitute for the one that used to support living cells but has now become diseased or partly destroyed—i.e., a new environment that is favorable to the "regeneration" of tissues and living cells. *Tissue engineering* is one of the approaches to that solution. It is based on the combination of engineering, knowledge and technology of biomaterials, and the life sciences. The "engineering" itself is a matter of the scaffold that provides the cells' living environment, in addition to the use of regulators (such as growth factors and morphogens) and the use of cells (such as stem cells).

Nanofibrous structures have been extensively studied as the 2-dimensional or 3-dimensional scaffolds that mimic the cell living environment for tissue regeneration. Nanofibrous structures provide temporary spaces with a tunable porosity in which cells can exchange metabolites and nutrients with their environment. This allows cellular functionality to be maintained, aids in the reconstruction of tissues, and helps the tailored mechanical properties to function as desired; the wound bed can be protected from collapsing, and mechanical mismatch between scaffolds and host tissues can be avoided (Hashi, Zhu, *et al.*, 2007). By replicating the host tissue matrices, nanofibrous structures are capable of regulating stem cell differentiation and promoting cell ingrowth (Xie, Willerth, *et al.*, 2009). Also, they can be fabricated as drug carriers capable of prolonged, sustained, and controllable release of therapeutic agents into wounds, substituting for the traditional direct injection of drugs that is sometimes problematic. More details about the application of nanofibers in tissue engineering can be found in Chapter 10.

While nanofibers are an enormous source of many useful applications, much of the development and design of nanofibers are still in the stage of laboratory experimentation and testing. *In vitro* and *in vivo* methods have been adopted to evaluate the performance of functionalized dressings, including their cytotoxicity (i.e., toxic effect on viable cells). *In vitro* tests refer to procedures conducted in a controlled environment outside of a living organism, usually involving usage of viable cells. For example, the antibacterial capacity of a drug-loaded nanofibrous dressing can be evaluated by having the dressing materials co-cultured with viable bacteria and measuring their capacity of inhibition. On the other hand, an *in vivo* procedure is performed within a living organism, either an animal or human being. For example, the healing capacity of a drug-loaded nanofibrous dressing can be further monitored after its application on the wounds of animals (e.g., mice, porcine) or human patients. *In vitro* methods usually provide better control on experimental conditions, and cost less than *in vivo* approaches. *In vivo* tests may involve ethics issues, especially in the cases when living creatures are the subjects. *In vivo* tests are essential, however, because *in vitro* tests can never reproduce the physiological environment in a living organism. A further discussion can be found in Chapters 9 and 10.

3.5. SUMMARY

This chapter is devoted to a discussion of the fabrication of nanofibers as a biomaterial, and the use of it as such. Several approaches to this fabrication have been included, focusing on the extracting of nanofibrils from natural materials by both mechanical and chemical means and electrospinning from a wide range of materials (both natural and synthetic). Of these, electrospinning has received greater attention for a number of reasons: it is convenient to operate, its processing parameters can be well controlled, and it is the most likely to reach the scale of mass, industrial production.

An adequate treatment of the subject should involve a discussion of production materials. Thus we have referred to a large variety of materials (i.e., natural and synthetic polymers) for nanofibers fabrication, including the choice and use of them, and a description of how their properties influence processing parameters and properties (biocompatibility, cytotoxicity, etc.) of the product.

We have also discussed the highly technical aspect of nanofibers' production and applications: modification towards functionalization of polymer nanofibers intended to improve their performance and function in biomedical applications. This purpose is achieved by incorporating such therapeutic agents as antibacterial agents and growth factors into the nanofibrous structures, so that the product will duly become capable of infection control, improving biocompatibility, promoting cell proliferation and differentiation, and, as a result of properly tailored orientation of the nanofibers, guiding cell growth in the course of tissue regeneration.

Polymeric nanofibers have found various applications in the biomedical field, such as use of nanofibrous affinity membranes in selective separation, functional wound dressings in wound care, and scaffolding materials for tissue repair and regeneration. We have cautioned that much of the nanofibers-related work has been performed in labs, a caution that will, we expect, function only to ignite greater endeavors towards their eventual clinical application.

3.6. REFERENCES

Altman, G.H., F. Diaz, *et al.* (2003). Silk-based biomaterials. *Biomaterials* **24**(3): 401–416.

Alvarez-Perez, M.A., V. Guarino, *et al.* (2010). Influence of gelatin cues in PCL electrospun membranes on nerve outgrowth. *Biomacromolecules* **11**(9): 2238–2246.

Atiyeh, B.S., M. Costagliola, *et al.* (2007). Effect of silver on burn wound infection control and healing: Review of the literature. *Burns* **33**(2): 139–148.

Barnes, C.P., S.A. Sell, *et al.* (2007). Nanofiber technology: designing the next generation of tissue engineering scaffolds. *Advanced Drug Delivery Reviews* **59**(14): 1413–1433.

Bhatnagar, A. and M. Sain. (2005). Processing of cellulose nanofiber-reinforced composites. *Journal of Reinforced Plastics and Composites* **24**(12): 1259–1268.

Boland, E.D., G.E. Wnek, *et al.* (2001). Tailoring tissue engineering scaffolds using electrostatic processing techniques: A study of poly(glycolic acid) electrospinning. *Journal of Macromolecular Science-Pure and Applied Chemistry* **38**(12): 1231–1243.

Buchko, C.J., L.C. Chen, *et al.* (1999). Processing and microstructural characterization of porous biocompatible protein polymer thin films. *Polymer* **40**(26): 7397–7407.

Casper, C.L., J.S. Stephens, *et al.* (2004). Controlling surface morphology of electrospun polystyrene fibers: Effect of humidity and molecular weight in the electrospinning process. *Macromolecules* **37**(2): 573–578.

Chen, J., B. Zhou, *et al.* (2011). PLLA-PEG-TCH-labeled bioactive molecule nanofibers for tissue engineering. *International Journal of Nanomedicine* **6**: 2533–2542.

Chen, J. P., G.Y. Chang, *et al.* (2008). Electrospun collagen/chitosan nanofibrous membrane as wound dressing. *Colloids and Surfaces A-Physicochemical and Engineering Aspects* **313**: 183–188.

Chen, Z.G., X.M. Mo, *et al.* (2008). Intermolecular interactions in electrospun collagen-chitosan complex nanofibers. *Carbohydrate Polymers* **72**(3): 410–418.

Chew, S.Y., R.F. Mi, *et al.* (2007). Aligned protein-polymer composite fibers enhance nerve regeneration: A potential tissue-engineering platform. *Advanced Functional Materials* **17**(8): 1288–1296.

Choi, J.S., S.W. Lee, *et al.* (2004). Effect of organosoluble salts on the nanofibrous structure of electrospun poly(3-hydroxybutyrate-co-3-hydroxyvalerate). *International Journal of Biological Macromolecules* **34**(4): 249–256.

Choi, J.S., K.W. Leong, *et al.* (2008). In vivo wound healing of diabetic ulcers using electrospun nanofibers immobilized with human epidermal growth factor (EGF). *Biomaterials* **29**(5): 587–596.

Corey, J.M., C.C. Gertz, *et al.* (2008). The design of electrospun PLLA nanofiber scaffolds compatible with serum-free growth of primary motor and sensory neurons. *Acta Biomaterialia* **4**(4): 863–875.

De Vrieze, S., T. Van Camp, *et al.* (2009). The effect of temperature and humidity on electrospinning. *Journal of Materials Science* **44**(5): 1357–1362.

Deitzel, J.M., J. Kleinmeyer, *et al.* (2001). The effect of processing variables on the morphology of electrospun nanofibers and textiles. *Polymer* **42**(1): 261–272.

Deitzel, J.M., J.D. Kleinmeyer, *et al.* (2001b). Controlled deposition of electrospun poly(ethylene oxide) fibers. *Polymer* **42**(19): 8163–8170.

Del Gaudio, C., A. Bianco, *et al.* (2009). Structural characterization and cell response evaluation of electrospun PCL membranes: micrometric versus submicrometric fibers. *Journal of Biomedical Materials Research Part A* **89A**(4): 1028–1039.

Desai, K., K. Kit, *et al.* (2008). Morphological and surface properties of electrospun chitosan nanofibers. *Biomacromolecules* **9**(3): 1000–1006.

Fallon, M.T., W. Shafer, *et al.* (1999). Use of cefazolin microspheres to treat localized methicillin-resistant Staphylococcus aureus infections in rats. *Journal of Surgical Research* **86**(1): 97–102.

Formhals, A. (1934). Process and apparatus for preparing artificial threads. US Patent 1,975,504.

Foster, L. and P. Moore. (1997). The application of a cellulose-based fibre dressing in surgical wounds. *J. Wound Care* **6**(10): 469–73.

Franklin, T.J., G.A. Snow, *et al.* (2005). Biochemistry and molecular biology of antimicrobial drug action. New York: Springer.

Frey, M.W. (2008). Electrospinning cellulose and cellulose derivatives. *Polymer Reviews* **48**(2): 378–391.

Gui-Bo, Y., Z. You-Zhu, *et al.* (2010). Study of the electrospun PLA/silk fibroin-gelatin composite nanofibrous scaffold for tissue engineering. *Journal of Biomedical Materials Research Part A* **93A**(1): 158–163.

Han, I., K.J. Shim, *et al.* (2007). Effect of poly(3-hydroxybutyrate-co-3-hydroxyvalerate) nanofiber matrices co-cultured with hair follicular epithelial and dermal cells for biological wound dressing. *Artificial Organs* **31**(11): 801–808.

Hartgerink, J.D., E. Beniash, *et al.* (2001). Self-assembly and mineralization of peptide-amphiphile nanofibers. *Science* **294**(5547): 1684–1688.

Hashi, C.K., Y. Zhu, *et al.* (2007). Antithrombogenic property of bone marrow mesenchymal stem cells in nanofibrous vascular grafts. *Proc. Natl. Acad. Sci. USA* **104**(29): 11915–20.

He, C.L., Z.M. Huang, *et al.* (2006). Coaxial electrospun poly(L-lactic acid) ultrafine fibers for sustained drug delivery. *Journal of Macromolecular Science Part B-Physics* **45**(4): 515–524.

He, L.M., S.S. Liao, *et al.* (2010). Synergistic effects of electrospun PLLA fiber dimension and pattern on neonatal mouse cerebellum C17.2 stem cells. *Acta Biomaterialia* **6**(8): 2960–2969.

Hong, K.H. (2007). Preparation and properties of electrospun poly(vinyl alcohol)/silver fiber web as wound dressings. *Polymer Engineering and Science* **47**(1): 43–49.

Hult, E.L., S. Yamanaka, *et al.* (2003). Aggregation of ribbons in bacterial cellulose induced by high pressure incubation. *Carbohydrate Polymers* **53**(1): 9–14.

Ignatova, M., N. Manolova, *et al.* (2009). Electrospun non-woven nanofibrous hybrid mats based on chitosan and PLA for wound-dressing applications. *Macromolecular Bioscience* **9**(1): 102–111.

Iguchi, M., S. Yamanaka, *et al.* (2000). Bacterial cellulose—a masterpiece of nature's arts. *Journal of Materials Science* **35**(2): 261–270.

Jacob, E., G. Cierny, *et al.* (1993). Evaluation of biodegradable cefazolin sodium microspheres for the prevention of infection in rabbits with experimental open tibial fractures stabilized with internal-fixation. *Journal of Orthopaedic Research* **11**(3): 404–411.

Jiang, Q.R., N. Reddy, *et al.* (2010). Cytocompatible cross-linking of electrospun zein fibers for the development of water-stable tissue engineering scaffolds. *Acta Biomaterialia* **6**(10): 4042–4051.

Jin, W.J., H.K. Lee, *et al.* (2005). Preparation of polymer nanofibers containing silver nanoparticles by using poly(N-vinylpyrrolidone). *Macromolecular Rapid Communications* **26**(24): 1903–1907.

Kalfa, D., A. Bel, *et al.* (2010). A polydioxanone electrospun valved patch to replace the right ventricular outflow tract in a growing lamb model. *Biomaterials* **31**(14): 4056–4063.

Khil, M.S., D.I. Cha, *et al.* (2003). Electrospun nanofibrous polyurethane membrane as wound dressing. *Journal of Biomedical Materials Research Part B-Applied Biomaterials* **67B**(2): 675–679.

Khil, M.S., H.Y. Kim, *et al.* (2005). Preparation of electrospun oxidized cellulose mats and their in vitro degradation behavior. *Macromolecular Research* **13**(1): 62–67.

Kim, C.H., J.W. Choi, *et al.* (1997). Synthesis of chitosan derivatives with quaternary ammonium salt and their antibacterial activity. *Polymer Bulletin* **38**(4): 387–393.

Kim, S.E., D.N. Heo, *et al.* (2009). Electrospun gelatin/polyurethane blended nanofibers for wound healing. *Biomedical Materials* **4**(4): 44106.

Lawrence, J.C. (1994). Dressings and wound infection. *Am. J. Surg.* **167**(1A): 21S–24S.

Lee, C.H., A. Singla, *et al.* (2001). Biomedical applications of collagen. *International Journal of Pharmaceutics* **221**(1–2): 1–22.

Li, D., Y.L. Wang, *et al.* (2003). Electrospinning of polymeric and ceramic nanofibers as uniaxially aligned arrays. *Nano Letters* **3**(8): 1167–1171.

Li, D., Y.L. Wang, *et al.* (2004). Electrospinning nanofibers as uniaxially aligned arrays and layer-by-layer stacked films. *Advanced Materials* **16**(4): 361–366.

Li, D. and Y.N. Xia. (2004). Direct fabrication of composite and ceramic hollow nanofibers by electrospinning. *Nano Letters* **4**(5): 933–938.

Liao, I.C., A.C.A. Wan, *et al.* (2005). Controlled release from fibers of polyelectrolyte complexes. *Journal of Controlled Release* **104**(2): 347–358.

Liu, H.Q. and Y.L. Hsieh. (2002). Ultrafine fibrous cellulose membranes from electrospinning of cellulose acetate. *Journal of Polymer Science Part B-Polymer Physics* **40**(18): 2119–2129.

Luu, Y.K., K. Kim, *et al.* (2003). Development of a nanostructured DNA delivery scaffold via electrospinning of PLGA and PLA-PEG block copolymers. *Journal of Controlled Release* **89**(2): 341–353.

Ma, P.X. and R.Y. Zhang. (1999). Synthetic nano-scale fibrous extracellular matrix. *Journal of Biomedical Materials Research* **46**(1): 60–72.

Ma, Z. and S. Ramakrishna. (2008). Electrospun regenerated cellulose nanofiber affinity membrane functionalized with protein A/G for IgG purification. *Journal of Membrane Science* **319**(1–2): 23–28.

Matthews, J.A., G.E. Wnek, *et al.* (2002). Electrospinning of collagen nanofibers. *Biomacromolecules* **3**(2): 232–238.

Megelski, S., J.S. Stephens, *et al.* (2002). Micro- and nanostructured surface morphology on electrospun polymer fibers. *Macromolecules* **35**(22): 8456–8466.

Min, B. M., G. Lee, *et al.* (2004). Electrospinning of silk fibroin nanofibers and its effect on the adhesion and spreading of normal human keratinocytes and fibroblasts *in vitro*. *Biomaterials* **25**(7–8): 1289–1297.

Miyamoto, K., M. Atarashi, *et al.* (2009). Creation of cross-linked electrospun isotypic-elastin fibers controlled cell-differentiation with new cross-linker. *International Journal of Biological Macromolecules* **45**(1): 33–41.

Muise-Helmericks, R.C., H. Buff, *et al.* (2009). Poly-N-acetylglucosamine nanofibers from a marine diatom promote wound healing and angiogenesis via an Akt1/Ets1-dependent pathway. *Wound Repair and Regeneration* **17**(2): A16.

Ohgo, K., C.H. Zhao, *et al.* (2003). Preparation of non-woven nanofibers of Bombyx mori silk, Samia cynthia ricini silk and recombinant hybrid silk with electrospinning method. *Polymer* **44**(3): 841–846.

Oksman, K., A.P. Mathew, *et al.* (2006). Manufacturing process of cellulose whiskers/polylactic acid nanocomposites. *Composites Science and Technology* **66**(15): 2776–2784.

Ondarcuhu, T. and C. Joachim. (1998). Drawing a single nanofibre over hundreds of microns. *Europhysics Letters* **42**(2): 215–220.

Oroudjev, E., J. Soares, *et al.* (2002). Segmented nanofibers of spider dragline silk: atomic force microscopy and single-molecule force spectroscopy. *Proceedings of the National Academy of Sciences of the United States of America* **99**: 6460–6465.

Paletta, J.R.J., S. Bockelmann, *et al.* (2010). RGD-functionalisation of PLLA nanofibers by surface coupling using plasma treatment: influence on stem cell differentiation. *Journal of Materials Science-Materials in Medicine* **21**(4): 1363–1369.

Park, J.Y., B.W. Han, *et al.* (2007). Preparation of electrospun porous ethyl cellulose fiber by THF/DMAc binary solvent system. *Journal of Industrial and Engineering Chemistry* **13**(6): 1002–1008.

Park, K.E., S. Park, *et al.* (2008). Preparation and characterization of sodium alginate/PEO and sodium alginate/PVA nanofiber. *Polymer-Korea* **32**(3): 206–212.

Patel, S., K. Kurpinski, *et al.* (2007). Bioactive nanofibers: synergistic effects of nanotopography and chemical signaling on cell guidance. *Nano Letters* **7**(7): 2122–2128.

Poon, V.K.M. and A. Burd. (2004). *In vitro* cytotoxity of silver: implication for clinical wound care. *Burns* **30**(2): 140–147.

Powell, H.M. and S.T. Boyce. (2009). Engineered human skin fabricated using electrospun collagen-PCL blends: morphogenesis and mechanical properties. *Tissue Engineering Part A* **15**(8): 2177–2187.

Ramakrishna, S. (2005). An introduction to electrospinning and nanofibers. Hackensack, NJ: World Scientific.

Ranganath, S.H. and C.H. Wang. (2008). Biodegradable microfiber implants delivering paclitaxel for post-surgical chemotherapy against malignant glioma. *Biomaterials* **29**(20): 2996–3003.

Schiffman, J.D. and C.L. Schauer. (2007). One-step electrospinning of cross-linked chitosan fibers. *Biomacromolecules* **8**(9): 2665–2667.

Schofer, M.D., U. Boudriot, *et al.* (2009). Influence of nanofibers on the growth and osteogenic differentiation of stem cells: a comparison of biological collagen nanofibers and synthetic PLLA fibers. *Journal of Materials Science-Materials in Medicine* **20**(3): 767–774.

Sell, S.A., M.J. McClure, *et al.* (2009). Electrospinning of collagen/biopolymers for regenerative medicine and cardiovascular tissue engineering. *Advanced Drug Delivery Reviews* **61**(12): 1007–1019.

Shai, A. and H.I. Maibach. (2005). Wound healing and ulcers of the skin. Berlin: Springer.

Shi, Q., N. Vitchuli, *et al.* (2011). One-step synthesis of silver nanoparticle-filled nylon 6 nanofibers and their antibacterial properties. *Journal of Materials Chemistry* **21**(28): 10330–10335.

Shukla, S., E. Brinley, *et al.* (2005). Electrospinning of hydroxypropyl cellulose fibers and their application in synthesis of nano and submicron tin oxide fibers. *Polymer* **46**(26): 12130–12145.

Siri, S. and S. Maensiri. (2010). Alternative biomaterials: natural, non-woven, fibroin-based silk nanofibers of weaver ants (Oecophylla smaragdina). *International Journal of Biological Macromolecules* **46**(5): 529–534.

Son, W.K., J.H. Youk, *et al.* (2004). Preparation of ultrafine oxidized cellulose mats via electrospinning. *Biomacromolecules* **5**(1): 197–201.

Stadelmann, W.K., A.G. Digenis, *et al.* (1998). Impediments to wound healing. *American Journal of Surgery* **176**(2A): 39s–47s.

Su, Y., X.Q. Li, *et al.* (2010). Fabrication and properties of PLLA-gelatin nanofibers by electrospinning. *Journal of Applied Polymer Science* **117**(1): 542–547.

Subramanian, A., D. Vu, *et al.* (2005). Preparation and evaluation of the electrospun chitosan/PEO fibers for potential applications in cartilage tissue engineering. *Journal of Biomaterials Science-Polymer Edition* **16**(7): 861–873.

Suwantong, O., P. Pavasant, *et al.* (2011). Electrospun zein fibrous membranes using glyoxal as cross-linking agent: preparation, characterization and potential for use in Biomedical applications. *Chiang Mai Journal of Science* **38**(1): 56–70.

Szentivanyi, A., U. Assmann, *et al.* (2009). Production of biohybrid protein/PEO scaffolds by electrospinning. *Materialwissenschaft Und Werkstofftechnik* **40**(1–2): 65–72.

Taniguchi, T. and K. Okamura. (1998). New films produced from microfibrillated natural fibres. *Polymer International* **47**(3): 291–294.

Verreck, G., I. Chun, *et al.* (2003). Incorporation of drugs in an amorphous state into electrospun nanofibers composed of a water-insoluble, nonbiodegradable polymer. *Journal of Controlled Release* **92**(3): 349–360.

Wang, B. and M. Sain. (2007). The effect of chemically coated nanofiber reinforcement on biopolymer based nanocomposites. *Bioresources* **2**(3): 371–388.

Wang, C., H.S. Chien, *et al.* (2007). Electrospinning of polyacrylonitrile solutions at elevated temperatures. *Macromolecules* **40**(22): 7973–7983.

Wang, Y.Z., H.J. Kim, *et al.* (2006). Stem cell-based tissue engineering with silk biomaterials. *Biomaterials* **27**(36): 6064–6082.

Wang, Y.Z., Y.X. Li, *et al.* (2006). A convenient route to polyvinyl pyrrolidone/silver nanocomposite by electrospinning. *Nanotechnology* **17**(13): 3304–3307.

Wnek, G.E., M.E. Carr, *et al.* (2003). Electrospinning of nanofiber fibrinogen structures. *Nano Letters* **3**(2): 213–216.

Woerdeman, D.L., P. Ye, *et al.* (2005). Electrospun fibers from wheat protein: Investigation of the interplay between molecular structure and the fluid dynamics of the electrospinning process. *Biomacromolecules* **6**(2): 707–712.

Xie, J., S.M. Willerth, *et al.* (2009). The differentiation of embryonic stem cells seeded on electrospun nanofibers into neural lineages. *Biomaterials* **30**(3): 354–62.

Xu, J., J.H. Zhang, *et al.* (2009). Preparation of chitosan/PLA blend micro/nanofibers by electrospinning. *Materials Letters* **63**(8): 658–660.

Xu, S.S., J. Zhang, *et al.* (2008). Electrospinning of native cellulose from nonvolatile solvent system. *Polymer* **49**(12): 2911–2917.

Xu, X.L., L.X. Yang, *et al.* (2005). Ultrafine medicated fibers electrospun from W/O emulsions. *Journal of Controlled Release* **108**(1): 33–42.

Xu, X.L., W. Zhong, *et al.* (2010). Electrospun PEG-PLA nanofibrous membrane for sustained release of hydrophilic antibiotics. *Journal of Applied Polymer Science* **118**(1): 588–595.

Yang, F., R. Murugan, *et al.* (2005). Electrospinning of nano/micro scale poly(L-lactic acid) aligned fibers and their potential in neural tissue engineering. *Biomaterials* **26**(15): 2603–2610.

Yeom, C.K. and K.H. Lee. (1996). Pervaporation separation of water-acetic acid mixtures through poly(vinyl alcohol) membranes crosslinked with glutaraldehyde. *Journal of Membrane Science* **109**(2): 257–265.

Zhang, Y.Z., X. Wang, *et al.* (2006). Coaxial electrospinning of (fluorescein isothiocyanate-conjugated bovine serum albumin)-encapsulated poly(epsilon-caprolactone) nanofibers for sustained release. *Biomacromolecules* **7**(4): 1049–1057.

Zhao, Y., X.Y. Cao, *et al.* (2007). Bio-mimic multichannel microtubes by a facile method. *Journal of the American Chemical Society* **129**(4): 764–765.

Zhong, S.P., W.E. Teo, *et al.* (2006). An aligned nanofibrous collagen scaffold by electrospinning and its effects on in vitro fibroblast culture. *Journal of Biomedical Materials Research Part A* **79A**(3): 456–463.

Zhou, Y.S., D.Z. Yang, *et al.* (2008). Electrospun water-soluble carboxyethyl chitosan/poly(vinyl alcohol) nanofibrous membrane as potential wound dressing for skin regeneration. *Biomacromolecules* **9**(1): 349–354.

Zimniewska, M., R. Kozlowski, *et al.* (2008). Nanolignin modified linen fabric as a multifunctional product. *Molecular Crystals and Liquid Crystals* **484**: 409–416.

CHAPTER 4

Textiles as a Source of Comfort and Healthcare Problems

A large barrier organ, the skin protects the human body from external hazards (heat, cold, chemicals, mechanical forces, etc.) and helps maintain its integrity. Clothing usually comprises a system of textiles, and provides an extra barrier to offer the aesthetic, thermophysiological, and sensorial comfort for the wearer, in addition to doing much of the protection that the skin is capable of. However, these vital benefits are not offered without running risks: direct contact of the skin with textiles may engender interactions, and these interactions can cause inconvenience, damage or disease to the body; or they may produce *discomfort*. Use of healthcare and medical textiles involves similar risks, leads to similar problems, and requires similar considerations and efforts to prevent such problems and, above all, to secure good comfort.

The level of comfort is a vital concern in the design and development of any textile product to be applied next to the human skin. This concern is even more critical for the various medical and healthcare textile products, because the skin they will be in contact with is, as a rule, fragile, or is already damaged or diseased. For example, diaper rash is a common skin disease suffered by babies, and therefore the prevention of which is the major concern in the development of diaper products, because a diaper that fails to be *comfortable* for the baby to wear is good for nothing, notwithstanding its many other merits. The comfort of protective clothing (e.g., a surgeon's uniform) is important for the wearer to perform procedures to the best of their ability, contributing to both the comfort of the wearer and the health and life of someone else. For wound care textile products, the level of comfort is not only a measure of the physical comfort to be experienced by the person who bears the wound, but also intrinsically related to the efficiency of the product to assist the wound healing process. Indeed, while comfortable clothing

69

may border on extravagance, the comfort from a medical and healthcare textile product is never something extra.

Although an extremely simple word, *comfort* is complex or even "nebulous" to define. In the case of the comfort that a textile product can provide, a relevant definition can be "a pleasant state of physiological, psychological and physical harmony between a human being and the environment" (Slater, 1985). In that situation, comfort consists of three aspects:

1. Comfort as an *aesthetic appeal,* especially in the case of "clothing", which contributes to the overall charm of the individual who wears it. This aspect of comfort is largely psychological in nature, and the effort to gain or improve such appeal is typically found in the trade of fashion design. This book can therefore do without a discussion about it, because the theme of this book is technical textiles.
2. Comfort as a *thermophysiological benefit,* which secures a proper level of warmth and wetness as a result of the transport of heat and moisture through a system of fabrics. If well-designed, such a system is expected to keep the wearer warm in the cold, and cool in the heat, and maintain breathability and permeability in all cases. See Section 4.1.
3. Comfort as a *sensorial satisfaction,* which is related to the elicitation of various sensations (e.g., pain, prickle and itch) when a textile product is in contact with the skin. These sensations are reactions of the skin to the textiles or, more often than not, to the elements brought along with the textiles, such as chemicals and agents (e.g., dyes and finishing agents) incorporated into the textile product. They are engendered also by mechanical forces, including pressure and friction, as a result of the contact between the skin and fabric. See Section 4.2.

Textiles have nothing to do with comfort or problems unless they are placed on or near to the skin, forming a textile-skin system. Thermophysiological comfort and sensorial comfort are the result of the textile-skin *contact.* As such they are not independent, but work together to enhance or reduce the comfort levels of a product, or even to cause such skin problems as blistering and ulceration, as will be discussed in Section 4.3.

4.1. MICROCLIMATE AND THERMOPHYSIOLOGICAL COMFORT

Extremely open to the environment, textiles (or "fabrics", typically in the form of "clothing") in the textile-skin system give rise to a

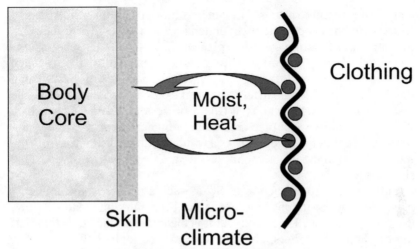

FIGURE 4.1. *Microclimate in the skin-fabric system.*

microclimate (Figure 4.1) to influence and be influenced by such factors as exchange of heat and flow of micro-space airstream between the skin and textiles, expressed by such environmental parameters as temperature and humidity (Cena and Clark, 1981). The significance of the microclimate is that (1) it directly influences comfort, and (2) such comfort can be obtained in the course of product design by referring to microclimate-related properties of the textile materials (e.g., moisture and heat transport), and by regulating physiological and environmental conditions in the use of textile products. Since this comfort is heat-physiology-related, it is tagged "thermophysiological".

4.1.1. Stratum Corneum and Transepidermal Water Loss

Human skin contains a stratified tissue composed of four layers, which from top to bottom are the stratum corneum (SC), the viable epidermis, the dermis and the subcutis. SC consists of multiple layers of keratinized cells (corneocytes), which are dead cell layers originating from the underlying basal layer. It is the most superficial layer of the skin and is in direct contact with the fabric.

SC plays an important role in maintaining the skin's clinical appearance due to its water-retaining capacity. Water travels from within the skin towards the outer environment in two manners. One is the active transport of water known as *sweating,* which involves primarily liquid water exuded by sweat glands in the skin. The evaporation of sweat from the skin is of a cooling mechanism, as energy is consumed to turn water from liquid to vapor. The other is more of an insensible loss of water: from the deeper, highly hydrated layers of the epidermis and dermis, a passive flux of water takes place towards the more superficial SC layers, which have a relatively low water content. This is the so-called transepidermal water loss (TEWL), which is a parameter for evaluating the function of SC as a barrier to prevent excessive water loss (Agache and Humbert, 2004). The TEWL is a process of diffusion, in which water vapor moves from the area under a higher vapor pressure to another that is under a lower one. As a result, it can be estimated from the measurement of the water vapor pressure gradient non-invasively at the skin surface.

Fulfillment of the function of SC as such a barrier is so complex a phenomenon that its physiology has not been fully understood. However, it has been well accepted that it is the intercellular lipids (consisting of cholesterol esters, cholesterol, saturated long-chain fatty acids and ceramides) of the SC that contribute vitally to that fulfillment, and that an increase in the environmental temperature or relative humidity usually leads to an elevated TEWL (Agache and Humbert, 2004).

4.1.2. The Impact of Textiles on Human Thermoregulation

Normal humans maintain a core body temperature of about 37°C. A variation from the core temperature beyond 5°C is usually fatal. The body maintains its temperature by means of thermoregulation, i.e., keeping a balance between the rates of heat production and heat loss to the environment.

The ambient temperature in our living environment may vary between –50 to 50°C. For humans to feel comfortable, however, a fairly narrow variation of surface temperature (and humidity) must be maintained in the air immediately surrounding the body. The range of ambient temperature within which basal metabolic rate is minimal and constant is called the *thermoneutral zone,* which has been found to be between 28–30°C for a human being that is naked and quiet. Obviously, clothing is the most important means of regulating body temperature and controlling heat loss. In other words, a system of fabrics, especially clothing, functions also to expand the thermoneutral zone. Autonomic physiological responses may occur when temperature falls beyond that zone: in the cold, vasoconstriction (i.e., contraction of blood vessels) helps restrain heat loss and shivering (usually unconscious) increases heat production from within the body. In the heat, on the other hand, vasodilation (i.e., dilation of blood vessels) and sweat both increase heat loss. This physiological mechanism, which as a rule cannot operate effectively for long, constitutes the last line of defense. Prolonged exposure to an environment of very high or low temperature may lead to hyperthermia (heat stroke) or hypothermia, which can be fatal.

The mechanism for heat (*S*) to be stored in and lost from the human body is expressed in the following equation:

$$S = M(\pm W) - E \pm D \pm C \pm R \qquad (4.1)$$

which correlates the several factors:

M represents the metabolic heat production, and *W* is the external work accomplished. Since these are factors that usually cannot be regulated by a system of fabrics, they will not be discussed further in this book. The following four factors, on the other hand, can be influenced, and are explained as follows:

E (evaporative heat loss) indicates the portion of heat that is dissipated by means of perspiration. There are two types of perspiration: the sensible perspiration or sweat and the insensible perspiration already denoted as TEWL. Perspiration depends on relative humidity, i.e., the higher the relative humidity, the lower the rate of perspiration. As a result, it is essential for a system of fabrics to be efficient enough to regulate the dissipation of water (in the form of both vapor and liquid) to the outer environment, so as to keep a relatively dry microclimate between the skin and the fabric. When the opposite is the case, an excess of liquid will collect in the fabric, making it as wet and sticky as to adhere to the skin, resulting in discomfort and further blocking the sweat glands.

D (heat lost/gained by conduction) is used to denote that, when two material media or objects are in direct contact, conduction of heat occurs from the one with a higher temperature to the other, until both reach an identical temperature. The efficiency of heat transfer through a material by conduction is called its thermal conductivity (*k*), which can be defined as the heat loss (*Q*, in watts, or *W*) through a unit thickness (*L*, in m) in the direction normal to a unit area (*A*, in m^2) of the material due to the unit temperature gradient (ΔT, in Kelvin, or K):

$$k(W.m^{-1}.K^{-1}) = \frac{Q \times L}{A \times \Delta T} \qquad (4.2)$$

Table 4.1 shows thermal conductivity of different materials. It indicates that textile fibers are much lower in thermal conductivity as compared to the other material classes, and explains why fiber materials can be used as good insulators to keep us warm. The thermal conductivity of fibers is also lower than that of water and much higher than that of still air, which is why a damp or wet piece of fabric or clothing can be cold to the touch. On the other hand, a system of fabrics with a large

TABLE 4.1. Thermal Conductivity (W.m⁻¹.K⁻¹) of Different Materials
(Cardarelli, 2008).

	Diamond	Copper	Glass (sodalime)	Water	Nylon	Air (still)
Thermal conductivity	900	401	1.4	0.58	0.25	0.024
Relative to air	375,000	16,708	58.3	24.2	10.4	1

amount of entrapped still air will provide excellent insulation, which explains, for example, why hollow fibers with still air entrapped in each individual fiber have been developed as filling materials for winter jackets and sleeping bags. The down of birds, a layer of fine feathers found under the tougher exterior feathers, is a natural fibrous material of a loose structure, with which the material allows the entrapment of large amounts of still air, and is therefore regarded as an excellent insulation material. It is also well known that a multiple-layered system of fabrics usually results in greater body heat retention than a single-layered one; although the two systems may have an identical thickness, they differ from each other because different amounts of air are entrapped and held still to slow down heat conduction.

C (Heat lost/gained by convection) refers to the motion of a liquid or gas that carries energy from a warmer region to a cooler one. Usually a fabric structure with a high porosity allows more efficient heat transfer by convection.

R (Heat lost/gained by radiation) refers to energy that is radiated or transmitted in the form of rays or waves or particles. Radiation does not require the presence of an intervening medium; it occurs within a vacuum. Similarly, a fabric with a more open structure allows more efficient heat transfer by radiation.

In general, a system of fabrics that allows more ventilation is noted for its greater heat loss by both convection and radiation in warm weather. This effect can be achieved by structural design of the fabric, making it thinner, sheerer or more porous (e.g., using knits). The same effect can be attained by wearing-loose fitting fabrics, or an assembly. On the other hand, thick fabrics of close structures are related to minimized heat loss.

4.1.3. The Impact of Fabric on the Transport of Vapor/Liquid Water

Transport of water (in the form of vapor or liquid) takes place following a number of paths from the microclimate through a system of fabrics. Water thus released is either dissipated into the environment or retained by the fiber.

Water vapor usually dissipates by diffusion—namely, the water molecules move from the area of a higher vapor pressure to the area of a lower vapor pressure, driven by a vapor pressure gradient, until equilibrium is reached (when vapor pressures of the two areas become identical). Obviously, the rate of water vapor diffusion or dissipation decreases as environmental humidity (i.e., environmental vapor pressure) increases.

When a piece of fabric is placed over the skin, water vapor in the microclimate will first diffuse into the void space of the fabric, including the interstice between the yarns, between the fibers, and the void space inside the fiber, and then make its way to the outer environment. The type of fiber is closely related to (if not "determines") the transport of water. Usually, a fabric containing hydrophilic fibers has a higher rate of water vapor diffusion than the fabric with a similar structure but composed of hydrophobic fibers. Fibers or fabrics that allow the transport of water vapor from the microclimate to the outer environment are known as *breathable* fibers or fabrics. Breathability is a requirement for most textile products to regulate humidity in the microclimate.

Liquid water can be retained by the fabric in three different manners; water thus held in the fabric is referred to as:

1. *Absorbed water,* which refers to water molecules held within the fibers. A fiber is composed of a large number of polymer chains that may run through different regions of different packing densities (Figure 2.3). Polymer chains either pack tightly in an orderly fashion in the crystalline regions, or distribute loosely in a disordered pattern in the amorphous regions. Water molecules can enter a hydrophilic polymer system (e.g., cellulose and wool) in its spacious amorphous regions and be held tenaciously via hydrogen bonding. Absorbed water is usually not felt by the skin. The space in the crystalline regions, however, is too small to allow the penetration of water molecules.

2. *Adsorbed water,* which is the water held on the surface of a fiber. Hydrophilic fibers may hold the water more tenaciously than hydrophobic fibers, because hydrogen bonding can form between the fiber polymer and water. Water adsorption onto a fiber surface is affected by the *wetting* capacity (i.e., wettability) of a fiber material. Surface area of a fibrous structure is another important factor for water adsorption, i.e., the larger the surface area, the greater the amount of water adsorbed. It is known that fine fibers have a higher surface-to-volume ratio (i.e., amount of surface area per unit volume of a material) or surface-to-mass ratio (i.e., amount of surface area per unit mass of a material). As a result, micro- or even nanofibers are superior in applications where higher capacities of liquid adsorption are required.

3. *Imbibed water,* which is held in the interstices between fibers of the fabric. The amount of imbibed water a fabric can hold is related to its capacity of wicking as a result of spontaneous wetting, as discussed in greater details in the following box. In addition to the factors that affect wettability of a fibrous structure, the amount of capillaries in the structure also influences its capacity for wicking. A fibrous structure composed of fine fibers presents a larger amount of capillaries than the one that consists of thick fibers but is equal to the former in fiber mass or volume. Accordingly, micro- or nanofibers are also suitable for applications where a large capacity of wicking is essential.

Concept & Theory: What is Wetting?

The term "wetting" is usually used to describe the displacement of a solid-air interface with a solid-liquid interface. When a small liquid droplet is put in contact with a flat solid surface, two distinct equilibrium regimes may be found: partial wetting with a finite contact angle θ, or complete wetting with a zero contact angle (de Gennes, 1985), as shown in Figure 4.2.

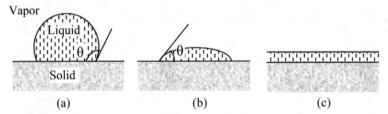

(a)   (b)   (c)

Figure 4.2. A small liquid droplet in equilibrium over a horizontal surface: (a) partial wetting, mostly non wetting, (b) partial wetting, mostly wetting, (c) complete wetting.

The forces in equilibrium at a solid-liquid boundary are commonly described by the Young's equation:

$$\gamma_{SV} - \gamma_{SL} - \gamma_{LV} \cos\theta = 0 \qquad (4.3)$$

where γ_{SV}, γ_{SL}, and γ_{LV} denotes, respectively, the solid/vapor, solid/liquid and liquid/vapor interfacial tensions, and θ is the equilibrium contact angle.

The parameter that distinguishes partial wetting and complete wetting is the so-called spreading parameter, S, which is a measure of the difference between the surface energy (per unit area) of the substrate when it is dry and that when it is wet:

$$S = [E_{substrate}]_{dry} - [E_{substrate}]_{wet} \qquad (4.4)$$

or

$$S = \gamma_{So} - (\gamma_{SL} - \gamma_{LV}) \qquad (4.5)$$

where γ_{So} is the surface tension of a vapor-free or "dry" solid surface.

If the parameter S is positive, the liquid will spread completely in order to lower its surface energy ($\theta = 0$). The final outcome is a film of nano-scale thickness resulting from the competition between molecular and capillary forces.

If the parameter S is negative, the drop will not spread out; at equilibrium, a spherical cap resting on the substrate forms, with a contact angle θ. A liquid is said to be "mostly wetting" when $\theta \leq \pi/2$, and "mostly non-wetting" when $\theta > \pi/2$ (de Gennes, Brochard-Wyart, *et al.*, 2004). In contact with water, a surface is usually called "hydrophilic" when $\theta \leq \pi/2$, and "hydrophobic" when $\theta > \pi/2$.

Wetting of fibers can be dramatically different from wetting on a flat surface due to the geometry of its cylindrical shape. A liquid that fully wets a material in the form of a smooth, planar surface may not wet the same material when on a smooth fiber surface. Wetting of fibrous materials is an even more complex process since it involves interaction between a liquid and a porous medium of a curved, intricate and tortuous structure, and with a soft and rough surface, instead of a simply solid and smooth surface. Literature is available for readers who wish to know more about the phenomenon (Pan and Zhong, 2006).

Concept & Theory: What is Wicking?

Wicking is the spontaneous flow of a liquid in a porous substrate, driven by capillary forces. As capillary forces are caused by wetting, wicking is a result of spontaneous wetting in a capillary system (Kissa, 1996).

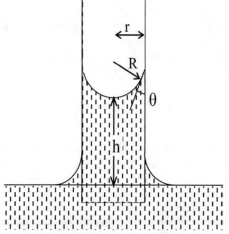

Figure 4.3. Wicking in a capillary.

A meniscus is formed in the simplest case of wicking (i.e., wicking occurring in a single capillary tube), as shown in Figure 4.3 The surface tension of the liquid causes a pressure difference across the curved liquid/vapor interface. The value for the pressure difference of a spherical surface was independently deduced in 1805 by Thomas Young (1773–1829) and Pierre Simon de Laplace (1749–1827), and is represented in the Young-Laplace equation (Adamson and Gast 1997):

$$\Delta P = \gamma_{LV}\left(\frac{1}{R_1} + \frac{1}{R_2}\right) \tag{4.6}$$

For a capillary with a circular cross section, the radii of the curved interface R_1 and R_2 are equal. Thus:

$$\Delta P = 2\gamma_{LV}/R \tag{4.7}$$

where

$$R = r/\cos\theta \tag{4.8}$$

and r is the capillary radius.

Most textile processes are time limited, so the kinetics of wicking becomes very important. The classical Washburn-Lucas equation (Washburn, 1921) describes the liquid's velocity, dh/dt, moving up or down in a perpendicular capillary with the radius r, neglecting the inertia of the liquid column.

$$\frac{dh}{dt} = \frac{r\gamma\cos\theta}{4\eta h} \tag{4.9}$$

where η is the viscosity of liquid, γ the surface tension and ρ the density of liquid.

The Washburn equation was used in the studies of wicking dynamics in fibrous structures, which led to the establishment of an empirical equation stating that the wicking height of liquid in a fiber or yarn was proportional to the square root of the time (Minor, 1959):

$$h = W_c t^{1/2} = \left(\frac{r\gamma\cos\theta}{2\eta}t\right)^{1/2} \tag{4.10}$$

This empirical equation provides a simple approach to correlate the wicking capacity of a fibrous structure with its specifications. Simple as it is, it has several limitations. According to Equation (4.10), the height of the liquid front will keep rising with time; actually, however, the liquid column will cease to rise after a certain period of time due to the balance of surface tension and gravity; also, the equation incorrectly assumes a constant advancing contact angle for the moving liquid front. Wicking is also affected by the morphology of fibrous assemblies. A fibrous structure is never a perfect capillary, but is changeable due to the swelling of the fiber (if hydrophilic), and can therefore further complicate the problem.

4.1.4. Product Development for Improved Comfort: Cases

Textile product development involves the designing and engineering of such components of textiles as fiber material, fabric structure, and finishing.

Product Development Question 4.1

How can we improve thermophysiological comfort by the design and development of FIBER materials?

Suggested answer: The interstices between fibers are important wicking channels (capillaries) for water to be carried away from the microclimate. The morphology of the fibers, therefore, has an impact on their wicking capacity. Fibers with unique engineered micro-channel cross sections have been developed, including fibers with kidney-bean, trilobal and multi-channel cross sections (Figure 4.4). These micro channels effectively expedite the transport of moisture through the fabric to maintain a dry microclimate next to the human skin. A well-known example is the Coolmax® fabric.

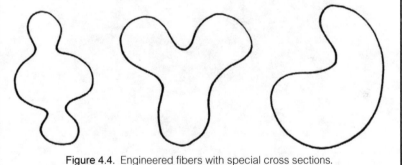

Figure 4.4. Engineered fibers with special cross sections.

Product Development Question 4.2

How can we improve thermophysiological comfort by the design and development of FABRIC structure?

Suggested answer: A fabric structure that speeds up the moisture transfer from the microclimate to the outer environment is always desired. An example is the Polartec® Power Dry® fabrics. It is a bi-component knit structure composed of polyester fibers: A brushed inner surface is responsible for moving moisture away from the skin, while an outer porous surface (i.e., Pointelle) draws moisture and spreads it over a wide area so that the fabric will dry quickly.

Product Development Question 4.3

How can we improve thermophysiological comfort by the design and development of special FINISH/TREATMENT?

Suggested answer: Take Outlast® technology for example. It involves the incorporation of phase change materials (PCMs) into clothing. These PCMs are capable of absorbing and storing excessive heat generated by the body and releasing the stored heat back to the body as needed. The PCMs are usually packed into a large number of micro-capsules that contain a polymer as the shell and the PCMs in the core. The durable protective polymer shell will keep stable during various textile processing procedures. Then these micro-capsules can be incorporated directly into the fibers during a spinning process [Figure 4.5(a)], or incorporated into the fabrics during the finishing processes [Figure 4.5(b)]. This technology was originally developed by NASA (National Aeronautics and Space Administration) for astronaut suits for extreme temperatures in outer space. A more detailed discussion about this finishing method using a smart material can be found in Chapter 11.

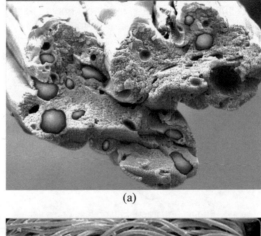

(a)

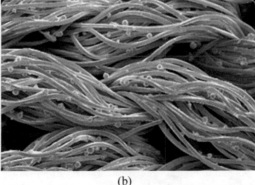

(b)

Figure 4.4. Engineered fibers/fabrics incorporated with PCMs (with permission from the Outlast Technologies, Inc.): (a) Viscose rayon fibers incorporated with PCMs, (b) A fabric finished with PCMs.

4.2. TEXTILE/SKIN INTERACTION AND SENSORIAL COMFORT

The interactions between textiles and human skin may lead to discomfort or reactions. Irritation of the skin is a well-known instance of the skin's reaction to textiles (or, to be specific, to such substances as chemicals incorporated into the textiles during textile processes) as a result of the textile-skin contact and friction. Since factors for such discomfort can be identified, it is possible to bring about the good sensorial comfort by removing the undesirable factors and fully utilizing the desirable ones.

4.2.1. Skin Irritation Caused by Chemicals

Numerous chemicals may be incorporated into the textile products during various processes, ranging from fiber formation, spinning, fabric construction to dyeing and finishing. These chemicals, when in contact with the skin, may cause allergic contact dermatitis (ACD), a well-known dermatological problem.

Among problematic chemicals, dyes may be the most notorious. Thirty-five dyes, mainly those that are termed as *disperse dyes* and are *anthraquinone* or *azo* in structure, may cause allergic contact dermatitis (Hatch and Maibach, 1985; 1995). However, the representation of ACD prevalence—the amount of ACD cases that occur in a population—varies enormously from one study to the next (Hatch and Maibach, 2000); most of these studies were conducted in Europe, primarily in Italy. All of the above-mentioned tests were performed by placing a dye (mostly a disperse one) of unknown purity (instead of a dyed fabric) directly on the skin. Accordingly, the term "textile-dye ACD", in contrast to "color textile ACD", was adopted in such studies, because the latter involves more complicated factors, such as dye molecules transferred or released from textiles to the skin and perspiration fastness of the dyes. It was also reported that dyes to which patients were patch-test positive were infrequently identified in the fabric suspected of having caused skin problems (Hatch, Motschi, *et al.*, 2003). This means that further investigation is desired in the diagnosis and management of colored-textile allergic contact dermatitis.

As for chemicals used for textile finishing, some of those used on fabrics to improve performance characteristics have been found to cause irritation, or allergic contact dermatitis. The most significant findings are concerned with formaldehyde and N-methylol compounds for durable press fabrics. Textile formaldehyde resins for durable press finish was often the focus, because formaldehyde released from the resin was believed to be the causal agent.

A detailed documentation of textile chemicals that have been reported to cause dermatitis can be found in a handbook by Kanerva (2000). However, it is a difficult task to define and predict the extent of skin problems caused by textile-associated chemicals; as SKIN problems, they have to be influenced by the variation of the skin's sensitivity and capacity of absorption from one patient to another, and to be influenced by the amount of pressure and friction exerted on the skin, transfer of irritant chemicals from textiles to the skin, and synergy of sweating. There will, as a result, be such complexities as the fact that a chemical can be harmful for one person, but not for another.

4.2.2. Skin Reactions Caused by Physical Contact

Physical contact between a fabric and the skin can lead to a feeling of itching or prickling. The mechanisms of such interactions are summarized in Figure 4.6. They denote that the discomfort originates from both the normal force (i.e., pressure) and shear force (friction) at the skin/fabric interface during the contact of the two surfaces. It should be noted that such a reaction or *inflammation* is not an allergic response, but an irritant one, and usually subsides and diminishes after the source fabric is removed, unless the contact is so prolonged as to cause physical damage to the skin tissues. Proceedings of a case of itching/prickling are listed as follows:

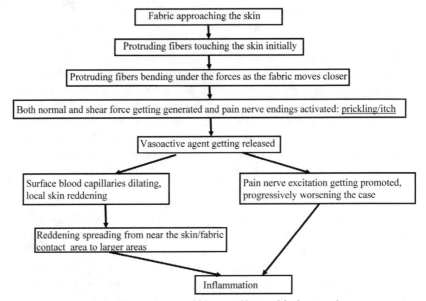

FIGURE 4.6. *The mechanism of fabric prickling and further complications.*

The normal force or pressure can be generated from the bending of protruding fibers as they approach the skin. Obviously, a soft fiber (with a low stiffness) is less prickly than a rigid one (with a high stiffness), because a smaller force is required to bend it. Fibers at the lower end of stiffness include wool, viscose, acetate, acrylic and olefin. Since stiffness of a fiber increases with the decrease of its length, fabrics composed of a filament induce less prickliness than fabrics containing a staple fiber of the same type. Fiber size, among the fiber specifications, has the greatest impact on the stiffness, and consequently on the prickliness a fabric may induce. Generally, doubling a fiber's diameter leads to a 16-fold rise in stiffness. The pressure imposed by a piece of fabric on the skin also varies depending on the fabric weight, fit and elasticity. The weight of the fabric (usually expressed in mass per unit area) determines the amount of burden that will be loaded on the skin. A piece of fabric that fits tightly will apply a higher pressure on the skin than the one that fits loosely.

The frictional force (f) between the skin and the fabric is a function of normal force (P), as shown in the simple Coulomb's law:

$$f \leq \mu P \qquad (4.11)$$

where μ is the frictional coefficient, and the maximum frictional force ($f_{max} = \mu P$) occurs when the fabric is sliding across the skin.

The frictional coefficient can be affected by the roughness/smoothness of either the fabric or skin—i.e., irregularities in a surface. Usually a glabrous skin or finger causes less friction than a hairy skin or forearm. The roughness of a fabric depends on the amplitude and frequency of protruding points, ridges and/or dots in a fabric structure. The surface roughness of the constituent fibers may affect the roughness of the fabric. For example, the surface of the wool fiber is characterized by a layer of scales, which contributes to the roughness of wool fiber and fabrics. The roughness of a fiber/fabric increases dramatically with the increase of the size of the fiber or yarn. Such loose fabric structure as knit, which contains large numbers of yarn loops, may have a relatively high roughness. Woven fabrics with lower interlacing frequencies, like satin fabrics, are known for their surface smoothness.

Some finishing processes can also be employed to improve the surface smoothness and reduce prickling induced by fabrics. For example, fabrics become smoother coming out of such physical finishing processes as *glazing* or *polishing,* where a surface layer of starch, wax, or resin is applied onto the fabric. In addition, several mechanical finishing processes (e.g., schreinerizing) enhance the smoothness of fabrics as a result of pressing the fabrics between cylinders. Greater details about such finishes can be found in Chapter 2.

As mentioned above, both pressure and friction play important roles in determining the level of comfort expected of fabrics. The pressure imposed on the skin can be regulated by the fabric restraint and elasticity. The skin stretches during dynamic movements, especially around the joints. For example, when one changes his/her position from standing to sitting, the skin at the knee goes through strains/stretches—approximately 20% horizontally and 40% vertically. A full bending of one's elbow leads to even larger strains/stretches: about 28% horizontally and 50% vertically (Li and Layton, 2001). When the skin stretches, the fabric worn next to the skin will also undergo stretching and/or slipping to accommodate changes caused by the movement of the skin. In either situation, frictional forces occur: static friction in the former and kinetic in the latter. It is therefore important that, in order for a piece of fabric to "fit", fabric elasticity and smoothness be fully considered in the design and development of a textile product so as to provide optimum sensorial comfort.

Fabric fitness is affected by the ratio of its size to the size of the body (or a *part* of the body) and by the specification of the "end" use, which can be accommodated in the course of product design. Thus clothing to be used by a hospitalized patient may vastly differ from what is for a sportsman to wear; in the latter case, the clothing (i.e., *sportswear*) may be designed to be closely fit to reduce resisting force during body movement. Even in the same hospital, the inpatients may not wear the same type of clothing. Thus the *pressure garment* is designed to be closely fitting so that an appropriate amount of pressure will be applied to the body of, say, a patient with a severe burn wound as a temporary substitute for the damaged skin. In the design of a closely fitting garment, a higher level of sensorial comfort is demanded, as a larger skin area will be in contact with the garment and be subjected to pressure and friction.

To better understand how the above factors influence sensorial comfort, four different scenarios can be presented as follows:

1. A fabric of high elasticity and rough surface (e.g., a wool knit) usually has a high friction against the skin. However, the high elasticity also lends the fabric a higher tendency to stretch. During the body movement, if the force required to extend the fabric along with the stretched skin is smaller than the maximum frictional force (kinetic frictional force), the fabric will stretch to accommodate the strain of the skin rather than slide against the skin. The level of comfort provided by such a fabric is then acceptable. It should be noted that, if the garment does not closely fit the wearer, he will not be able to take full advantage of the high elasticity, but will be subjected to the high frictional force as the fabric tends to slip across the skin.

2. A fabric of high elasticity and smooth surface (e.g., a nylon/spandex knit for the closely fitting pressure garment, which has been further reinforced with a layer of medical grade silicone elastomer sheet), provides an appropriate amount of pressure and minimum friction and, as a result, the least disturbance and a high level of comfort to the injured skin.

3. A fabric of low elasticity and smooth surface, like a polyester satin, is prone to slip against the skin rather than stretch with the skin. As the surface is smooth, the kinetic frictional force will be relatively low, and the fabric will still be quite comfortable. Such a fabric is usually designed to fit the wearer loosely so that it will not hinder movement of the wearer.

4. A fabric of low elasticity and rough surface, such as a linen woven fabric, leads to a larger amount of friction against the skin and results in discomfort.

4.2.3. The Coupling of Thermophysiological and Sensorial Comfort

Although most skin reactions are induced directly by physical contact and/or mechanical forces, resulting in sensorial comfort, factors that relate to thermophysiological comfort are just as important; they combine to account for the overall comfort that is expected of textile products.

The humidity in the microclimate influences the moisture content of the skin, and further impacts on its interaction with fabrics. On the one hand, an excess of moisture in the skin may cause the stratum corneum (SC) to soften, making it more penetrable by the protruding fibers on the fabric surface, thus making the skin more vulnerable to damage caused by mechanical forces. As revealed in research studies, both the frictional coefficient and abrasion damage of the skin as a result of wearing diapers will increase with the increase of the moisture content of the skin (Zimmerer, Lawson, *et al.*, 1986). This phenomenon is even more prominent for the "hairy" skin than for the "glabrous". Recent research data suggest further that moisture content of the skin may be more influential than fiber type or fabric construction parameters in determining the nature and intensity of fabric-to-skin friction (Gwosdow, Stevens, *et al.*, 1986; Kenins, 1994). If liquid water is condensed from moisture in a highly humid microclimate, the fabric may adhere to the skin to further increase its friction against the skin. When the skin is excessively dry, on the other hand, there will be cracks in the skin that allow bacterial invasion. To make things worse, these cracks will develop into new irregularities on the surface of the skin to increase its roughness.

Similarly, an increase of temperature in the microclimate will lead to larger amounts of perspiration to result in increased local humidity, and there will then unfold the same scenario described previously.

4.3. TYPES OF FIBER AS RELATED TO COMFORT

Fiber materials vary in their capacities to yield and maintain thermophysiological comfort. Such fibers as wool, cotton, rayon and polypropylene fibers, which are frequently used in products worn next to the skin, will be discussed in this section. Refer also to structures and properties of these fiber materials, which have already been discussed in Chapter 2.

4.3.1. Wool Fiber

A "hygroscopic" fiber, wool has the highest capacity in terms of water absorption among commonly used fibers. It absorbs large amounts of moisture without causing a wet feel. Wool is also the highest regarding its heat of wetting (i.e., heat that is released from the absorption of water molecules into the amorphous region of the fiber), which enables wool fiber to remain warm in a cold and damp environment, all as a result of containing hydrophilic functional groups (i.e., primary amine/–NH_2 and carboxyl/–COOH) in its polymeric structure. It is also characterized by a high percentage of amorphous region (70–75%) in its fine structure (Hatch 1993). These structural features contribute to its high absorbency as well as its tenacity in holding water. To put it in simpler words, it takes a long time to dry out a wool fabric.

The wool fiber is covered by a very thin layer of wax-like substance called *epicuticle,* which contains numerous microscopic pores, making the fiber breathable (i.e., allowing water vapor to be absorbed into the fiber) and yet water repellent (i.e., preventing liquid water from getting into the interior of a fiber). As a result, a wool fabric may shed water in misty rains, but will not do so in a heavy rain. This epicuticle, on the other hand, can be easily damaged by frictional forces during the end use of a wool fabric.

Another structural feature of the wool fiber is its three-dimensional (3D) *crimps*—i.e., waves, twists, or curls along the fiber length. Presence of these 3D crimps not only results in the high elasticity of the wool fiber, but also contributes to the highly porous structure of wool yarns and fabrics, which further account for the large amounts of still air to be held therein. It is this void space, which represents as much as two-thirds of the volume of a wool fabric, that explains the excellent insulation of wool fabrics in cold weather.

Wool fiber is generally appreciated for its excellent thermophysi-ological comfort, as discussed in the above. In terms of sensorial comfort, however, the wool fabric is related to certain reactions. Wool fibers, especially those termed as short and/or coarse, are known for the likelihood of causing itching or prickling sensations. The protective scales that cover the surface of the wool fiber may contribute to the itching feeling, too. In addition, some people are *allergic* to wool or, precisely, to the substance *lanolin* (known also as *wool alcohols* or *wool fat*) in the wool. Wool lanolin has been identified as one of the many agents that cause immunologic contact urticaria.

Concept & Theory: What is Contact Urticaria?

The contact urticaria or the contact urticaria syndrome (CUS) refers to immediate inflammatory reactions that appear usually within minutes after contact with the eliciting substance. CUS can be either immunologic or nonimmunologic, according to its underlying mechanisms. Wool lanolin has been classified as the agent that leads to immunologic CUS, which occurs to people who have previously become sensitized to the causative agent. Specifically, wool lanolin penetrates the epidermis of the skin to react with the specific antibody (i.e., Immunoglobulin E [IgE] molecules) that occurs on the surface of some leukocytes (i.e., white blood cells). As a result, vasoactive substances (e.g., histamine) are released to elicit cutaneous symptoms, such as erythema (i.e., redness or rash on the skin) and edema (i.e., swelling caused by fluid retention and accumulation) (Marzulli, Zhai, *et al.*, 2008).

4.3.2. Cotton and Rayon

Cotton is a hydrophilic cellulosic fiber. The plentiful hydroxyl groups in the molecular structure of the cotton fiber contribute to its high capacity for water absorption. A cotton fiber contains multiple layers or walls, between which water can be absorbed and held. In addition, the cotton fiber has a very special morphology due to its kidney-bean-shaped cross-section and natural twists along the length. These features account for the high percentage of void space in cotton yarns or fabrics, which further results in their high wicking capacity. Generally, cotton is considered to be a comfortable fiber, as it quickly absorbs the moisture in the microclimate and passes it to the outer environment to keep the surface of the skin dry. On the other hand, cotton is able to hold its contained water tight because of its hydrophilic functional groups; because of this, when a cotton fabric gets wet, it will be difficult to dry.

Its high level of sensorial comfort is largely owing to the tapered ends of the cotton fiber, which render the fiber comfortable to the touch. This high level of comfort is also related to the size of the cotton fiber. Namely, the coarser the cotton fiber (indicating a larger diameter), the stiffer the cotton fiber will be, and, accordingly, the more harsh the cotton fabric will feel. The cellulose-based cotton fiber is not related to any allergic reaction. In addition, the cotton fabric has a small electrical buildup even at a low humidity, which causes it to be a good material for comfortable wear in dry weather.

Rayon, also known as viscose, is regenerated cellulose and therefore has a molecular structure similar to that of cotton—they share the identical repeating unit in their constituting polymers. Rayon has, however, a lower degree of polymerization and a higher percentage of amorphous region than cotton. As a result, rayon has a very high capacity of water absorption, even higher than cotton, ranking second only to wool among the commonly-used fibers. It is also high in heat of wetting, comparable to wool. For these reasons rayon is considered to be a fiber of good thermophysiological comfort. In terms of sensorial comfort, rayon fibers are soft and comfortable to the touch. It also has a low electrical buildup. Admired for these qualities, rayon is frequently used in healthcare and medical textile products that require contact comfort and absorption, such as wipes and bandages.

4.3.3. Polypropylene

Polypropylene (PP) is a synthetic fiber that has found much application in the healthcare and medical sectors due to its special properties. PP fiber is known for its zero absorbency but a high wicking capacity. As a result, PP fabrics can quickly transport the moisture or liquid water away from the microclimate to keep the skin dry. Since PP fabrics do not easily get wet, they are admired for their thermal insulation, and the PP fiber has found applications not only in active sportswear, underwear and socks, but also in coverstocks for absorptive hygiene products.

In terms of sensorial comfort, PP fiber is of the lowest density, and a lightweight fabric tends to impose less burden or pressure on the skin, especially during active movement. As a non-polar polymer, PP electrons can hardly travel to the fiber surface to cause electrostatic buildup. This feature of PP fibers, with their zero absorption also considered, contributes much to the comfort they will provide in low humidity. PP fibers have not been reported to cause any undesirable skin reactions. As a thermoplastic synthetic fiber, it can be extruded directly into spunbonded nonwoven fabrics without using any chemical agents. For these reasons, PP fibers have been dominant in medical textile products that require a dry, chemical-free and static-free, next-to-skin surface. The topsheet for disposable hygiene products (e.g., diapers and sanitary napkins) is a good example of such applications.

4.4. TEXTILE-RELATED HEALTHCARE PROBLEMS

Prolonged or extensive contact combined with pressure, friction, or shear between fabric and the skin may lead to serious problems or injuries, such as friction blisters and pressure ulcers. It may be unrealistic to think of ultimate solutions, but increased awareness and knowledge about these problems are certainly beneficial.

4.4.1. Friction Blister

Friction blistering is a prevalent skin problem associated with sports and vigorous activities. It can be critical if it occurs during athletic competitions or military missions, when reduced performance or mobility is costly, injurious, or fatal.

Blisters result from frictional forces that mechanically separate epidermal cells at the level of the stratum spinosum. Hydrostatic pressure causes the area of separation to become filled with a fluid that is similar in composition to plasma but has a lower protein level. It is more likely for blisters to form in skin areas (e.g., palms of the hands or soles of the feet) that are characteristic of a thick horny layer held tightly to underlying structures (Knapik, Reynolds, *et al.*, 1995).

Friction blistering is a concern in the design and development of textile products (especially socks) for sports and military purposes. Generally, efforts have been concentrated on such remedies as pressure relief and/or friction control. Measures that can be utilized to reduce pressure include the use of more resilient socks and liners in shoes as a cushion. However, a cushion liner should not be so thick that it can affect the mobility of the wearers. Where friction control is necessary, lubrication can be used to reduce the coefficient of friction; also, antiperspirant can be applied to reduce skin hydration and subsequently bring down the friction coefficient. Fabrics of a high transport of moisture or a large wicking capacity are adopted to lower the humidity of the microclimate so as to lower skin hydration. However, the friction coefficient should not be so small as to adversely affect the wearer's ability to come to a standstill and/or move on without the fabric sliding when the wearer needs to perform these acts.

To date, however, it is still difficult to predict the prevalence or severity of friction blistering, not to mention articulating an approach to prevent it. The cause may lie in the dramatic variation of skin conditions (surface roughness, hydration, adhesion between skin layers, etc.) among individuals, or at different anatomic sites of the same person.

4.4.2. Pressure Ulcer

Pressure ulcer, known also as bedsore, decubitus ulcer, or pressure sore, is defined as "localized injury to the skin and/or underlying tissue, usually over a bony prominence, as a result of pressure, or pressure in combination with shear" (EPUAP and NPUAP, 2009). It presents a significant health-care threat to hospitalized patients. Approximately 1 million hospitalized and nursing home patients are diagnosed with pressure ulcers and about 60,000 die as a result of pressure ulcer complications annually (Bergstrom, 1997). Related costs have been estimated to exceed $1 billion annually in the United States (Moore, 1998; Beckrich and Aronovitch, 1999).

Etiologically, formation of a pressure ulcer is the occurrence of occlusion and thrombosis (i.e., formation of a blood clot inside a blood vessel, obstructing the flow of blood through the circulatory system) of capillaries, when compressive and/or shear/friction forces reach a threshold (i.e., a certain level of force intensity and duration) (Figure 4.7). This will be followed by tissue anoxia (i.e., deficiency in the level of oxygen) that is signaled first by the release of toxic metabolites and ultimately by cell death and tissue necrosis (i.e., the state of dying) (Keller, Wille, *et al.*, 2002).

Some of the major factors in the formation of pressure ulcers are related to the use of textile products (Maklebust and Sieggreen, 2001; Morison, 2001). A good understanding of these factors may help us arrive at decisions about the use of some products, and the disuse of some others. They are (1) pressure, (2) friction, and (3) level of moisture in the microclimate.

A capillary perfusion pressure (e.g., 32 mm Hg at the arteriolar end and 12 mm Hg at the venous end) (Maklebust and Sieggreen, 2001) on the human body will, generally, continue maintaining a patency (i.e., the quality or state of being open or unobstructed) of capillary vessels and, as a result, will not disturb the regular supply of oxygen and nutrients to the tissues. An external pressure greater than what is stated in the above critical figures, if prolonged, may cause cell and/or tissue death as a result of a restricted supply of blood to the spot subjected to the pressure. Bony areas of the body are especially vulnerable to such complications.

Garment fit and fabric elasticity are important factors in determining the amount of pressure to be applied to the skin, as discussed in the previous section. Use of medically appropriate fabrics (clothing and

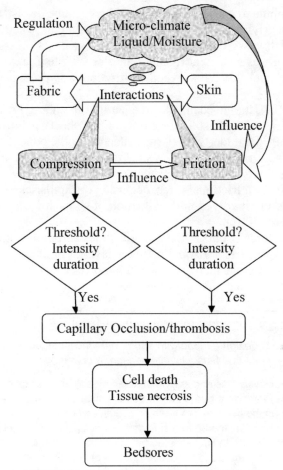

FIGURE 4.7. *Formation of bedsores and related factors.*

beddings) alone may not suffice to reduce pressure experienced by the patient; other solutions, such as repositioning, use of pillows/cushions/ foam wedges, low-pressure mattresses or seats, help attain that purpose. An especially efficient means is wearing socks specially designed and developed for the purpose of pressure ulcer prevention and treatment. For example, wearing padded hosiery may decrease the risk of ulceration as a result of reduced plantar pressures. These socks, when worn with suitable shoes, may be an acceptable, inexpensive addition to the existing methods of preventing the high-risk, insensitive diabetic foot ulceration.

These means play even more significant roles in cases where pressure and body motion are involved—namely, cases where pressure and friction combine to cause the problem, which can be devastating to the skin and underlying tissues. It was demonstrated that, when both pressure and friction were applied on the skin of swine, a pressure as low as 45 mmHg was sufficient to cause an ulcer, while a pressure of 290 mmHg was likely to do so when no friction was present (Dinsdale, 1974).

Friction (i.e., the mechanical force parallel to an area) occurs when the body is pulled against a fabric (e.g., a bed sheet), a situation when the body pulls the underlying tissues attached to the bone in one direction while the surface skin tissues stick to the sheet and remain stationary. Such a force may obstruct, tear or stretch blood vessels. In the presence of such a frictional force, occlusion of capillaries may occur at half the pressure involved in the situation of no such force (Maklebust and Sieggreen, 2001).

Frictional force occurs when a fabric slides across the skin, causing the damage known as *abrasion* to the top layer(s) of the skin. Such erosion of surface tissues increases the likelihood of causing damage in the deeper tissues, which have survived the first round of devastation.

Product Development Question 4.4

How to design a fabric with appropriate frictional properties that help alleviate bedsore problems?

Suggested answer: This end can be attained by, say, the design of a double-layer woven fabric as a bed sheet material, which ensures different friction coefficients on the two sides of the fabric (Snycerski and Frontczak-Wasiak, 2004). To be specific, the bottom side of the sheet will be given a higher friction coefficient so as to limit slipping between the sheet and the underlying bedding materials intended to reduce bed sheet wrinkling, and a lower friction coefficient given to the top side so as to allow the patient to make easier, smoother position changes.

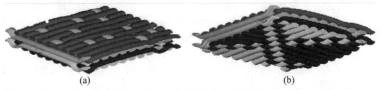

(a)   (b)

Figure 4.9. A design of bed sheet for friction relief ((Snycerski and Frontczak-Wasiak, 2004)—Reprint with permission from the Autex Research Journal): (a) The top side of the bed sheet is a satin weave that provides smoothness, which allows easier and smoother position changes for patients, (b) The bottom side of the bed sheet is a structure with a high frequency of yarn interlacing to provide a high frictional coefficient, which limits the slip between the bed sheet and underlying bedding materials and, therefore, reduces bed sheet wrinkling.

Fabric surface smoothness and stiffness/flexibility are important factors for the frictional force to be experienced by the patient who uses such fabric. A more detailed discussion can be found in the previous section.

An appropriate level of moisture should be maintained in the microclimate to prevent or reduce pressure ulceration. Too low a level may lead to greater vulnerability of the skin to cracking, which will lead to invasion of microorganisms. Conversely, too high a level (e.g., as a result of incontinence and/or perspiration) may cause skin maceration that will further result in lower tissue tolerance to shear stress and friction (Keller, Wille, *et al.*, 2002). On the other hand, moisture may create favorable conditions for the growth of microorganisms. Infection caused thereby is a major complication that impedes wound healing, for example. The clothing and bedding system plays an important role in moderating the level of moisture to maintain a healthier microclimate near the skin surface.

It is believed that the role textiles play in the formation and prevention of pressure ulceration and other skin problems is probably underestimated. This role has not been subjected to comprehensive study, especially when considering the fact that textile properties can largely influence such factors as pressure, shear/friction, and skin moisture content, and that the wise control of these can increase the likelihood of having them contribute only to textile efficiency and comfort. Larger efforts to make a change may begin with a better understanding about them.

4.5. SUMMARY

Skin provides the first, critical defense against external hazards. It is then aided and reinforced by a buffering system of fabrics, which helps maintain human health and the normal functions of the body by means of producing and sustaining thermal and sensorial comfort, in addition to preventing environmental risks (from macro-solids to microorganisms) to which the naked skin is vulnerable. A failure to do these, or doing these unwisely or inefficiently, can lead to various problems, from thermophysiological discomfort and irritation to injuries, such as blisters and pressure ulcers. As always, the best that can be done is the largest supply of comfort and suppression of problems.

Thermophysiological comfort is a function of desirable conditions in the microclimate as represented by temperature and humidity, via the transport of heat and moisture through the system of fabrics. Textile structures and properties can be designed to influence the: (1) amount of heat obtained or dissipated from the microclimate and human body, specifically via evaporation, conduction, convection and radiation; (2) amount of moisture that transports through the fabric via diffusion; and (3) amount of liquid water taken up by the fabric system in three different manners: (a) absorbed into the amorphous region of the polymer structure; (b) adsorbed onto the surface of the fiber; and/or (c) imbibed into the interstices in the fibers and yarns.

Sensorial comfort is the desirable result of the elicitation of sensations when the skin is physically in contact with a system of textiles. It requires the elimination of any itching, prickling feelings or skin reactions, induced usually by chemicals or allergens. Mechanical forces (pressure and friction) also cause discomfort. Pressure can be regulated with regard to fit and elasticity of fabrics, while friction can be reduced by properly handling fabric surface smoothness. These particulars should be taken into account in the design and development of textile materials and products. Thus, to be specific, it is largely the alleviation or removal of those problems that brings about the desired sensorial comfort.

These two types of comfort (or the two components of the ONE comfort) are not independent, so it is essential to take well-incorporated measures so as to have the most comfort possible. The worst problems against such comfort—skin blistering and pressure ulceration—are given the most attention in this chapter. Increased knowledge about them will reinforce the fight against them.

Textile comfort is the type of comfort textile researchers and healthcare people *can afford*. Namely, it can be derived in the course of product design and fabrication by referring to such properties of the textile materials as moisture and heat transport on the one hand and, on the other, by pretreating undesirable factors that would lead to problems, and in the use of textile products by regulating physiological and environmental conditions. It is in this sense that it is worth talking about comfort and problems.

4.6. REFERENCES

Adamson, A.W. and A.P. Gast. (1997). Physical chemistry of surfaces. New York: Wiley.

Agache, P.G. and P. Humbert. (2004). Measuring the skin: non-invasive investigations, physiology, normal constants. New York: Springer.

Beckrich, K. and S.A. Aronovitch. (1999). Hospital-acquired pressure ulcers: a comparison of costs in medical vs. surgical patients. *Nurs. Econ.* **17**(5): 263–71.

Bergstrom, N.I. (1997). Strategies for preventing pressure ulcers. *Clin. Geriatr. Med.* **13**(3): 437–54.

Cardarelli, F. (2008). Materials handbook: a concise desktop reference, 2nd Ed. London: Springer.

Cena, K. and J.A. Clark. (1981). Bioengineering, thermal physiology, and comfort. New York: Elsevier Scientific Pub. Co.

de Gennes, P.-G., F. Brochard-Wyart, *et al.* (2004). Capillarity and wetting phenomena: drops, bubbles, pearls, waves. New York: Springer.

de Gennes, P.-G. (1985). Wetting—statics and dynamics. *Reviews of Modern Physics* **57**(3): 827–863.

Dinsdale, S.M. (1974). Decubitus ulcers: role of pressure and friction in causation. *Arch. Phys. Med. Rehabil.* **55**(4): 147–52.

EPUAP and NPUAP. (2009). Treatment of pressure ulcers: quick reference guide. Washington, DC: European Pressure Ulcer Advisory Panel and National Pressure Ulcer Advisory Panel.

Gwosdow, A.R., J.C. Stevens, *et al.* (1986). Skin friction and fabric sensations in neutral and warm environments. *Textile Research Journal* **56**(9): 574–580.

Hatch, K.L. (1993). Textile science. Minneapolis/Saint Paul, West Pub.

Hatch, K.L. and H.I. Maibach. (1985). Textile fiber dermatitis. Contact Dermatitis **12**(1): 1–11.

Hatch, K.L. and H.I. Maibach. (1995). Textile dye dermatitis. *J. Am. Acad. Dermatol.* **32**(4): 631–9.

Hatch, K.L. and H.I. Maibach. (2000). Textile dye allergic contact dermatitis prevalence. *Contact Dermatitis* **42**(4): 187–195.

Hatch, K.L., H. Motschi, *et al.* (2003). Disperse dyes in fabrics of patients patch-test-positive to disperse dyes. *Am. J. Contact Dermat.* **14**(4): 205–12.

Kanerva, L. (2000). Handbook of occupational dermatology. New York: Springer.

Keller, B.P., J. Wille, *et al.* (2002). Pressure ulcers in intensive care patients: a review of risks and prevention. *Intensive Care Med.* 28(10): 1379–88.

Kenins, P. (1994). Influence of fiber-type and moisture on measured fabric-to-skin friction. *Textile Research Journal* **64**(12): 722–728.

Kissa, E. (1996). Wetting and wicking. *Textile Research Journal* **66**(10): 660–668.

Knapik, J.J., K.L. Reynolds, *et al.* (1995). Friction blisters. Pathophysiology, prevention and treatment. *Sports Med.* **20**(3): 136–47.

Li, Y. and J.M. Layton. (2001). The science of clothing comfort : a critical appreciation of recent developments. Manchester: Textile Institute International.

Maklebust, J. and M. Sieggreen. (2001). Pressure ulcers: guidelines for prevention and management, 3rd ed. Pennsylvania: Springhouse.

Marzulli, F.N., H. Zhai, *et al.* (2008). Marzulli and Maibach's dermatotoxicology. Boca Raton, FL: CRC Press.

Minor, F.W. (1959). The migration of liquids in textile assemblies, Part II. *Textile Research Journal* **29**: 931.

Minor, F.W. (1959). The migration of liquids in textile assemblies, Part III. *Textile Research Journal* **29**: 941.

Moore, J.D., Jr. (1998). Bedsores: $1 billion burden. N.Y. peer review organization tries education to stop a preventable problem. *Mod. Healthc.* **28**(29): 43.

Morison, M.J., ed. (2001). The prevention and treatment of pressure ulcers. London: Harcourt Publishers Limited.

Pan, N. and W. Zhong. (2006). Fluid transport phenomena in fibrous materials. Cambridge, England: Woodhead Publishing.

Slater, K. (1985). Human comfort. Springfield, Ill.: C.C. Thomas.

Snycerski, M. and I. Frontczak-Wasiak. (2004). A functional woven fabric with controlled friction coefficients preventing bedsores. *AUTEX Research Journal* **4**(3): 137–142.

Washburn, E.W. (1921). The dynamics of capillary flow. *Physical Review* **17**: 273–283.

Zimmerer, R.E., K.D. Lawson, *et al.* (1986). The effects of wearing diapers on skin. *Pediatr. Dermatol.* **3**(2): 95–101.

CHAPTER 5

Biocompatibility, Bioresorbability, and Biostability: Solutions and Beyond

TEXTILES for the medical and healthcare sectors can generally be divided into two categories: those for external uses and those for internal uses. Medical textiles for external uses include disposable hygiene products (see Chapter 6), protective products (Chapter 7) and wound care products (Chapter 8). These are usually used in direct contact with the skin and therefore require a high level of comfort (see Chapter 4). On the other hand, medical textiles for internal uses refer to implantable, extracorporeal devices (e.g., artificial kidney, which is placed outside of the human body but still in direct contact with human blood) and scaffolding materials for tissue engineering (Chapters 9 and 10). Wound dressings for deep wounds have interactions with internal tissues of the body and therefore can also be considered products for internal uses. Biocompatibility and bioresorbability (or biostability) are the most important criteria for evaluating a biotextile material or any fiber/textile product that will react with a biological system in its end uses.

5.1. BIOCOMPATIBILITY

Defined as "the ability of a material to perform with an appropriate host response in a specific application" (Williams, 1987), biocompatibility is the term used to evaluate the ability of a biomaterial (e.g., a biotextile) to elicit benign responses from the cells, tissues and organs of the patient who has received an implanted foreign material. The human body has a defense (i.e., the immune) system that counteracts invasion by entities from outside the body, including infectious agents (such as viruses, bacteria and parasites), inert agents (like splinters and implants) and tumor cells. In other words, the immune system is a system of cells, tissues and their products (e.g., signal molecules) that recognizes, attacks and destroys what is foreign to the body (Mak and Saunders, 2006). For example, under the circumstance of infection or injury, a response of inflammation is activated: immune cells flux into and accumulate at the site of attack or injury to guard against infection and promote recovery. However, such a defense response may also be the result of implantation and may compromise the normal functions of the implanted biotextile device or material in the human body.

Biocompatibility involves the interactions between the implanted materials (or a device made from them) and host tissues. All aspects of the material properties, including mechanical, chemical, pharmacological and surface properties, may impact on such interactions (Park and Lakes, 2007). The effect of implanted materials on the host cells or tissues at the biomaterials/tissue interface may include blood-material interactions, toxicity, inflammation, infection, foreign body reaction and tumorigenesis (Ratner, Hoffman *et al.*, 2004).

5.1.1. The Blood-material Interaction

When an injury to a blood vessel occurs, a hemostasis process will be activated to stop bleeding. However, the same process may cause negative effects when an artificial graft is implanted in contact with blood. Such a process involves platelet adhesion to artificial surfaces (or to the injured blood vessel), platelet aggregation to form plugs (or initial blockage of bleeding in the injured vessel), and formation of a blood clot or thrombus (or blood coagulation in the injured vessel). In a native vessel, the system has inhibition mechanisms to avoid massive clot formation once the coagulation is initiated, and the blood clot at the injured site can be later removed by fibrinolysis after healing occurs, which is a process involving the digestion of the blood clot by enzymes and the release of soluble digestion products into the circulating blood. When an artificial graft surface is exposed to the blood, however, an imbalance between the activation and inhibition processes can cause excessive thrombus formation and inflammatory responses. Such blood-material interactions and the resulting thrombosis have limited the application of many biomaterials as blood-contacting devices or implants.

As a parameter for evaluating the suitability of a material as a blood-contacting device, blood compatibility can be defined as "the property of a material or device that permits it to function in contact with blood without inducing adverse reactions" (Ratner, Hoffman, *et al.*, 2004). The adverse reactions that can be induced by a non-blood compatible material usually include the formation of a clot or thrombus. The thrombus may affect the normal function of a blood-contacting device; the detached thrombus (e.g., from an artificial heart valve) can enter the blood circulation and, when traveling to the brain, may lead to a stroke. Minimization of these reactions is vital for the design and development of biomedical grafts.

Three factors determine the blood-biomaterial interaction: the blood, the flow of blood, and the blood-contacting surface of the material (Ratner, Hoffman, *et al.*, 2004).

First, the nature of the blood (e.g., species, health, gender and age of the blood donor) and the ways in which the blood has been handled (e.g., the time interval at which the blood has been handled *in vitro* and the temperature at which the blood has been kept in storage) can have important influences on the blood-material interaction.

Second, the wall shear rate (i.e., the flow velocity gradient, or the slope of the velocity at the surface) can affect the platelet transportation and formation of thrombosis. For example, the initial attachment of platelets to a graft surface increases with the wall shear rate. Specifically, at a small wall shear rate (e.g., in a vein), the adhesion of platelets to the material surface depends more on the availability of platelets (i.e., their transport from the blood to the material surface) than the properties of the material's surface; at a high wall shear rate (e.g., in an artery), on the other hand, the platelets' adhesion can be affected by both the transport rate of platelets and properties of the material surface.

Lastly, properties of the blood-contacting surface of a material can have an important impact on the initial events, including the deposition of blood protein and platelets on the material's surface. However, how these events may affect the later formation of thrombosis remains unclear due to complexity of the phenomena. Although a variety of material surface parameters (e.g., charge, roughness, hydrophilicity, polarity) have been studied for their correlation with formation of thrombosis or blood compatibility of materials, there has been no consensus on labeling or ranking various biomaterials for their blood compatibility (Schaub, Kameneva, *et al.*, 1999; Sefton, Sawyer, *et al.*, 2001).

Since it is difficult to determine blood compatibility of a biomaterial from its surface properties, evaluation of the blood-material interaction (*in vitro* and *in vivo*) is essential for the development of any blood-contacting grafts or devices. Generally, blood is allowed to flush through a tube made of the material to be tested, either *in vitro* or *in vivo*. The blood coming out of the testing system and the tube (i.e., the material) can then be evaluated, for example, for the amount of thrombi that have been formed and the behavior of the platelets (Sefton, Gemmell, *et al.*, 2000).

5.1.2. Inflammation

Inflammation is generally defined as "the reaction of vascularized living tissue to local injury" (Ratner, Hoffman, *et al.*, 2004)—a basic way in which the body reacts to infection, irritation or other injuries, with symptoms such as redness, swelling and pain. It is now recognized as a type of nonspecific immune response. The reaction usually tends to counteract, alleviate or shield the injurious agent or process. It also triggers a series of complex events that may help heal the injured tissue and/or form scar tissue.

Closely related to the blood-material interaction, the inflammatory response is characterized by exudation of fluid and plasma proteins, and the accumulation of these liquids in the body tissue, which leads to swelling (known as edema). At the same time, leukocytes (white blood cells) emigrate to, and accumulate at, the injury site. The major role of several types of leukocytes (neutrophils and macrophages) is to phago-cytose microorganisms and foreign materials; that is, they usually recognize, attach to, engulf, kill and degrade these "invaders" as a defense mechanism. Similar attempts are made against implanted biomaterials. Because of the large size of an implant (much larger than a single cell), it may not be possible for the implant to be phagocytosed. However, leukocytes still recognize and attach to the surface of the implant, and will release chemicals (e.g., enzymes) as an effort to degrade the bio-material.

On the other hand, the physical and chemical properties of a bioma-terial may lead to a prolonged inflammatory response. For example, inflammation can be induced by debris detached from an implant (e.g., ligament prosthesis) due to abrasion/wear and by degradation products of a biodegradable biomaterial (e.g., acids produced by the degradation of PGA).

5.1.3. Foreign Body Reaction

After being implanted, most biomaterials elicit a foreign body reac-tion (FBR), which may persist at the tissue-material interface for the lifetime of the implant. FBR to a biomaterial may involve macrophages (a type of white blood cell that ingests foreign material), foreign body giant cells (formed from the coalescence of macrophages) and granula-tion tissues (a tissue containing a large number of pink tiny granules, which are actually newly-formed, young blood vessels). These cells/tis-sues can adhere to the material's surface to different degrees, depending on the surface and structure of the implanted biomaterial. For a bioma-terial with a flat and smooth surface (e.g., breast prosthesis), FBR may involve only a flat structure of a couple of layers of macrophages. For a graft with a relatively rough surface (e.g., ePTFE vascular graft), FBR can involve layers of macrophages and foreign body giant cells. For a prosthesis with a rough surface (e.g., one in a fabric structure), FBR will involve macrophages, foreign body giant cells and various degrees of granulation tissues (Ratner, Hoffman, *et al.*, 2004).

The final healing response to a biomaterial, several weeks after im-

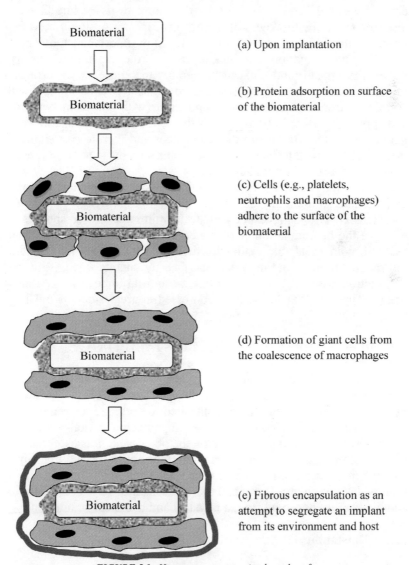

FIGURE 5.1. Host responses to an implanted graft.

plantation, is usually fibrosis or fibrous encapsulation. An acellular fibrous capsule that has formed around a biomaterial is composed of densely compacted collagen, which is on top of the cells and/or granulation tissues produced by FBR. This fibrous capsule can segregate an implant from its environment and host, and may impede its normal function. Thickness of the fibrous layer depends on several factors. Generally, the more chemically inert a material, the thinner the fibrous capsule will be. The motion and fit at the implant-tissue interface can also impact on the thickness of the fibrous capsule. A highly inert material, if implanted in such a way as to allow interfacial movement, can cause the formation of a thick layer of fibrous capsule, which may loosen the implant and make it vulnerable to failure. As a result, an implant made of a porous material has advantages over an implant with a smooth surface in that a porous material (with sufficient pore size and appropriate distributions) allows the penetration and attachment of newly grown cells/tissues to its void spaces and therefore strengthens the implant-tissue interface against complex stresses to prevent loosening of the implant (Long, 2008).

As a summary of the above discussion, a sketch of the host response to a biomaterial upon implantation is shown in Figure 5.1.

Extensive efforts have been made to minimize host responses or enhance the biocompatibility of materials in the design and development of biomaterials/biotextiles for their medical applications, including modification of the material's surface by chemical (e.g., grafting of functional groups) or physical (e.g., anti-thrombogenic coatings) means. These approaches will be addressed in greater details in Chapters 9 and 10.

5.2. BIORESORBABILITY AND BIOSTABILITY

For a bioresorbable implant, such as a resorbable suture or a scaffold for tissue repair, it is important that the process of its being absorbed by the body can be predicted or controlled to optimize the remodeling of host tissues. For a non-absorbable implant, like a non-absorbable suture or a polyester vascular graft on the other hand, it is essential that the implant remain stable and functional during its service life. Since an implant functions under a mechanical load and in an environment of liquids that are chemical in nature, a discussion of its bioresorbability and biostability has to be from a physical and chemical standpoint.

5.2.1. Biostability

Biostability is the term to describe the abilities of a biomaterial to maintain its original dimensions, mechanical and chemical properties during an extended period of time, preferably for the rest of a patient's life, under a hostile biological environment (Sumanasinghe and King, 2003). The characterization of materials, especially their mechanical and chemical properties, is therefore important for choosing a material for a particular purpose.

Mechanical properties of a biomedical implant are of great concern because it is constantly subjected to different types of loadings depending on its location of implantation and may therefore be deformed, broken and/or wear out to lead to the failure of the implantation.

For a material subjected to a mechanical load F (Newtons, N), the stress σ (Pascal, Pa) is defined as a force per unit cross sectional area $A(m^2)$:

$$\sigma = F/A \qquad (5.1)$$

For a textile material (e.g., fibers, yarns) that has a small cross-sectional area and long length, the stress is more often expressed as grams per denier (g/den) or newtons per tex (N/tex). Denier and tex are two parameters to describe the size of a textile material. Tex is defined as the number of grams per one kilometer length of a fiber or yarn, while denier is defined as the number of grams per nine kilometer length of a fiber or yarn.

$$\text{Tex} = \text{Weight (g)}/\text{Length (km)} \qquad (5.2a)$$

$$\text{Denier} = \text{Weight (g)}/[9 \times \text{Length(km)}] \qquad (5.2b)$$

The load in Equation (5.1) can be a tension, compression, shear (as shown in Figure 5.2) or a combination of them. The deformation of a material as a result of a load is referred to as strain ε:

$$\varepsilon = (L - L_0)/L_0 \qquad (5.3)$$

where L and L_0 are deformed length and original length of the material, respectively.

During a mechanical strength testing of a material sample, a *stress-strain curve* can be produced to show the relationship between a gradually increasing stress applied on the material and the resulting strain. A number of mechanical properties of the material can be derived from this stress-strain curve, as discussed below and instanced by a tensile stress-strain curve (Figure 5.3).

The first segment of a stress-strain curve is usually a straight line, the

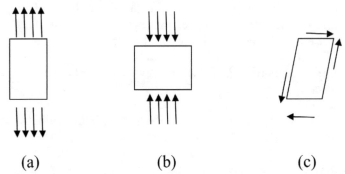

FIGURE 5.2. *Three types of loads on a material: (a) tension, (b) compression and (c) shear.*

slope of which is referred to as the *initial modulus* (*Young's modulus* or *modulus of elasticity*) of the material indicative of the *stiffness* of a material, or of how easily a material is extended under a small stress. The higher the modulus, the stiffer a material is. In this initial segment, changes of the strain are proportional to the stress applied. When we say that a material is in its *elastic region* we mean that, when the applied stress is removed, it will return to its original shape.

At the *yield point,* the stress-strain curve flattens, and the material enters its *plastic region.* After the yield point, a material undergoes permanent deformation—that is, when the stress is removed, the material will not return to its original shape. The stress corresponding to the

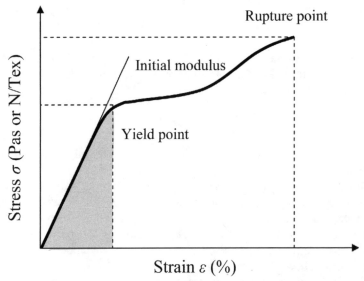

FIGURE 5.3. *A typical tensile stress-strain curve of a textile fiber.*

yield point is called *yield strength.* It is important in the design of an implant that its yield strength should be higher than the load level to which it will be subjected. A ligament prosthesis, for example, will undergo permanent deformation if subjected to a load higher than its yield strength. As a result, its capacity to sustain further load will be significantly reduced, which may lead to failure of the implant.

Resilience is the capacity of a material to absorb energy when it is elastically deformed and, upon removal of the stress, to have the energy recovered. A parameter to describe such a property, the *modulus of resilience* corresponds to the area under the stress-strain curve up to the yield point, shown as the shaded area in Figure 5.3.

At the *fracture point,* a material reaches the maximum stress (i.e., *tensile strength* or *breaking tenacity*) it may sustain and breaks. The elongation of the material at this point is known as the *breaking elongation.* The total amount of work (or energy) required to break the material is referred to as the *work of rupture* or *toughness,* represented by the area under its stress-strain curve up to the fracture point.

The stress-strain curve provides information on the mechanical behavior of a material in a quasi-static situation (i.e., at a small rate of strain). However, an implant will usually be subjected to a repeated (cyclic) load during its service life; even if such a load is considerably below its breaking strength and yield strength, the implant can fail after a period of time. This is known as *dynamic* (cyclic) *fatigue.* The applied load can be axial (tension-compression), flexural (bending) or torsional (twisting). An S-N curve can be used to describe the fatigue behavior of a material, as shown in Figure 5.4. Obviously, the stress required to break the material decreases with increased numbers of cycles of load.

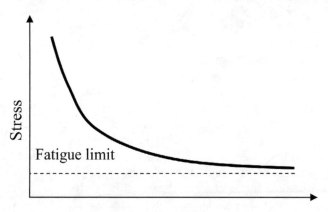

Number of cycles to failure

FIGURE 5.4. *A typical S-N curve.*

The *fatigue limit* is the stress below which a material can endure an infinite number of cycles before failure. Implants that may be subjected to fatigue include vascular grafts (which are exposed to pulsating flow loadings).

Besides their tensile properties, flexural behaviors of polymer or fibrous materials are also critical for their biomedical applications. *Flexural stiffness* is the parameter used to describe the resistance of a material to bending. *Flexibility* of a fiber is represented by the number of times a fiber can be bent without fracture. Flexural properties are important for handling the implants during surgery and for the performance of a material after it has been implanted. For example, a flexible suture is easier to handle and knot. Some materials may have high tensile strength but poor flexibility: carbon fibers, for instance, have much higher tensile strength than other commonly used textile fibers, but can be broken once it is subjected to bending or folding. Comparatively, a polyester fiber can endure 437,000 bends before fracture (Hatch, 1993).

In addition to breaking or fracture, there are other manners in which an implant fails. For example, an implanted vascular graft may go through *abrasion* with its neighboring tissues, resulting in surface damage or causing material to be scraped away from the surface to lead to local damage (e.g., leaking) or damage to the surrounding tissue due to debris from the worn graft. As a result, *abrasion resistance* is also an important mechanical property of a biomaterial.

Creep is the slow, gradual and permanent deformation of a material due to the application of a constant stress, which may be below the yield strength of the material. An implanted graft may experience such a stress and exhibit creep. For a vascular graft, for instance, application of long-term radial stress may result in dilation (expansion in its diameter); a ligament prosthesis, which is under constant tension, may display undesirable elongation. The creep effect is detrimental to implants because it can render them less (or no longer) functional.

Due to their *chemical properties,* materials vary in their reactivity to chemicals and resistance to degradation by chemicals. Implanted materials are usually expected to be inert; that is, they should not chemically affect or be affected by the host environment.

Constantly exposed to body fluid in the host environment, an implant's functionality depends on its resistance to hydrolysis, a chemical decomposition due to which a compound (e.g., polymer) is split into other compounds by reacting with water. Hydrolysis is the most frequently encountered degradation experienced by implants. A variety of polymers, including polyesters (e.g., PET), polysaccharides (e.g., cellulose), polyamides (e.g., nylon), and polyacetals can be degraded by hydrolysis (Hamid, Amin, *et al.*, 1992).

A popular polyester for biomedical end uses, PET (polyethylene tere-phthalate) is produced by an esterification reaction, which involves the reaction of an alcohol (ethylene glycol) with an acid (terephthalic acid) that has been treated for the elimination of water, as shown in Figure 5.5. This reaction is reversible with the long-term exposure of PET to water. The existence of either acids or bases may further accelerate the hydrolytic reaction. The general mechanisms of hydrolytic degradation of polyester at different pH values vary, as shown in Figure 5.6. In an acidic environment, the addition of a proton (H^+) to an oxygen atom of the ester group increases the likelihood of its reaction with water, result-ing in the scission of the ester bond and the production of a hydroxyl and carboxyl groups; under the alkaline condition, on the other hand, it is the hydroxide anion that attacks the ester group to break it, due to the production of a hydroxyl and carboxyl groups. Such hydrolytic deg-radation leads to polymer chain scission and weakens the mechanical properties and performance of a PET implant (Hosseini, Taheri, *et al.*, 2007; Pethrick, 2010).

Similarly, the polyamides, which are produced from the reaction be-tween an acid and an amide having been treated for the elimination of water (Figure 5.7), are also susceptible to hydrolytic degradation as a reverse reaction. The existence of acids accelerates the hydrolytic reac-tion (Pethrick, 2010).

Polysaccharides (e.g., cellulose) can be degraded by hydrolysis at the glycosidic bonds (which are the links between the six-member rings), as shown in Figure 5.8. The acidic environment accelerates the hydro-lytic reaction.

Polytetrafluoroethylene (PTFE) and polyolefin (e.g., Polypropylene)

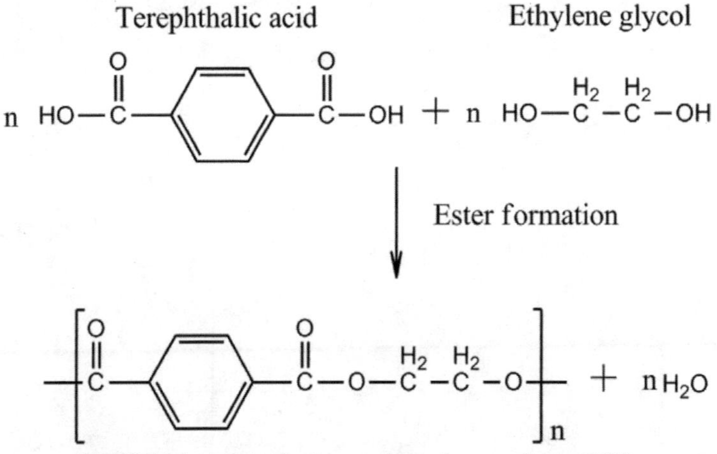

FIGURE 5.5. *An esterification reaction to form a polyester (PET).*

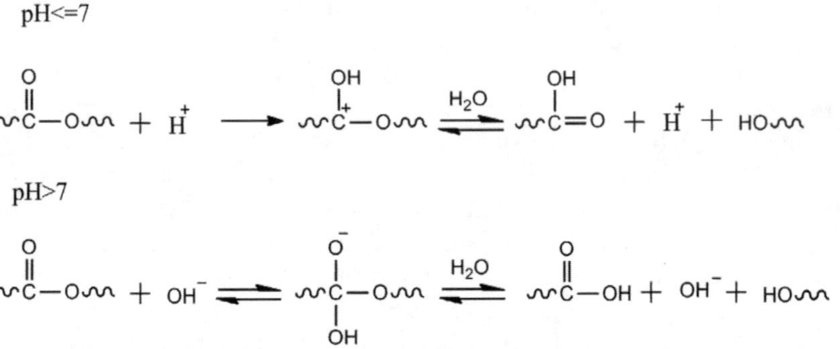

pH<=7

$$\text{\textapprox} C-O\text{\textapprox} + \overset{+}{H} \longrightarrow \text{\textapprox}\overset{OH}{\underset{+}{C}}-O\text{\textapprox} \overset{H_2O}{\rightleftharpoons} \text{\textapprox}C{=}O + \overset{+}{H} + HO\text{\textapprox}$$

pH>7

$$\text{\textapprox}\overset{O}{C}-O\text{\textapprox} + OH^- \rightleftharpoons \text{\textapprox}\overset{\overset{\bar{O}}{|}}{\underset{OH}{C}}-O\text{\textapprox} \overset{H_2O}{\rightleftharpoons} \text{\textapprox}C-OH + OH^- + HO\text{\textapprox}$$

FIGURE 5.6. *Hydrolytic scission of an ester bond under different pH conditions.*

are two polymers with zero absorbency of water and are more resistant to biological environment. They are, however, more vulnerable to mechanical problems or failure.

5.2.2. Bioresorbability

In some situations, there is the need for the temporary presence of a device or implant that does not have to be surgically removed when they are no longer needed. For example, sutures are needed to close the incision into a heart after an open heart surgery until the wound has healed. From a tissue engineering approach, a temporary scaffold is needed to support cell proliferation and tissue remodeling, and is then expected to disappear after the complete regeneration of the tissue. Degradable biomaterials and implants are useful for such applications.

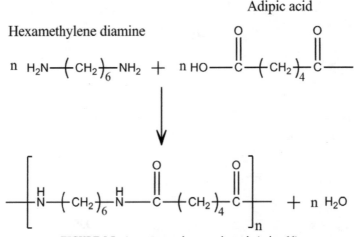

FIGURE 5.7. *A reaction to form a polyamide (nylon 66).*

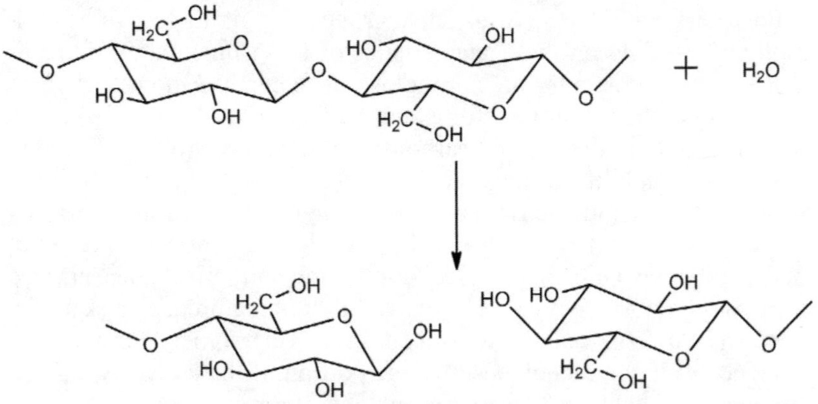

FIGURE 5.8. *Hydrolysis of cellulose.*

Biodegradation, bioabsorption and *bioresorption* are some of the terms in existing literature to describe materials that will eventually disappear after being implanted into a living organism. They are slightly different from each other but have been used almost interchangeably. The term "biodegradation" refers to a chemical process in which long-chain polymers are cleaved in a biological environment, resulting in molecules with smaller sizes. The terms "bioabsorption" and "bioresorption" are used interchangeably, indicating that a polymer and/or its degradation products can be removed by the cellular activity (e.g., phagocytosis) in a physiological condition (Ratner, Hoffman, *et al.*, 2004).

There are several mechanisms whereby these biodegradable polymers can be broken down *in vivo*. Hydrolysis, as previously mentioned, is the most common one. Oxidizing agents and enzymes can be secreted by cells to digest materials. Structural defects (e.g., cracks) can produce new surfaces to accelerate the degradation process.

Hydrolyzable polymers are vulnerable to degradation in a biological environment when in contact with body fluid. The susceptibility of a polymer material to hydrolysis depends on the chemical structure, morphology, and size of the material, and is related to the nature of the environment where it functions.

It is now known that it is due to the existence of some functional groups that polymers are susceptible to hydrolysis. These functional groups include carbonyls bonded to oxygen, nitrogen or sulfur (i.e., esters, amides, urethanes, carbonates and anhydrides), ether, acetal, nitrile, phosphonate, sulfonate and sulfonamide. Table 5.1 shows the hydrolysis reactions of these functional groups and examples of polymers containing these functional groups.

Polymers containing hydrolysable groups exhibit degrees of degradability, depending on the characteristics of these functional groups as well as other molecular or morphological features. Among polymers containing carbonyl groups, for example, their hydrolysis rates can be ranked as: anhydrides>esters>carbonates> (the other groups). The high hydrolytic instability of polyanhydrides has actually limited their applications in degradable implants; aliphatic (i.e., non-aromatic) polyanhydrides, for instance, can be degraded in a number of days. Still, their good *in vivo* biocompatibility allows polyanhydrides to be applied in cases where relatively short-term stability is required. For example, they can be used as vehicles for drug delivery via microencapsulation or nanoencapsulation techniques. A large portion of the currently studied degradable synthetic polymers for implants are polyesters.

The hydrolysis rate of a bulk polymer material is strongly dependent on the ability of water molecules that will enter the polymer matrix. Consequently, the hydrolysis rate of polymers increases with an increase in the percentage of hydrolysable groups in their backbone or side chains, or with an increase of polar groups that improve the hydrophilicity of the polymers, or with an increase of surface-to-volume ratio. On the other hand, the rate of hydrolysis decreases with the increase of hydrophobic groups (e.g., hydrocarbon or fluorocarbon), cross-linking density, and degree of crystallinity. In a biological environment, ions (e.g., H^+, OH^-) and enzymes in extracellular fluids may act as catalysts for hydrolysis reactions.

For several decades, numerous biodegradable synthetic polymers have been studied and introduced for their potential application in biomedical implants. However, in most cases, their applications are limited by their performance *in vivo*. Biodegradable materials have to meet more stringent requirements than non-degradable materials in regard to biocompatibility. Namely, not only a biodegradable material itself but also its degradation products and subsequent metabolites should be such as to never cause any major host response or toxicity. To date, only a limited number of synthetic polymers (e.g., polylactic acid, polyglycolic acid, polydioxanone, polycaprolactone, or the copolymers of these base materials) have been developed for medical implants to be used clinically. Their properties in terms of biodegradability and *in vivo* biocompatibility, as well as their major biomedical applications, are listed in Table 5.2.

Natural polymers (e.g., collagen, gelatin, hyaluronic acid), as compared with synthetic ones, have the advantage that they are similar or identical to some macromolecular substances existing in the native tissues, and therefore can be accepted in a more "friendly" manner. In other words, they are more biocompatible and will induce host responses

TABLE 5.1. Functional Groups Susceptible to Hydrolysis in Polymers
(Ratner, Hoffman, et al., 2004).

Hydrolysis Reactions	Examples

Hydrolysis Reactions

$$-\overset{\overset{O}{\|}}{C}-R- \quad \xrightarrow[\text{H}^+,\ \text{OH}^-\ \text{or enzyme}]{\text{H}_2\text{O}} \quad -\overset{\overset{O}{\|}}{C}-OH \ + \ H-R-$$

R=O, NH, S

$$-R-\overset{\overset{O}{\|}}{C}-R'- \quad \xrightarrow[\text{H}^+,\ \text{OH}^-\ \text{or enzyme}]{\text{H}_2\text{O}} \quad -R-\overset{\overset{O}{\|}}{C}-OH + H-R'-$$

$$\downarrow$$

$$-R-H \ + \ CO_2 \ + \ H-R'-$$

R=O, NH, S
R'=O, NH, S

$$-\overset{\overset{O}{\|}}{C}-R-\overset{\overset{O}{\|}}{C}- \quad \xrightarrow[\text{H}^+,\ \text{OH}^-\ \text{or enzyme}]{\text{H}_2\text{O}} \quad -\overset{\overset{O}{\|}}{C}-OH \ + \ RH-\overset{\overset{O}{\|}}{C}-$$

R=O, NH, S

$$-O-\overset{\overset{H_2}{}}{C}-O- \quad \xrightarrow[\text{H}^+]{\text{H}_2\text{O}} \quad -OH + \overset{\overset{O}{\|}}{CH_2} + HO-$$
Acetal

$$-\overset{\overset{H_2}{}}{C}-O-\overset{\overset{H_2}{}}{C}- \quad \xrightarrow[\text{H}^+]{\text{H}_2\text{O}} \quad -\overset{\overset{H_2}{}}{C}-OH + HO-\overset{\overset{H_2}{}}{C}-$$
Ether

$$-\overset{|}{\underset{\underset{C\equiv N}{|}}{CH}}- \quad \xrightarrow[\text{H}^+,\ \text{OH}^-]{\text{H}_2\text{O}} \quad -\overset{|}{\underset{\underset{NH_2}{|}}{\underset{C=O}{|}}{CH}}- \quad \xrightarrow{2\text{H}_2\text{O}} \quad -\overset{|}{\underset{\underset{OH}{|}}{\underset{C=O}{|}}{CH}}- + H_3N-OH$$
Nitrile

$$-OR-\overset{\overset{O}{\|}}{\underset{\underset{OR''}{|}}{P}}-OR'- \quad \xrightarrow[\text{H}^+,\ \text{OH}^-]{\text{H}_2\text{O}} \quad -R-OH + HO-\overset{\overset{O}{\|}}{\underset{\underset{OR''}{|}}{P}}-OH + HO-R'-$$
Phosphonate

$$-\overset{\overset{O}{\|}}{\underset{\underset{O}{\|}}{S}}-R- \quad \xrightarrow[\text{H}^+,\ \text{OH}^-]{\text{H}_2\text{O}} \quad -\overset{\overset{O}{\|}}{\underset{\underset{O}{\|}}{S}}-OH + HX-$$
Sulfonamide or sulfonate

$$-\overset{\overset{H_2}{}}{C}-\overset{\overset{C\equiv N}{|}}{\underset{\underset{OR}{|}}{\underset{C=O}{|}}{C}}-CH_2-\overset{\overset{C\equiv N}{|}}{\underset{\underset{OR}{|}}{\underset{C=O}{|}}{C}}- \quad \xrightarrow[\text{OH}^-]{\text{H}_2\text{O}} \quad -\overset{\overset{H_2}{}}{C}-\overset{\overset{C\equiv N}{|}}{\underset{\underset{OR}{|}}{\underset{C=O}{|}}{C}}-CH_2-OH + H\overset{\overset{C\equiv N}{|}}{\underset{\underset{OR}{|}}{\underset{C=O}{|}}{C}}-$$
Polycyanoacrylate

Examples

$$-\overset{\overset{O}{\|}}{C}-\overset{\overset{H}{|}}{N}- \quad \text{Amide}$$

$$-\overset{\overset{O}{\|}}{C}-S- \quad \text{Thioester}$$

$$-\overset{\overset{O}{\|}}{C}-O- \quad \text{Ester}$$

$$-\overset{\overset{H}{|}}{N}-\overset{\overset{O}{\|}}{C}-O- \quad \text{Urethane}$$

$$-\overset{\overset{H}{|}}{N}-\overset{\overset{O}{\|}}{C}-\overset{\overset{H}{|}}{N}- \quad \text{Urea}$$

$$-O-\overset{\overset{O}{\|}}{C}-O- \quad \text{Carbonate}$$

$$-\overset{\overset{O}{\|}}{C}-\overset{\overset{H}{|}}{N}-\overset{\overset{O}{\|}}{C}- \quad \text{Imide}$$

$$-\overset{\overset{O}{\|}}{C}-O-\overset{\overset{O}{\|}}{C}- \quad \text{Anhydride}$$

TABLE 5.2. *Properties and Biomedical Applications of Selected Biodegradable Polymers.*

Polymers	Properties	Applications	Unsolved Issues
Synthetic Polymers			
Polyglycolic acid (PGA)	A highly crystalline polyester, high rate of hydrolytic degradation (loses mechanical strength in 2-4 weeks), biocompatible	Sutures, bone fixation devices, scaffolds for tissue engineering	Most widely studied degradable synthetic polymers. Unresolved issues: poor substrate for *in vitro* cell growth; acidic degradation products, which may cause inflammatory response
Polylactic acid (PLA)	Biocompatible, hydrophobic, chiral molecule (i.e., a molecule not superimposable on its mirror image); see the following 3 stereoisomers:		
D-PLA (PDLA)	Semicrystalline	Less used	
L-PLA (PLLA)	Semicrystalline, low rate of degradation	Sutures, orthopedic devices, scaffolds for tissue engineering	
D, L-PLA	Amorphous, higher rate of degradation than PLLA	Drug delivery	
Copolymer of PGA and PLA	Reduced rate of degradation than PGA, biocompatible	Sutures, scaffolds for tissue engineering	
Polydioxanone (PDS)	Degrade to low-toxicity monomers *in vivo*	Sutures	
Polycaprolactone (PCL)	A semicrystalline polymer; degrades at a rate lower than PLA, remains stable for over 1 year; nontoxic and biocompatible	Long-term drug delivery, wound closure	
Polyanhydrides	High degradation rate, excellent in vivo biocompatibility	Short-term drug delivery	
Natural Polymers			
Collagen	Biocompatible, degraded by natural occurring enzymes, degradation rate controllable by crosslinking	Wound closure, artificial skin, vascular grafts, drug delivery, scaffolds for tissue engineering	Lower mechanical strength than synthetic polymers
Gelatin	Biocompatible and bioresorbable	Drug delivery, scaffolds for tissue engineering	
Hyaluronic acid	Biocompatible and bioresorbable	Scaffolds for tissue engineering	

to a lesser degree. Another important feature of natural polymers is that they can be degraded by naturally occurring enzymes, ensuring that they will eventually be absorbed in a physiological environment, usually via normal metabolic processes. The most frequently used natural polymer for biomedical applications (collagen) is normally degraded by mammalian collagenases. In addition, the rate of their degradation or biostability can be controlled by chemical crosslinking. Properties and biomedical application of some commonly used natural polymers are also shown in Table 5.2.

5.3. SUMMARY

Biocompatibility, biostability and bioresorbability (and several like terms) are the most vital properties of any biomaterial. This discussion appears rather "theoretical" at times (covering, for example, material mechanics), but on the whole is extremely practical. Narratively, the discussion is organized along two lines: (1) factors that cause problems with biocompatibility, biostability, and bioresorbability; (2) how a clarification of such problems can lead to the wise choice and use of biomaterials or biotextiles, discussed from the standpoint of application.

One source of the problems is the insertion (*implantation*) of a foreign material (or device) into the body, which causes such general problems as the various *reactions* between the material and body fluids, such as the reaction between a foreign material and blood (a major body fluid) and inflammation (a reaction of the body to infection, irritation, etc., as caused, in this case, by the placement of a foreign material), and such specific problems as degradation of the implant caused by body fluids through the natural phenomenon *hydrolysis*. It is interesting that some of these problems are not entirely "bad": hydrolysis and the related degradation, for example, are not adverse actions and have to be considered or utilized in the case of using absorbable implants, because they aid *bioabsorption* to increase the bioresorbability of an implant.

All of these problems, general or specific, appear as a "response" (*host response*)—i.e., a performance of the body to counteract the placement of a foreign body, often as part of its vital *defense mechanism*. Thus we know nature of the problem (a natural biological phenomenon) and cause of the problem (a foreign material). Since we can do nothing about what is *natural,* we know the ONE thing we can do: use materials that will induce minimal problematic host response, or as much of a "benign" response as possible. To that end, studies have been performed and research and development efforts made. And this chapter reveals what is already known and what can be done, all as a result of these studies and efforts.

Hence we resume the old task—the task of textile materials. Generally, efforts are made towards minimization of host responses, especially those that are "adverse" or produce adverse effects. For instance, by knowing that hydrolytic degradation leads to polymer chain scission and weakens the mechanical properties and performance of a PET implant, we know it is important to guard against using such materials. (Most of the "what to do" and "what to use" particulars have been discussed in previous chapters or will be discussed in subsequent chapters.)

Some of the "problems" are not natural; mechanical failure of an implant, for example, is not all related to the natural host response. Hence *mechanical properties* of biomaterials are included in the discussion, for the same purpose of knowing what to do and use. For instance, we speak of the *fatigue limit,* the point beyond which there is danger of the failure of an implant; the pinpointing of that point certainly helps prevent such failure.

All the related studies, and research and development endeavors based on them, are performed towards this end: a clarification of, and decision on, the use of textile materials that are of the best biocompatibility, biostability, or bioresorbability.

5.4. REFERENCES

Hamid, S.H., M.B. Amin, *et al.* (1992). Handbook of polymer degradation. New York: M. Dekker.

Hatch, K.L. (1993). Textile science. Minneapolis/Saint Paul: West Pub.

Hosseini, S.S., S. Taheri, *et al.* (2007). Hydrolytic degradation of poly(ethylene terephthalate). *Journal of Applied Polymer Science* **103**(4): 2304–2309.

Long, P.H. (2008). Medical devices in orthopedic applications. *Toxicologic Pathology* **36**(1): 85–91.

Mak, T.W. and M.E. Saunders (2006). The immune response: basic and clinical principles. Boston: Elsevier/Academic.

Park, J.B. and R.S. Lakes (2007). Biomaterials: an introduction. New York: Springer.

Pethrick, R.A. (2010). Polymer science and technology for scientists and engineers. Dunbeath: Whittles Pub.

Ratner, B.D., A.S. Hoffman, *et al.* (2004). Biomaterials science: an introduction to materials in medicine. Boston: Elsevier Academic Press.

Schaub, R.D., M.V. Kameneva, *et al.* (1999). Assessing acute platelet adhesion on opaque metallic and polymeric biomaterials with fiber optic microscopy. *Journal of Biomedical Materials Research* **49**(4): 460–468.

Sefton, M.V., C.H. Gemmell, *et al.* (2000). What really is blood compatibility? *Journal of Biomaterials Science-Polymer Edition* 11(11): 1165–1182.

Sefton, M.V., A. Sawyer, *et al.* (2001). Does surface chemistry affect thrombogenicity of surface modified polymers? *Journal of Biomedical Materials Research* **55**(4): 447–459.

Sumanasinghe, R.D. and M.W. King (2003). New trends in biotextiles—the challenge of tissue engineering. Journal of Textile and Apparel, Technology and Management **3**(2).

Williams, D.F. (1987). Blood compatibility. Boca Raton, Fla.: CRC Press.

Williams, D.F. (1987). Definitions in Biomaterials: Proceedings of a Consensus Conference of the European Society for Biomaterials, Chester, England. New York: Elsevier.

Wise, D. L. (2000). Biomaterials and bioengineering handbook. New York: Marcel Dekker.

Part II
Applications

CHAPTER 6

Disposable Hygiene Textiles

MOST of the hygiene products are disposables or single-use items. They are typically diapers, sanitary napkins, tampons, incontinence products, panty shields and wipes. These end uses require the utilization of materials and/or structures that are: (1) highly absorptive so as to receive, absorb and retain fluid or solid waste; (2) comfortable to the fragile or sensitive skin of those who use these products; and (3) of low cost. As a result, most of them are made from nonwovens, which are highly porous in structure and are relatively inexpensive to produce.

This chapter will start with the simple yet important product, the diaper, a well-known example of a disposable absorbent product.

6.1. THE DIAPER

The diaper is the largest of all hygiene product sectors in terms of value, with a $30 billion global market and almost 8% growth in 2008 (Kondej, 2010).

The diaper bears a tale. It has a history of evolution and development, mirroring lifestyles of the human race and progressing as a product in the various ages and societies. Ancient people used leaves, animal skins and other natural resources for diapers. Crude as it was, the early diaper was among the first objects to establish human dignity, and to distinguish man from animals. Even for the ancients, healthiness (*hygiene*) and comfort were the major concerns in identifying diaper materials and using diapers. In the many centuries to come, diapers had styles and varied from nation to nation, although the old concerns continued.

It was not until the 1800s when the diaper became a textile product composed of cotton or linen cloth. It had been a tradition in many regions of the world that diapers were made from used cotton quilts or

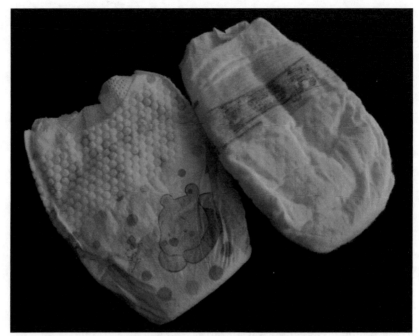

FIGURE 6.1. *Modern disposable diapers.*

clothes, because they were the most comfortable (e.g., very soft after repeated washing), healthy (e.g., rarely causing any diaper rash), and of course economical. A cloth diaper was usually folded to fit a baby and held in place with safety pins. These reusable diapers required great energy and time in boiling and drying for the purpose of hygiene, not to mention that the safety pins constituted a risk of safety to the baby. Today, commercially available diapers are used and immediately committed to waste bags. Convenient as they are, these disposable diapers raise environmental concerns (see Section 6.3), leading to a continuous debate over disposable versus cloth diapers.

The first disposable diaper appeared in the 1940s as layers of creped cellulose tissues held in a rubber pant. These early-stage disposable diapers were bulky, with high cost and low capacity in absorbance. Since then, untiring efforts have been made to design, develop, and fabricate diapers that are thinner, less likely to leak, more absorbent, more comfortable, and less expensive. Fluff pulp, for its higher efficiency of absorption and lower cost, replaced the cellulose tissues as the absorbent component in the 1950s. The introduction of diapers made by machines and produced industrially enlarged production and reduced cost. The adoption of super-absorbent polymers (SAP) in the 1980s led to a breakthrough in the development of diapers, bringing about a 50%

reduction in weight among other improvements. Today, the diaper continues to be a product under continuous development, demonstrated by such facts as mounting patents granted annually on further improved function and greater comfort of this small but enormously important product.

6.1.1. The Anatomy of a Typical Modern Diaper

A typical modern diaper has a multi-layered structure, from top to bottom at a cross section, composed of: (1) a porous nonwoven top-sheet; (2) an acquisition/distribution layer; (3) an absorbent/storage layer; and (4) a laminate back sheet. Each layer has its own function, achieved by choices of the material and structure.

The *top-sheet,* the layer that is placed next to the skin of the baby, is also referred to as *cover, coverstock, coversheet* or *facing*. It functions to allow the body's fluid to flow through, to maintain a comfortable touch to the skin, and to retain the structural integrity of the absorbent core.

Before the 1970s, hydrophilic fibers such as rayon were the dominant material for the top-sheet, as it was generally accepted at the time that the diaper top-sheet should be absorbent. As a result of this belief, many of the design considerations, including choices of the fabric structure and binders, were based on the objective to obtain maximum absorbency. The last few decades witnessed a reversal, however. The current belief is that it is more comfortable and healthy to have a dry surface in contact with the skin because a wet surface next to the skin may promote bacteria proliferation and make the skin more vulnerable to frictional damages.

Consequently, the polypropylene fiber came to be preferred as the material for the diaper top-sheet. Polypropylene is known for its zero absorbency, an essential advantage in keeping a dry surface next to the skin. As a thermoplastic fiber, polypropylene allows the fabrication of a nonwoven sheet (highly porous in structure) through thermal bonding, which eliminates the use of any adhesive chemicals (including formaldehyde) that may cause a toxic effect when in contact with the skin.

A typical diaper top-sheet is made of a composite structure containing both spunbonded (S) and meltblown (M) fabric layers. Arrangement of the layers can be SMS, SMMS or SSMMS. A meltblown layer is a dense web containing microfibers; its small pore sizes can effectively prevent the loss of superabsorbent particles embedded in the absorbent core. Since the meltblown fabric is usually low in mechanical strength, it is usually sandwiched between spunbonded fabrics, which contain thicker filaments (Chatterjee and Gupta, 2002).

The *acquisition/distribution layer* of the diaper, also known as the surge layer, is supposed to be able to repeatedly receive the liquid and hold it temporarily, to improve the liquid distribution in the diaper and to allow the liquid to pass through quickly and smoothly to the absorbent core.

A typical acquisition/distribution layer between the coverstock and absorbent core is usually composed of multiple sublayers (Chatterjee and Gupta, 2002), as shown in Figure 6.2, and consists of: (1) a top sublayer made from the thickest fibers with the lowest density, largest pore size and highest porosity among the sublayers; (2) a middle sublayer made from finer fibers with higher density, smaller pore size and lower porosity than the top sublayer; and (3) a bottom sublayer made from the finest fibers with the highest density, smallest pore size and lowest porosity among the sublayers. This multilayered structure gives rise to a density gradient, bringing into play this law: the smaller the size of a pore (capillary), the larger the capacity of wicking. As a result, this gradient in wicking capacity effectively causes the liquid to move in the radius direction toward the upper sublayer(s) to alleviate the flooding in the zone that repeatedly receives the urine and also enhances utilization of the underlying absorbent layer.

Materials for this acquisition/distribution layer are usually hydrophobic fibers (such as polypropylene) and hydrophilic fibers (such as cross-linked cellulose fibers). Diaper designers use different combinations of these two types of fibers to provide optimum distribution of the liquid.

The *absorbent core,* also referred to as the storage or retention layer, is the most important functional component of the diaper. It receives and retains most of the liquid. It contains both fluff pulp (cellulose) and the so called *superabsorbent* polymers (SAPs), which are designed to take up liquid tens to hundreds of times of their own weight. The in-

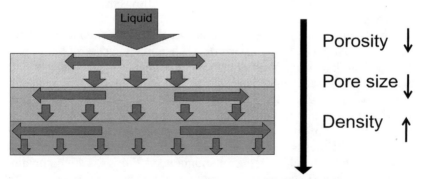

FIGURE 6.2. *A typical acquisition layer consisting of multiple sublayers.*

troduction of superabsorbent polymers in diaper products in the 1980s greatly reduced the weight and thickness of the diaper. More detailed information about SAPs will be given in the next section.

The *back-sheet,* i.e., the bottom layer of a diaper, exists to prevent leakage, keep the diaper cloth layer that is next to the skin dry and, preferably, breathable. This layer is usually made of a hydrophobic polyethylene (PE) film, or of a PE film plus a PE nonwoven sheet in a laminate structure.

Product Development Question 6.1

For a laminate back-sheet, which material should be placed on the back of the diaper, the PE film or the nonwoven sheet?

Suggested answer: It does not make any difference to a baby which one faces the back of the diaper, either the film or the nonwoven sheet. However, it DOES make a difference to the mother, the one who makes the decision on purchase. When the mother is holding the baby in her arm, especially during the summer when the baby wears no extra cloth other than the diaper, the enhanced perspiration caused by the close contact between the occlusive PE film and the skin is very unpleasant. The adoption of a porous nonwoven sheet on the back of the diaper, however, may alleviate or eliminate the problem. That explains why most of the diapers on market are using the nonwoven sheet as the bottom sheet in a diaper, and the PE film just above to seal any leakage of liquid from the diaper.

In addition, the diaper comprises *elastic folds,* placed between the two lateral edges of the diaper, which are there to prevent side leakage of liquid. These folds are made to stand up from the surface of a diaper. As a result, they are called the *standing leg cuffs* or *standup cuffs.* The material and structure used for these cuffs are similar to the material and structure for the top-sheet—that is, polypropylene fibers of an SMS composite structure. The spunbonded layers provide strength and stability to the structure, while the dense meltblown layer renders the material waterproof and breathable.

In some designs, a *secondary facing* is introduced immediately beneath the top-sheet. It is expected to promote rapid transfer of liquid from the top-sheet to the adjacent acquisition layer. This secondary facing may have a rough surface that faces the top-sheet and a smooth surface that faces the acquisition layer. The liquid tends to travel from the rough side to the smooth side as a result of wicking. This layer can be especially beneficial for diapers with standing leg cuffs, which may cause the top-sheet to be pulled away from the underlying layers during the end use (Chatterjee and Gupta, 2002).

6.1.2. Superabsorbent Polymers

A critical component for the absorbent core of a diaper, superabsorbent polymers (SAPs) are a group of cross-linked hydrophilic polymers able to absorb large volumes of water and aqueous solutions (up to hundreds of times of their original weight) in a short period of time and to retain them under a slight mechanical pressure. The SAPs can be either modified natural polymers (cellulose or starch) or synthetic polymers (polyacrylamide or polyacrylate polymers). Figure 6.3 illustrates the structures of a typical cellulose-based SAP (Sodium carboxymethyl cellulose/CMC) and a synthetic SAP (Sodium polyacrylate).

One characteristic in common between sodium CMC and sodium polyacrylate is that they both have the ionizable hydrophilic group on each repeat unit; i.e., the carboxyl group ($-COO^-$). They are both cross-linked; namely, their polymer chains are joined at certain points by small molecules, which give rise to a network structure as shown in Figure 6.4 (a). When large amounts of water molecules diffuse into the network of the polymer chains of the SAPs in the form of particles, they quickly form stable hydrogen bonds with the carboxyl groups. As a result, the coiled polymer network expands to accommodate the water uptake, and the SAP particles swell into the state of a gel, as shown in Figure 6.4 (b).

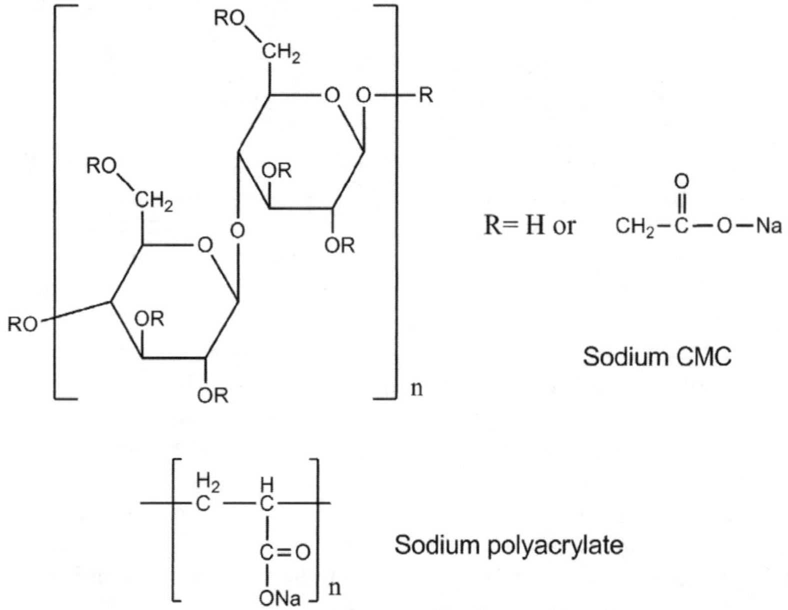

FIGURE 6.3. *Structures of typical SAPs: sodium CMC and sodium polyacrylate.*

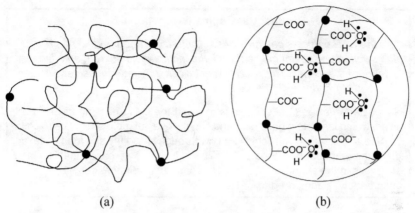

FIGURE 6.4. *The SAP polymer network: (a) when it is dry; (b) when it is wet and swollen.*

Cross-links between polymer chains limit the swelling of SAPs and prevent them from being dissolved in water. The degree of cross-linking has a direct effect on the level of the swelling of SAPs, as well as the strength of the gel. Generally, the higher the cross-linking density,

---

Product Development Question 6.2

Diapers are always subjected to pressure in use. How can the absorbing capacity of the SAPs be improved without sacrificing their absorbance against pressure?

Suggested answer: Different ways can be employed to handle the problem. One approach is to reduce the pressure applied on the SAP particles: Fluff pulps are usually used as a matrix of the SAP particles to distribute the pressure applied. The other approach is to increase the resistance of the SAP particles to mechanical pressure. For example, the SAP particles can be designed to have different cross-linking density between the shell and core areas, so as to have a highly cross-linked shell and moderately cross-linked core, as shown in Figure 6.5. As a result, the moderately cross-linked core contributes to a good capacity of absorbency, while the highly cross-linked shell provides a strong shield to prevent liquid from being squeezed out.

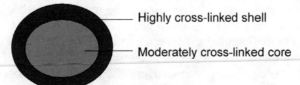

Highly cross-linked shell

Moderately cross-linked core

Figure 6.5. A design for SAP particle with increased resistance to mechanical pressure.

Product Development Question 6.3

As the SAP particles can quickly swell into a gel upon uptake of a liquid, the swollen masses of gel can block the incoming liquid from entering the interior of the diaper. This so-called gel block may lead to leak and longer contact of urine with the skin of a baby. How to solve the problem?

Suggested answer: One solution is to avoid the close packing of SAP particles, which leads to a gel block. Again, cellulose fluff pulp should be used to provide a matrix in which liquid can flow through smoothly and then be taken up by the embedded SAP particles. This is the second reason that fluff pulp still exists in the absorbent layer of the commercial diapers despite its lower absorbency as compared to SAPs.

---

the higher the gel strength, but the lower the swelling and absorbing capacity. In other words, a decrease in cross-linking density may result in an increase of the absorbing capacity but a decrease in gel strength against pressure.

6.1.3. Diaper Rash or Dermatitis

Diaper rash (or dermatitis) is the term used to describe any inflammatory eruption of the skin occurring in the diaper area as a consequence of disruption of the barrier function of the fragile skin through prolonged contact with feces and urine (Atherton, 2004; Scheinfeld, 2005). It causes irritation or pain to infants, as well as anxiety to parents and caregivers.

Diaper rash can be ascribed to a combination of factors, including urine, feces, wetness of the skin and mechanical force (pressure and friction) applied to the skin. These factors are also correlated (Scheinfeld, 2005): urine not only increases the wetness, but also raises pH value in the diaper area, both of which lead to increased risk of diaper rash. The prolonged contact of the vulnerable skin of infants with liquid in the diaper makes it more fragile and susceptible to frictional damage. The increased wetness and pH value also cripple the barrier function of the skin (see Chapter 4), causing it to be more vulnerable to irritant chemical penetration and bacterial growth. In addition, fecal enzymes are erosive to the integrity of the epidermis. Microorganisms in the feces may also increase the risk of infection in the diaper area.

To alleviate or eliminate diaper rashes, an ideal diaper should be highly absorbent (so as to keep the skin dry), and soft to the touch (to reduce pressure and friction). Extensive efforts have been devoted to the design and development of diaper products that meet such demands.

Disposable diapers containing SAPs and hydrophobic coverstocks usually maintain a drier skin, while cloth diapers may provide a more gentle touch. However, general practice suggests that disposable diapers are associated with a higher risk of diaper rash than cloth diapers, as a result of the following:

Firstly, cloth diapers (usually composed of hydrophilic natural or regenerated fibers) provide a more gentle touch to the infants' skin than the coverstocks (made of polypropylene fibers) of the disposables. Secondly, since cloth diapers are less absorbent, parents or caregivers will change them more frequently than they would when dealing with disposables, so that it is less likely to have the negative impact of the wet surface of a diaper. Finally, when cloth diapers are frequently changed, they will be more breathable and will result in less heat accumulation in the diaper area of the skin, which will increase comfort and reduce the risk of skin rash.

When such a comparison became known and understood, extensive research and development began. The good news is that much of the efforts towards improvement were led by manufacturers of the disposables. Approaches they have tried and found effective include the adoption of a breathable back sheet (Akin, Spraker, *et al.*, 2001), or a topsheet impregnated with substances that may prevent diaper rash, such as petrolatum, zinc oxide, stearyl alcohol, aloe vera extract or a combination of these ingredients (Odio, O'Connor, *et al.*, 2000; Baldwin, Odio, *et al.*, 2001).

Issues about diaper rash fall into the scope of textile comfort, a detailed discussion of which is given in Chapter 4.

6.2. OTHER DISPOSABLE HYGIENE TEXTILES

Other disposable hygiene textiles include sanitary napkins, tampons, incontinence products, panty shields and wipes. A lot of these products have similar requirements (to be absorbent, etc.) and structures as diapers. However, they are different from each other in that they are expected to absorb different types of fluids and/or different amounts of them. Some of these hygiene products will be discussed briefly in this section.

6.2.1. Sanitary Napkins

The trend in the development of sanitary napkin products is largely similar to that for diapers. The general goal in the design and development is to make the product more comfortable (i.e., thinner and softer) and/or efficient (more absorbent and/or less likely to leak). A sanitary napkin has a multi-layered structure similar to that of the diaper. It is usually composed of three layers: the top-sheet, the absorbent layer, and the back-sheet.

The *top-sheet* of a sanitary napkin should be hydrophobic, porous and soft, and can be expected to quickly transfer menstrual blood from its surface to the central absorbent layer and stop the back flow of the fluid. To achieve this goal, a nonwoven structure containing multiple sub-layers with a pore size gradient (similar to what is shown in Figure 6.2) is often used. It is also important that this top-sheet be comfortable to the touch and able to maintain its integrity when it is wet. This nonwoven sheet can be polypropylene or polyethylene fibers that are thermal bonded or entangled by water jets. Chemical bonding agents are usually avoided to eliminate possible allergic issues when the sheet is in contact with the skin. The top-sheet of a napkin is usually lighter than that of a diaper, as it handles a fluid that is of a lesser quantity but higher viscosity.

The *absorbent layer* is made from superabsorbent polymers embedded in a cellulose matrix. This is the layer where the transferred blood is absorbed and stored. The absorbent layer in a napkin is thinner than that in the diaper because a smaller amount of fluid is expected to be dealt with. Another consumer requirement for the napkin is that it must be highly flexible to favor daily activities. As a result, there has been a trend for designers to give the absorbent core an *anatomical* shape.

In order to prevent blood leakage, the *back-sheet* is usually made of polyethylene film. Its bottom (or outer surface) is usually coated with a layer of sensitive adhesive so as to affix the napkin to the undergarment.

6.2.2. Adult Incontinence Products

It is estimated that unexpected leakage of urine, a disorder caused by an *overactive* bladder, affects 33 million people in the U.S. 1/3 of them have urinary incontinence, or suffer from involuntary discharge of large amounts of urine that leads to physical or emotional distress (McIntyre, 2010). Elderly people are more vulnerable to this disorder, due to malfunctions of the pelvic and abdominal muscles and of the diaphragm and/or control nerves. These realities have made the adult incontinence products a growing demand in the market. The materials and structural features for the adult incontinence products are similar to those for baby diapers.

6.2.3. Absorbent Wipes

Absorbent wipes are widely used in home, industrial and institutional (including medical and healthcare) sectors for picking up either aqueous or oil-based waste liquid. Hydrophilic fibers, such as cotton, rayon or wood pulp, are often used for handling aqueous waste, while hydrophobic fibers, like polyester, polyolefin and nylon, are more suitable in treating oil-based waste. Currently, the majority of such wipes on the market is made from nonwoven structures. Cellulose-based hydrophilic wipes are usually processed via latex bonding of wet-laid or dry-laid webs. Hydrophobic wipes can be produced from melt blown webs and applied in a wide variety of end uses that range from the cleaning of indoor surfaces to the pick-up of oil spills in a water body. Spunlace nonwoven fabrics are produced by water jet entanglement, which is a binder-free approach suitable for both cellulose-based and synthetic fibers.

6.3. ENVIRONMENTAL ISSUES

The use of disposable diapers has become a fashion only in the last couple of decades. Use of similar disposable products has a similar history. The greatest recommendation of these products is their *disposability,* from which is derived their advantage: convenience in use. A lesser advantage is their relatively low cost; for many people, to use disposable diapers is a means of economy. According to Webster's Third New International Dictionary, *disposable* means "capable of being disposed of easily; especially designed to be thrown away after use with only negligible loss." It is these advantages that have moved more and more people to the use of disposable products, until there is an environmental consequence. It is, indeed, their disposability that is to blame.

To speak of the diaper alone: a daily consumption of 6 pieces makes up an annual demand for over 2,000 diapers for a single baby. Thus, Americans alone consume 16 to 18 billion single-use diapers annually (Lehrburger, 1988). Huge amounts of this disposable product end up in landfills in North America, and in incinerators in European countries. It takes up to 500 years for a single diaper to degrade in a landfill (Lehrburger, 1988), while tons of them emit large amounts of fumes and carbon dioxide in the incinerators. This innocent baby diaper, among many other disposable products, is therefore to blame for adding fuel to burning environmental issues. To alleviate the burden of these disposable products on our environment, different approaches have been created and proposed, as briefly discussed in the following.

Some people have recently proposed *returning* to the use of reusable cloth diapers. Modern people have gone a long journey towards the development of a cloth diaper that has a stylish look and satisfactory performance as compared to those used by their great grandmothers. A typical cloth diaper is illustrated in Figure 6.6. Such a diaper is usually made from natural fibers. An average advertisement on behalf of the reusable cloth diaper is that it is much more breathable and comfortable and, as a result, greatly reduces the incidences of diaper rash or dermatitis, in addition to the many environmental advantages. However, there are counter arguments that it takes time and energy to have the cloth diaper washed and dried, which would largely counteract its environmental benefits. And, since the usage of cloth diapers means giving up the convenience—a result of the disposability—and since it is usually women who have to have the burden of the returned *inconvenience,* there is the feminist fear that the young, working mothers may not love the old-time cloth diaper. This fear brings forward a larger fear: will they BUY such a diaper?

Another approach is to render disposable products *degradable.* Fibers or plastics that are used for these products are supposed to maintain the same performance and properties as their non-degradable peers for their service life or shelf life, until degradability is activated by one or more triggers, including heat, pressure, UV light, or a combination of

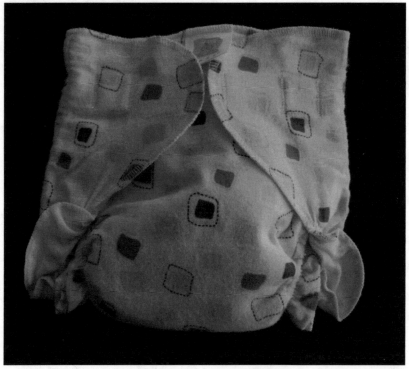

FIGURE 6.6. A typical modern cloth diaper.

them. By degradation, the long chain polymers of the fibers/plastics will be broken down or cut into smaller pieces with lower molecular weight within a relatively short period of time (say, a few years instead of centuries), with the final destiny of turning completely into carbon dioxide, water and biomass as a part of a normal bio-cycle. Such goals can be achieved by adding plastic additives during fabrication of the products.

6.4. SUMMARY

The design and development of diapers and other disposable hygiene products have come a long way and are still attracting extensive efforts, as reflected from the large numbers of patents granted in the last few decades concerning absorbent hygiene products. Most of these disposable products have a composite structure composed of multiple layers, each of which is has a unique design and performs a specific function. Because of their isotropic structure, high permeability and low cost, nonwoven fabrics have predominantly been the material for these products. A prominent milestone, the introduction of superabsorbent polymers contributed to reducing the volume and thickness of a product, increasing its capacity, and improving its performance. Efforts to be made in the future will, like always, be devoted to the development of textile products that are of: (1) better function (especially in terms of absorbency); (2) greater comfort (e.g., better fit to the body, lighter in weight, and more pleasant to the touch); and (3) relatively low cost.

Serious problems have been found with disposable products, and new milestones revealed, especially in the direction of developing new, environmentally friendly products. They are expected to be just as efficient as, or even better than, their predecessors, in addition to the likelihood of giving a lesser, or preferably *benign,* environmental impact.

A Debated Topic for Reflection: Disposable vs. Cloth Diapers

Hints: The debate over the choice of disposable or cloth diapers has seemed endless, but each choice has been allowed its advantages and disadvantages. Table 6.1 contains a comparison of disposable and cloth diapers. Most of the contents of the table have been discussed in this chapter. What is already obvious is that the disposable diapers have better performance (mostly because of the adoption of superabsorbent polymers) and can be used more conveniently than cloth diapers, but may provide less comfort and lead to higher risks of diaper rash than cloth diapers. In addition to these relatively "well-accepted" views that have often been quoted by advocates on both sides, there are less settled arguments on economic and environmental grounds, as listed in the table below.

TABLE 6.1. A Summary of Comparison Between Disposable
and Cloth Diapers.

		Disposable Diapers	Cloth Diapers
Performance	Absorption capacity	High	Low
	Leakage	Less	More
Comfort	Keeping the skin dry	Better	Less
	Breathability	Less	Better
	Softness	Less	Better
	Higher risk of diaper rash	Yes	No
Convenience	Frequencies of changing	Low	High
	Need for wash/dry	No	Yes
Cost	For purchase	Varies*	Varies*
	For maintenance	No	Yes
Environmental impact	From production	High	Low
	From maintenance	No	Yes
	During disposal	High	Low

*There have been diverse opinions on the costs and environmental impact associated with disposable and cloth diapers (Rockney, Culpepper, et al., 1991).

Supporters for cloth diapers made a calculation for a San Francisco Bay Area family that have used both disposable and cloth diapers:

(1) For disposables, it is estimated that each baby (< 2 years old) consumes 6,000 pieces per year and the average cost per piece is 25.5 cents. Thus the family's annual expenses are about $1,600.

(2) For cloth diapers, each baby needs about 6 dozen (72) diapers. The total cost may vary from $300 (for the basic type, which includes only prefolds and covers) to over $1,000 (for the more advanced type, which contains organic cotton fitted diapers and wool covers). It can be seen that even the most luxurious choice of cloth diapers costs less than disposables. Most of these may last for a couple of years, and may further cut down the long-term cost. If the family is willing to have the DIY (do-it-yourself) cloth diapers, they can save more.

However, advocates of disposable diapers dispute such calculations. Proctor and Gamble (P&G) Co., the disposable product giant, publicized its study to defend disposable diapers in 1990 (Little, 1990). It points out that there are factors that equalize the costs of cloth and disposable diapers, including the need of using double cloth diapering occasionally to increase absorbency, the readily available discount coupons for disposables, and the decreased frequency of diaper changes due to increased capacity of newly developed disposable diapers. The report also indicates that laundering a cloth diaper over the course of its lifetime consumes up to six times the water used to manufacture a single-use diaper. In addition, the study concludes that laundering cloth diapers produces nearly ten times the water pollution created in manufacturing disposables.

The P&G report was followed by an immediate rebuttal, criticizing the potential biases in the data and assumptions upon which it is based. It suggests that the central issue lies in the relative impacts of different environmental consequences of the two choices: disposables generate 90 times the solid waste produced by using cloth diapers, while laundering cloth diapers consumes 2~6 times the amount of water as required in the production and use of disposables (Tryens 1990; Rockney, Culpepper, *et al.*, 1991).

To date, while the debate over disposables and cloth diapers is far from over, the reality is that disposable diapers continue to dominate the consumer market, and most of the mothers and caregivers enjoy using the former, mostly for the CONVENIENCE.

6.5. REFERENCES

—. "Real diaper association—diaper facts." Retrieved Feb 2, 2011, from http://www.realdiaperassociation.org/diaperfacts.php.

Akin, F., M. Spraker, *et al.* (2001). Effects of breathable disposable diapers: reduced prevalence of Candida and common diaper dermatitis." *Pediatric Dermatology* 18(4): 282–290.

Atherton, D.J. (2004). A review of the pathophysiology, prevention and treatment of irritant diaper dermatitis. *Curr. Med. Res. Opin.* 20(5): 645–9.

Baldwin, S., M.R. Odio, et al. (2001). Skin benefits from continuous topical administration of a zinc oxide/petrolatum formulation by a novel disposable diaper. *Journal of the European Academy of Dermatology and Venereology* 15: 5–11.

Chatterjee, P.K. and B.S. Gupta (2002). Absorbent technology. Oxford: Elsevier Science.

Kondej, M. (2010). Diaper sales remain strong. *Nonwovens Industry.* 41: 28–32.

Lehrburger, C. (1988). Diapers in the waste stream: a review of waste management and public policy issues. Sheffield, MA: National Association of Diaper Services.

Little, A.D. (1990). Disposable versus reusable diapers: health, environmental and economic comparisons. Cincinnati:Procter and Gamble Co.

McIntyre, K. (2010). The evolution of adult incontinence. *Nonwovens Industry.* 41: 46–48.

Odio, M.R., R.J. O'Connor, *et al.* (2000). Continuous topical administration of a petrolatum formulation by a novel disposable diaper—1. Effect on skin surface microtopography. *Dermatology* 200(3): 232–237.

Rockney, R.M., L. Culpepper, et al. (1991). Diaper choice—too costly to bury. *Clinical Pediatrics* 30(8): 472–477.

Scheinfeld, N. (2005). Diaper dermatitis: a review and brief survey of eruptions of the diaper area. *Am. J. Clin. Dermatol.* 6(5): 273–81.

Tryens, J. (1990). Review of Arthur D. Little, Inc.'s Disposable versus reusable diapers. Washington, D.C.: Center for Policy Alternatives.

CHAPTER 7

Healthcare Protective Textiles

HUMANS have increasingly become conscious of the many *hazards,* natural and man-made, that they may or may not be able to foresee. These hazards include exposure to extremely high or low temperatures, insect bites, microorganisms, accidental fires, toxic chemicals, and nuclear radiation. In response, humans have developed significant solutions to protect themselves from these hazards. These solutions include articles or devices that are waterproof, bulletproof, fireproof, or dust-impermeable, to name a few.

Thus we speak of *protective textiles,* one of such means of protection. Generally, protective textiles or protective textile products function by a variety of mechanisms to form a barrier between the user and a hazard. The hazards that usually occur in medical/healthcare facilities to such people as hospitalized patients and those who attend to them (doctors, nurses, etc.) are: (1) microorganisms that cause disease as well as infection to spread the disease to more people; (2) fire that causes loss of health and lives; and (3) electrostatic charge, which can be a nuisance sometimes, especially to such people as hospitalized patients.

This chapter is devoted to the various types of protective textiles used in these places, and to the many mechanisms, materials and approaches that combine to make the textiles and their products protective.

Since most of these protective textile products are used next to the skin, comfort is a major concern in the development and use of such products. A detailed discussion about textile comfort has already been given in Chapter 5. Comfort, as a concept in textile science, may mean more than is usually found in the word. Direct contact and interactions between textiles and the skin may cause reactions or even damage and disease, and may lead to skin irritation and intolerance caused by textiles, dermatitis caused by chemicals (e.g., dyes and finishes) and physi-

135

cal contact/friction. When we have—or are advised—to wear a piece of clothing or other product (e.g., a mask) that is "protective", we expect that it will be so "comfortable" as never to cause these problems to us. Now it is clear that such comfort can be derived from proper designs of the microclimate between clothing and the skin, which ensures thermo-physiological comfort as well as sensorial comfort that necessarily goes with protective clothing. Comfort as a requirement for the design and de-velopment of protective textiles will be discussed further in this chapter.

7.1. TEXTILES FOR INFECTION CONTROL

In recent years, there has been an increasing awareness of infectious disease such as SARS (severe acute respiratory syndrome), bird flu, H1N1 swine flu and multi-drug resistant tuberculosis. They may pose even more serious problems in healthcare facilities, where there is a population of patients with infectious conditions or compromised health status. Nosocomial infection—that is, infection acquired in healthcare facilities—is a growing problem. It is estimated that 5–10% of hospi-talized patients acquire nosocomial infections. Annually in the United States, it affects about 2 million patients, leads to around 90,000 deaths, and accounts for a patient care cost of $4.5–5.7 billion (Burke, 2003). However, these infections can be largely avoided by taking appropriate measures in hygiene and infection control, including the utilization of protective textiles against pathogens.

Since pathogenic microorganisms such as viruses, bacteria and fungi may transmit disease through air, liquid and/or solid media (such as fabrics); various protective textiles have been developed for the making of barrier/defense devices against these hazards. They are used in respi-ratory masks, surgical gowns, drapes, and mats. According to how they work, they can be categorized into physical barriers or biocide-treated textiles, as expounded in the following sections.

7.1.1. Textiles as Physical Barrier

A large number of pathogens can be transmitted via air or liquid (blood or body fluid). Some protective textiles function by serving as a physical barrier to block the penetration of airborne pathogens and biological bloods that may carry pathogens.

7.1.1.1. Protective Respirators

Respirators, or face masks, are one of the most frequently used pro-tective devices in healthcare facilities and other locations with airborne hazards. Protective respiratory masks are worn by healthcare workers attending patients with airborne infectious diseases, or emergency personnel responding to biological accidents. To date, most of these respirators for biodefense in the healthcare sectors are disposable products. Different types of respirators are available to provide different levels of protection.

Surgical masks are primarily used to trap respiratory secretions (which may include bacteria and viruses) expelled by the wearer and prevent disease transmission to others (Johnson, Druce, *et al.*, 2009). A typical surgical mask is shown in Figure 7.1(a). They may be used by people who have acquired a transmitted disease, or by surgeons con-

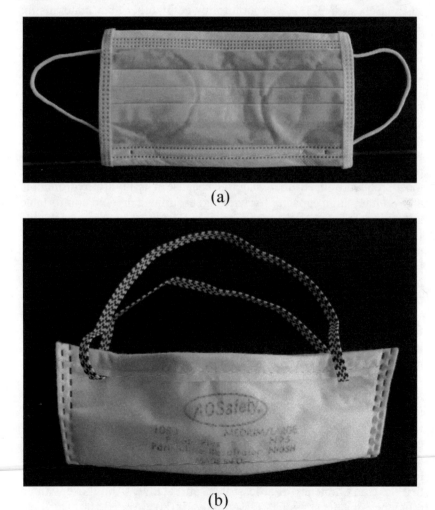

(a)

(b)

FIGURE 7.1. *Respirators: (a) A surgical mask, (b) A N95 respirator.*

ducting surgical procedures so as to protect the environment from the wearer. They can also provide protection to the wearer when more effective respirators are needed but not yet available (Derrick and Gomersall, 2005).

Introduced in 1918, early reusable surgical masks were made of multi-layered cotton gauze. With a larger number of layers, the protective capacity of the masks may increase, but their breathability and comfort level are compromised. In the 1960s, disposable masks became available. The disposable mask was made of fine glass fiber nonwoven mat, and was proven to have a capacity of deterring bacteria and viruses (Belkin, 1997). It was soon followed by other fiber materials for surgical masks. A comparative study was conducted, revealing that the relative efficiency of the masks made of different fiber materials are, in descending order, polypropylene fibers, polyester-rayon fibers, glass fiber mats and cellulose (paper) (Madsen and Madsen, 1967).

Glass fibers are seldom used nowadays, because they cause prickliness and skin reactions when coming in contact with the skin. Currently, surgical masks are mostly disposable and are usually composed of three nonwoven layers—a cover web, a filter layer, and a shell. The cover web is the layer that is adjacent to the skin; it is made of a spun-bonded polypropylene or air-laid cellulose nonwoven mat. Polypropylene is the most frequently-used fiber material because it is highly hydrophobic and yet has a high capacity for wicking, ensuring a dry and comfortable microclimate between the mask and face. The filter layer is responsible for most of the protection tasks. It is composed of melt-blown polypropylene nonwoven mat so as to have a high filtration capacity to deter hazardous aerosol particles, microorganisms and body fluids. The shell is to support the filter layer, and can be made of a spun-bonded polypropylene or air-laid cellulose nonwoven mat (Chen and Willeke, 1992).

N95 respirators are becoming well-known to more and more people for their bio-protection capacity, since the recent world outbreaks of pandemic diseases such as SARS, influenza and AIDS (acquired immune deficiency syndrome or acquired immunodeficiency syndrome).

N95 respirators are named after a rating system of US NIOSH (National Institute for Occupational Safety and Health). In 1995, NIOSH issued 42 CFR Part 84, "Respiratory Protective Devices", for certifying air-purifying particulate respirators. Under this regulation, NIOSH certifies nine classes of filters with three levels of filter efficiency and three levels of filter degradation resistance in each class. Respirator filters that deter at least 95% of the challenge aerosol are rated 95. Those that have an efficiency of at least 99% are rated 99. And those with an efficiency of at least 99.97% (essentially 100%) are rated 100. The three efficiency levels (95, 99 and 99.97%) are tested using the most penetrating particle size, about 0.1–0.3 μm aerodynamic diameter. In addition to the numerical code, respirator filters are also rated as N, R, or P according to their capacity of protection against oil aerosols. Respirators are rated N if they are not resistant to oil, R if somewhat resistant to oil, and P if strongly resistant to oil. (NIOSH, 1995). Therefore, the alphanumerical code N95 refers to a protective respirator that filters at least 95% of airborne particles but is NOT resistant to oil.

A typical N95 mask may consist of 4 to 5 nonwoven layers, in which 2 to 3 filter layers are sandwiched between two outer protective layers. The filter layers, which are responsible for most of the protective function, are made of meltblown thin sheet containing ultrafine Polypropylene fibers densely packed together. The mask usually comes with a nose-clip that can be adjusted to conform to the contour of the wearer's face, so that the leaking of hazardous particles between the mask and face can be minimized.

Some N95 masks also include *electret fibers,* which are filter-forming fibers that carry an electric charge, produced by corona charging (Vanturnhout, Hoeneveld, *et al.*, 1981). The charged fibrous filters capture hazardous particles and microorganisms via electrostatic attraction in addition to mechanical actions. One advantage of this type of filter is that it is more breathable because it is less dense than the conventional fibrous filter without losing its efficiency in capturing hazardous particles or microorganisms. However, the efficiency of such electrets filters degrades over time from exposure to aerosols (Moyer and Bergman, 2000).

N95 respirators are the most commonly used protective respirators against transmitted disease or biohazards (Qian, Willeke, *et al.*, 1998) because it is easy to apply, the unit cost is relatively low (typically around $1.00), and since it is disposable, it does not require any cleaning and maintenance. However, there are residual concerns about the efficiency of N95 masks in their bio-protective applications. One of them is whether they will constitute a "secondary infection risk".

Many pathogens will survive for hours or even days after being trapped on fibrous media, resulting in the risk of secondary infection. Specifically, as protective respirators tend to be used throughout a work shift before being discarded, sneezing and coughing may free the trapped pathogens and cause them to be re-suspended in the air, not to mention that mechanical handling such as contact and compression of fibrous materials can lead to mechanical transfer of pathogens to other media, which in turn become new sources of secondary infection to people who have access to these contaminated media (Reponen, Wang, *et al.*, 1999). This secondary infection risk has posed new challenges to the product development of bio-protective respirators.

Concepts & Theories: Mechanisms of Aerosol Deposition on Fibrous Filters

Deposition of aerosol particles on fibrous filters during aerosol filtration is caused by mechanical capture and/or electrical attraction. Mechanisms of mechanical capture comprise interception, inertial impaction, diffusion deposition, and gravitational settling (Brown, 1993).

Collection by *interception* occurs when a particle moves along a gas streamline and happens to come within one particle radius of the surface of a fiber, as shown in Figure 7.2(a). The particle hits the fiber and is captured because of its finite size.

Inertial impaction of a particle on a fiber occurs when a particle, because of its inertia, is unable to adjust quickly enough to the abruptly changing streamlines in the vicinity of a fiber and crosses those streamlines to hit the fiber, as shown in Figure 7.2(b).

Diffusion deposition of a particle happens when the combined action of airflow and the random movement of a particle suspended in a fluid (Brownian motion) bring a small particle into contact with a fiber, as shown in Figure 7.2(c).

Gravitational settling refers to the deposition of a particle due to gravitational forces, as shown in Figure 7.2(d).

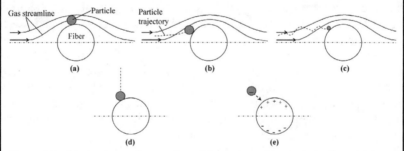

Figure 7.2. Mechanisms of aerosol particles captured by a single fiber: (a) interception, (b) inertial impaction, (c) diffusion deposition, (d) gravitational settling, (e) electrostatic attraction.

The relative contribution of diffusion and particle inertia to deposition are mainly related to particle diameter, gas velocity, and fiber diameter. In general, particle inertia makes a greater contribution for larger particles, while Brownian motion caused by thermal agitation plays a greater role for particles below 0.1 μm in diameter (Hinds, 1982). For particles in the medium size range, both particle inertia and thermal perturbations are relatively weak; as a result, the collection efficiency of a fibrous filter reaches a minimum value, as shown in Figure 7.3 (Hinds, 1982).

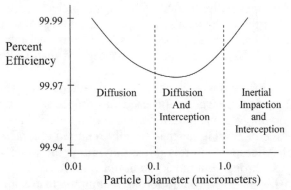

Figure 7.3.   Filter efficiency vs. particle size.

Application of electrostatic forces can significantly augment the collection efficiency of a fibrous filter, as shown in Figure 7.2(e). This is particularly useful for improving collection of particles in the medium size range, which are difficult to capture by other mechanical mechanisms (Wang, 2001). With the help of electrostatic force, a filter can achieve considerable collection efficiency at a lower packing density, thus reducing its resistance to the gas flow in the filter. However, the effects are insignificant unless the particles or fibers are highly charged.

A unique property of aerosol particles is that they will attach firmly to any surface (e.g., the surface of a fibrous filter) on which they have deposited. Also, aerosol particles adhere and form agglomerates when they come into contact with one another.

7.1.1.2. Waterproof and Breathable Textiles

Waterproof and breathable textiles are textile fabrics that prevent penetration of liquid water but allow the transmission of water vapor. Such fabrics have been used in sports and recreational textile products as well as in the healthcare sectors. The waterproof attribute keeps the user dry while the breathable attribute imparts comfort. The waterproof and breathable attribute can be engineered by using: (1) tightly woven fabrics; (2) microporous membranes, coatings or fabrics; (3) hydrophilic membranes (coatings); or (4) *smart* or *intelligent* polymers (Mukhopadhyay and Midha, 2008a; 2008b).

Both natural hydrophilic fibers, such as fine and long cotton fibers, and synthetic hydrophobic microfibers, such as polyester, nylon and acrylic fibers, have been used to construct *tightly woven fabrics* that are waterproof and breathable. Fabric structures used for this purpose include half-basket (i.e., oxford), plain (i.e., taffeta) and twill weaves.

These fabrics are usually treated with water-repellent finish, which can be silicones or fluorochemicals, and can be used for protective clothing in the medical/healthcare sectors. These tightly-woven fabrics usually have better breathability, but are less waterproof than coated or laminated fabrics.

A number of polymers, including polyurethane (PU) and poly-tetrafluoroethylene (PTFE), can be used to produce *microporous membranes or coatings*. A maximum pore size of no more than 2–3 μm for the membrane or coating layer is usually required to render the fabric waterproof. Micropores in this range may allow the water vapor molecules to pass through but block the liquid water.

The most well-known microporous membrane that can be used for waterproof and breathable textiles is expanded PTFE, invented in 1969 by Robert Gore and now known as Gore-Tex®. This membrane can be obtained by fast stretching PTFE membrane under high temperature, which produces numerous micropores in the membrane. Gore-Tex® is hydrophobic, chemically inert and smooth to the touch. It is used not only in protective medical gowns, but also in a variety of implanted devices (see Chapter 9). The expanded PTFE membranes are laminated to a face fabric or between an outer fabric and a liner fabric to make a waterproof and breathable laminated fabric.

PU is another frequently-used membrane material for microporous membranes or coatings, produced by a spray phase inversion process. This process involves dissolving PU in N,N-dimethylformamide (DMF) solvent. The PU solution and water (as a coagulant) are sprayed simultaneously and separately onto a collecting surface. This process leads to the exchange of water molecules and DMF molecules upon contact, and results in the formation of micropores in the coagulated PU membrane.

Waterproof and breathable fabrics containing microporous membranes can be used to make reusable medical gowns. Disposable protective gowns can also be made from *microporous fabrics* produced by *melt-blowing,* a process that produces nonwoven fabrics containing thermoplastic microfibers and micropores. The melt-blown microporous nonwoven layer(s) are usually further laminated to several other nonwoven layers for their end uses. For medical applications, it is the spun-bonded fabrics that are usually used in lamination with melt-blown fabrics, because of their low cost. Polypropylene is the most frequently used fiber material for this purpose because of its zero absorbency, high anti-static and wicking capacities. With the use of disposable medical gowns we can do without the sterilization process for medical gowns and be much relieved of the worry about cross-contamination; however, it increases the worry about the environment.

Waterproof and breathable textiles are also made from *hydrophilic (nonporous) membranes.* The membrane can be composed of an amphi-philic copolymer of polyester-polyether (Figure 7.4). The hydrophobic polyester segment (e.g., polyurethane) is water repellent, while the hydrophilic polyether segment (e.g., polyethylene oxide) allows the permeation of water vapor through the amorphous regions of the polymer film. Specifically, the ether groups (–O–) attract water molecules via reversible hydrogen bonds. Driven by a water vapor pressure gradient (i.e., the humidity or vapor pressure in the microclimate is usually higher than that in the outer environment, resulting in a vapor pressure gradient), these water molecules further diffuse through the film. Sympatex® is an example of a product made with hydrophilic membranes that are waterproof and breathable.

As compared to the microporous membrane, the hydrophilic membrane has both its advantages and disadvantages. Firstly, the microporous membrane may be contaminated by body oils, dirt, skincare lotions, and residual laundry detergent, which can block the pores and cause it to be less breathable. The micropores may also be enlarged as a result of stretching in the end uses or even in the laundry, so that the membrane will be less or no longer waterproof. The hydrophilic nonporous membrane is free from these shortcomings. However, the outer surface of the fabric may become wet after being exposed to large amounts of water or liquid, resulting in cold, clammy skin.

The last type of waterproof and breathable fabrics contains *smart* or *intelligent* polymer materials that can sense, react and/or adapt to environmental stimuli. These have found applications in a wide vari-

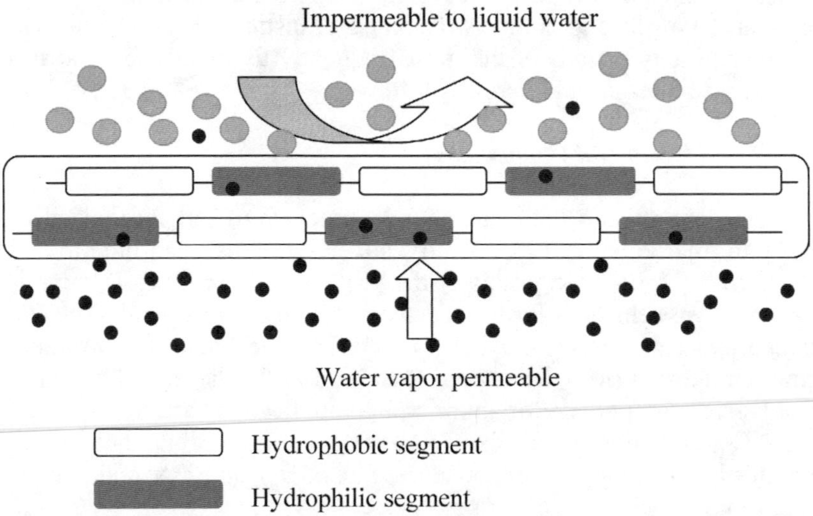

FIGURE 7.4. *Hydrophilic (nonporous) membranes made of amphiphilic copolymer.*

ety of textile products, such as protective devices that are waterproof and breathable. These smart fabrics will be waterproof and breathable either at a time of need or upon certain stimuli (e.g., the change of temperature). They have often been applied in the making of sports or foul weather survival clothing.

7.1.2. Antimicrobial Textiles

Textiles can be rendered "protective" by treating them with finishes that endow them with the function of microorganism inhibition. Inhibiting growth of microorganisms is important for many medical or healthcare textiles, especially those that will be reusable because textiles may form a microclimate fit for the growth of bacteria and fungi. Viruses can also be entrapped in the fine structures of textiles and may be further transferred to the outer environment via mechanical forces, resulting in secondary infections. These contaminated textiles, if not handled appropriately, may become a health threat to the user of textile products, or those around him or her.

As a solution to threats of secondary infection, antimicrobial finishes are applied to textiles. The finishing agents should be able to work effectively against a broad spectrum of microorganisms, while causing little toxicity or allergy to those who use the products. In addition, the finishes are expected to be durable to withstand various maintenance procedures, including washing, drying and pressing. Finally, the antimicrobial finishes should not adversely affect the quality (e.g., mechanical strength) and comfort properties (e.g., moisture transport, breathability and touch) of the end products (Gao and Cranston, 2008). The mechanisms and applications of the most frequently used antimicrobial finishes for textiles are discussed as follows.

7.1.2.1. Silver/metal Compounds

Some metals and their compounds have long been recognized as toxic to microorganisms. Generally, silver ions (Ag^+) can bind to and react with thiol (–SH) groups of the proteins and enzymes in the microorganism cells, and further inactivate the microorganisms. Ag^+ can also interact with bases in DNA (Deoxyribonucleic acid) to inhibit the microorganisms (McDonnell and Russell, 1999). The most frequently used silver compounds for antimicrobial applications are silver nitrate ($AgNO_3$) and silver sulfadiazine (AgSD). Other microbial metal compounds include copper compounds (e.g., $CuSO_4$), and Zinc compounds (e.g., $ZnSO_4$).

The silver/metal compounds can be incorporated into textile structures via different methods. For synthetic fibers, the silver particles can be incorporated into the polymer melt or solution before extrusion. As a result, these particles are embedded in the fibers after the spinning processes (Yeo, Lee, *et al.*, 2003). During the end uses of the silver-incorporated textiles, the silver particles will diffuse to the surface of the fibers and turn into silver ions when coming into contact with moisture. Alternatively, nano-silver colloids can be padded or coated onto the surface of both natural and synthetic fibers (Lee, Yeo, *et al.*, 2003). However, since no chemical bonds will form between the antimicrobial agent and fiber polymers, these finishes will not be stable enough, and the antimicrobial compound may leach out during the end uses or maintenance procedures (Kim, Park, *et al.*, 2011).

Silver/metal compounds can be incorporated only into natural fibers during the finishing process. Protein fibers, like silk and wool, have natural affinity to metal salts. These protein fibers have polar and ionizable groups (mostly free carboxyl groups/–COOH) on the side chains of the amino acids that constitute the fiber polymers. The weak acid group –COOH can be dissociated to carry negative charges (–COO⁻) in the presence of water, as shown in Equation (7.1), thereby enabling silk or wool fibers to bind such positive-charged molecules as metal ions and form complexes (Arai, Freddi, *et al.*, 2001). This characteristic of protein fibers has long been recognized as a mechanism to remove toxic chemicals. Wool fibers have been used to remove heavy metals; silk fabrics can be treated with metallic salts to increase the weight of the fabric and subsequently enlarge the body and cover of the fabric to give what is known as "weighted fabrics". However, the interaction between the protein polymers and metal ions is not stable and reversible, because the metal ions can be expelled from their binding sites due to the strong competition of hydrogen ions for the same binding sites, especially at a low pH environment. In order to enhance the binding between protein polymers and metal ions, wool or silk fibers are usually treated with tannic acid or acid anhydrides. Tannic acid can be physically adsorbed to the protein fiber substrate to provide extra negative-charged groups (Simpson, 1975). On the other hand, acid anhydrides induces acylation of protein fibers to supply acyl groups (–COR) that are also capable of binding metal ions (Arai, Freddi, *et al.*, 2001).

$$-COOH + H_2O \rightleftharpoons -COO^- + H_3O^+ \tag{7.1}$$

Cellulose fibers generally do not have functional groups that bind metal ions. However, a reduction in the size of silver particles to nanometers has been found to enhance the durability of the antibacterial treatment against washing, which may result from the deposition of silver nanoparticles into the molecular structure of the cellulosic fibers (El-Rafie, Mohamed, *et al.*, 2010; Ghosh, Yadav, *et al.*, 2010). Modification can also be applied to cellulose fibers to enhance the binding between the fiber polymers and antimicrobial metal compounds. For example, cellulose fibers can be treated with succinic anhydride to yield carboxyl groups, which will then bind themselves to metal ions (Nakashima, Sakagami, *et al.*, 2001).

7.1.2.2. *Quaternary Ammonium Compounds (QACs)*

QACs are cationic compounds that have been used both as active surface agents (cationic surfactants) and antiseptic agents. As shown in Figure 7.5, these compounds are positively charged at the N atoms in the solution. Usually, they are attached to microorganisms first via adsorption and penetration into the cell wall, and then by reacting with and disrupting the cell membranes and denaturing the proteins and nucleic acids, thus disintegrating cells of the bacteria (McDonnell and Russell, 1999). QACs can be applied to fibers/textiles via ionic interaction between the cationic QAC and anionic groups on the fiber surface. For example, QACs have been used to treat polyamides/nylon fibers that contain carboxyl ($-COO^-$) groups (Son and Sun, 2003). They have also been applied to acrylic fibers containing carboxyl or sulfonate ($-SO_2O^-$) groups (Cai and Sun, 2004). Similarly, wool fibers carry carboxyl groups that can be utilized to attract QACs (Zhao and Sun, 2007). Cotton fibers can be modified to create anionic sites (e.g., sulfonate groups) on the fabric surface to enhance their attraction to QACs (Son, Kim, *et al.*, 2006). However, it is due to this ionic interaction that the treatment results in diminished durability of the products during their end uses and maintenance.

An alternative approach is to develop polymerizable QAC monomers, followed by synthesis of polymeric QACs (Lu, Wu, *et al.*, 2007). This polymer contains the polyacrylate backbone and QAC side chains, which act as durable and laundry-resistant biocides. Intrinsically anti-

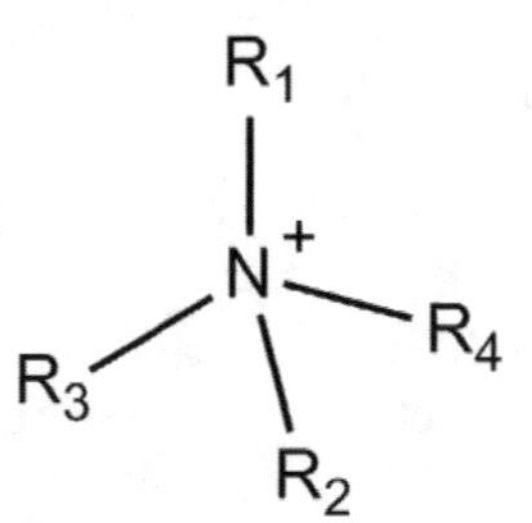

$$R_3 - \overset{\displaystyle R_1}{\underset{\displaystyle R_2}{\overset{|}{\underset{|}{N^+}}}} - R_4$$

FIGURE 7.5. *Structure of the quaternary ammonium compounds.*

bacterial, these polymers are potentially useful for the development of antibacterial textile products for healthcare and medical applications, although their fiber/fabric fabrications for textile products are yet to be developed and characterized.

7.1.2.3. N-halamines

N-halamines refer to a group of heterocyclic compounds com-posed of one or more pairs of covalently bonded nitrogen and halogen (N-X). Having been used effectively as water disinfectants for decades, N-halamines are broad spectrum biocides, inhibiting bacteria via a re-dox reaction to substitute hydrogen for the halogen (X) in the N-X in the presence of water. Subsequently, the X^+ ions may be bound to the microorganisms to hinder their enzymatic and metabolic processes, thereby destroying the microorganisms. As shown in Equations 7.2 and 7.3, this reaction is reversible, and will therefore enable the halogens to be recharged onto the polymer via the halogenation treatment. In this way, durable and regenerable antibacterial textiles can be produced via treatment with N–Halamine compounds. For example, textiles can be treated to bear N–Cl groups, which will deplete their active chlorine in the course of microorganism inhibition. On the other hand, the chlo-rines can be recharged by a simple chlorination procedure during the laundry process (i.e., bleaching) (Sun, Chen, *et al.*, 2001). After that, a reduction process (i.e., a treatment using sodium sulfite) may be neces-sary to remove the residual chlorine that has physically been adsorbed to the fabric surface to avoid any unpleasant odor and discoloring of the fabric (Li, 2003).

N-halamine compounds have been applied (usually via covalent bonding) to various fiber materials, including cotton (Sun and Xu, 1998), nylon (Lin, Winkelman, *et al.*, 2001), polyester fibers (Lin, Winkelmann, *et al.*, 2002) and polyester/cotton blends (Qian and Sun, 2004), so that the products will be "antibacterial" on the one hand, and "durable" and "refreshable" on the other. However, the N-halamine compounds may cause irritation to the skin and eyes, thus limiting their application in products that will be used next to the skin.

$$\rangle N-Cl + H_2O \rightleftharpoons \rangle N-H + Cl^+ + OH^- \qquad (7.2)$$

$$\rangle N-Cl \underset{\text{Bleach}}{\overset{\text{Kill bacteria}}{\rightleftharpoons}} \rangle N-H \qquad (7.3)$$

7.1.2.4. Chitosan

Chitosan is the deacetylated derivative of chitin (see Figure 3.5 for the structures of both chitin and chitosan), an abundantly occurring natural polysaccharide derived from crab and shrimp shells. Chitosan contains amino groups ($-NH_2$), which causes it to be a positively charged (i.e., cationic) polymer in an acidic environment. The cationic chitosan is capable of inhibiting the growth of microorganisms due to its adhesion between the cationic polymer and the negatively charged surface of the bacteria, as well as the further disruption of the cell membrane of the bacteria (Kim, Choi, et al., 1997; Franklin, Snow, et al., 2005). Chitosan is nontoxic, biocompatible and biodegradable, which are advantages over other antibacterial agents for textiles, although its antibacterial capacity is not as potent as the others. The antibacterial efficiency of chitosan depends on its chemical structure. Chitosan of a lower molecular weight may have a higher capacity of microbial inhibition; an increase in the degree of deacetylation means a larger number of amino groups on a molecule, which will further lead to a rise in its antimicrobial efficiency. Since the amino groups will become cationic in an acidic environment, the antimicrobial efficacy of chitosan is higher with a lower pH value (Lim and Hudson, 2003). There has also been the development of water-soluble chitosan derivatives, such as quaternized chitosan (Ignatova, Manolova, et al., 2007) and carboxymethyl chitosan (Gupta and Haile, 2007), which allow the chitosan to maintain its antibacterial activity in a wider range of pH values.

Chitosan can be incorporated into textiles by mixing it into the fiber spinning solutions (Ignatova, Manolova, et al., 2009). Alternatively, it is applied to cotton (Shin, Yoo, et al., 2001) and polypropylene (Shin, Yoo, et al., 1999) via finishing procedures, mostly the traditional pad-dry-cure method (Seong, Whang, et al., 2000). However, many factors have limited the application of chitosan as an antibacterial finish, such as its antimicrobial efficacy and the poor handle of the end textile products.

7.2. FLAME RETARDANT (FR) TEXTILES

Fire accidents not only cause destruction of properties but also lead to loss of health and lives. Hospitalized residents are especially vulnerable to burn injuries or fatalities because they are less able to evacuate during a fire than other people. Since most textile fibers are combustible, the various textile products (e.g., apparel, upholstery, bed linens, draperies and carpets) will only be extra fuel to spread the fire and worsen the damage. Availability of articles that will *retard* the fire is therefore more than a healthcare issue.

Understandably, laws and standards for textile flammability performance have been established around the world to regulate the manufacturing of textile products for certain end uses. For example, the US government issued the Federal Flammability of Clothing Textile Standard (Title 16CFR 1610) in 1954; the Canadian government released its Flammability Performance Requirements for Hospital Textiles (CAN/CGSB 4.162-M80) in 1980. These standards usually require that a *45° angle test* be used to determine if a textile fabric is acceptable. In such as test, the flame spread properties of a textile material are evaluated by imposing a flame of specific size for 1 second on a sample fabric that is held at an angle of 45°. A fabric sample is deemed acceptable if it does not ignite, or, if it ignites, it will not spread the flame beyond a certain distance (e.g., 5 inches/127 mm in the above standards), or the time of flame spread will be above a certain limit (e.g., 3.5 sec or more for smooth fabric as required in the U.S. standard and 7 sec or more as required by the Canadian standard for products such as patients' apparel and bed linens in hospitals).

According to these standards, it is obvious that textile products to be used in the hospital should be able to resist or inhibit the spread of flame after they have caught on fire. Such textiles are usually referred to as *flame retardant* (FR) or *flame-resistant* textiles. They are different from the so-called *fireproof* textiles, which will not catch fire when exposed to flame and can be used in such applications as firefighters' uniforms. Examples of fireproof textiles are the aramid and PBI fibers (details about them can be found in Chapter 2). Providing protection of higher levels, fireproof textiles are of much higher cost. The FR textiles will, however, provide a certain degree of safety by suppressing the spread of flame, but are of a relatively low cost.

7.2.1. Mechanism of Material Combustion

Fiber materials are different in their thermal properties. When subjected to elevated temperatures, a fiber material may first undergo the glass *transition temperature* (T_g), in which the fiber changes from a glassy state to a rubbery state; the thermoplastic fiber then goes through the *melting temperature* (T_m), in which the fiber changes from a solid to a liquid. If the temperature continues to rise to a certain point (*pyrolysis* or the *thermal decomposition temperature,* T_p), the fiber may decompose—that is, its polymer chains become fragmented. Beyond T_p, a fiber capable of combustion (i.e., *combustible*) ignites at the so-called *combustion or ignition temperature* (T_c). Not that all fiber materials will undergo the four temperatures. Generally, these temperatures will follow the sequence of $T_g < T_m < T_p < T_c$.

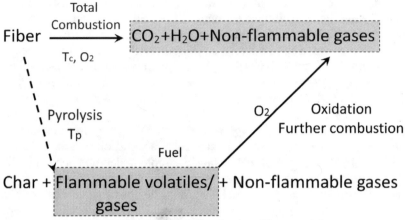

FIGURE 7.6. *Mechanism of combustion of fiber materials.*

The mechanism of the fiber material combustion is sketched in Figure 7.6. Under the ideal condition (i.e., at the combustion temperature and with oxygen), a fiber will experience total combustion, leaving behind carbon dioxide, water and non-flammable gases. More often than not, a fiber will be subjected to its pyrolysis temperature before the combustion one, and a pyrolysis reaction occurs instead of the total combustion. As a result, the fiber disintegrates into char, releasing both non-flammable and flammable gases. The flammable gases will spread to a wider area to fuel further combustion and expand the fire.

Another evaluator for fiber flammability is the limiting oxygen index (LOI), i.e., minimum oxygen concentration that supports the combustion of a fiber material. The normal concentration of oxygen in ambient air is about 21%. A material with a LOI below 21% is regarded as flammable; those with LOI above 21% are not flammable in normal air. The higher the LOI, the lower the flammability. Nevertheless, LOI is not the only ruler for material safety in fire. For example, the polyester fiber is low in LOI (20–21%) (Price, 1999), but it has a higher pyrolysis temperature (390°C) than most of the commonly used textile fibers (Hatch, 1993).

7.2.2. Development of Fire Retardant Textiles

According to the mechanism of fiber combustion described above, a fire (as a result of, say, the burning of textiles) can be extinguished by: (1) removing heat or applying cooling by using heat absorbing materials; (2) increasing the pyrolysis temperature as a result of using heat resistant materials; (3) preventing evaporation of the flammable gases;

and (4) eliminating oxygen from the combustion zone to stop combustion. These approaches will be discussed as follows.

7.2.2.1. Heat Absorbing Materials

Inorganic fillers are frequently used to render a polymer material flame retardant. The most widely used FR fillers are alumina trihydrate (ATH, $Al_2O_3 \cdot 3H_2O$) and magnesium hydroxide (MH, $Mg(OH)_2$) (Le Bras, 2005). The FR capacity of ATH is limited below 200°C, while MH remains stable above 300°C. At high temperatures, these FR fillers decompose endothermically; that is, they absorb large amounts of heat from the environment, releasing water at the same time to reduce the danger of fire. However, these FR fillers will not be effective unless they are heavily applied (typically a 60% loading). Therefore, it is wise to use them only in the treatment of textile products where a heavy coating is necessary and can be applied (e.g., in the production of carpets) (Weil and Levchik, 2009).

Recently, polymer-clay nanocomposites have been recognized as a new class of FR system. Clay is a fine-grained earthy material primarily composed of hydrated aluminum silicates. It has long been known for its excellent heat resistance. A polymer-clay nanocomposite usually consists of the spindle-shaped clay well dispersed in the matrix of a polymer in different forms (Figure 7.7). An attractive advantage of nanocomposites is that a low concentration (i.e., no more than 5% by weight) of dispersed clay can significantly improve performance of the polymer matrix, including its mechanical and flame resistant properties (Le Bras, 2005). Generally, it is believed that two mechanisms are involved in the enhancement of the FR performance for polymers. On the one hand, the degradation of a nanocomposite in high temperature burns away the polymer and leaves behind a multi-layered carbonaceous silicate char on the surface, which insulates the underlying material and slows down the release rate of the decomposition products, especially flammable volatiles (see also the following third mechanism "preventing evaporation") (Gilman, Jackson, *et al.*, 2000). On the other

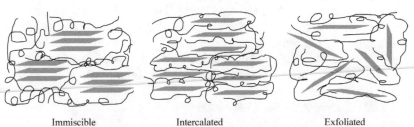

Immiscible   Intercalated   Exfoliated

FIGURE 7.7. *Polymer-clay nanocomposites of different kinds.*

hand, a small amount of iron in the clay can trap radicals generated by the combustion, so as to enhance the stability of the polymer (see the fourth mechanism "elimination of oxygen" below) (Zhu, Uhl, *et al.*, 2001). Still in the stage of laboratory development, this FR system is only potential at present, and more research and development efforts are needed before the polymer-clay nanocomposites can be applied in the production of any FR textiles that meet such performance-related requirements as comfort, flexibility, and a relatively low cost as well.

7.2.2.2. Inherent FR Fibers

Different fiber materials vary in their thermal properties; that is, they differ in decomposition temperatures. For example, wool decomposes at 230°C, cotton at 305°C, and nylon at 345°C. Polyester has the highest heat resistance among commonly used textile fibers with a decomposition temperature of 390°C (Hatch, 1993). As a result, polyester is frequently used in textile products (e.g., baby pajamas) that require a moderate level of FR, while any finishing chemicals are to be avoided out of concerns about skin irritation.

Although it has a low decomposition temperature, wool is regarded as the least flammable and combustible fiber, as it has an ignition temperature of 590°C as compared to polyester (560°C), cotton (400°C), nylon (532°C) and acrylic (530°C) (Hatch, 1993). Wool does not melt, and is thus free from the danger of adhering to the human skin to cause extra damage. In addition, wool burns slowly in a dry environment, smolders at a relatively high humidity of over 20%, and self-extinguishes when the flame source is removed. As a result, wool is a material with FR properties sufficient for most apparel purposes. But when it comes to institutional textiles (e.g., textiles used in healthcare facilities), where more stringent regulations are imposed, wool still needs to be treated with FR finishes.

Other high-performance fibers with high decomposition temperatures include the aramid fibers with a decomposition temperature of 430°C, the PBI fibers that decompose at 450°C, and the glass fibers that remain stable until 815°C (Hatch, 1993). These fibers do not burn, nor are they affected by fire. They are usually referred to as fireproof fibers and applied in high-end devices (e.g., firefighter's uniform). They are less likely to be used in medical/healthcare textiles because of their high cost and comfort-related issues (e.g., stiffness, prickling).

7.2.2.3. Materials for the Prevention of Flammable Volatiles

It can be seen from Figure 7.7 that a major cause of the spread of fire is the release of flammable volatiles as a result of polymer decomposition. These flammable volatiles quickly spread out and continue to burn once in contact with oxygen. The prevention of flammable volatiles thus helps prevent the fire from spreading to a larger area. A group of solid phase FR materials based on sulfur, phosphorous or boron have been developed for such as a purpose. Among them, phosphorous compounds are used most frequently.

Phosphorous-based flame retardants are frequently used in treating cellulosic fibers, either via the traditional pad-dry-cure wet finish process, or via chemical reactions to permanently affix the FR chemical to the cellulose fibers. When caught on fire, these phosphorous-based FR generates phosphorous pentoxide and phosphoric acid, resulting in dehydration of the cellulose to form stable non-volatile esters (Figure 7.8) at a temperature below its pyrolysis temperature. This in turn promotes the formation of a stable char to cut the burning fibers from the supply of oxygen, insulate them from heat, and prevent the release of flammable decomposition products to the combustion zone (Green, 1996).

Phosphorous-based FR has also been used to treat polyester fibers. Most of the currently available FR polyester products are composed of copolymers because they are more durable than the wet finished fabric, onto which the finishing chemicals are less permanently attached. Such copolymers comprise PET (polyethylene terephthalate) and an FR component, usually a phosphorous one. The functional phosphorous group occurs either on the main chain or on the side chain, as shown in Figure 7.9. Similarly, such phosphorous compounds promote formation of the char during the fire to suppress the spread of flame (Yang and Kim, 2007).

7.2.2.4. Materials for the Elimination of Oxygen

Combustion is supported by oxygen. An alternative approach to prevent combustion is to eliminate oxygen from the combustion zone. Similar to the mechanism of fire extinguishers containing carbon dioxide or carbon tetrachloride, a group of vapor-phase flame retardants, mostly halogenated compounds (e.g., bromide compounds), have been

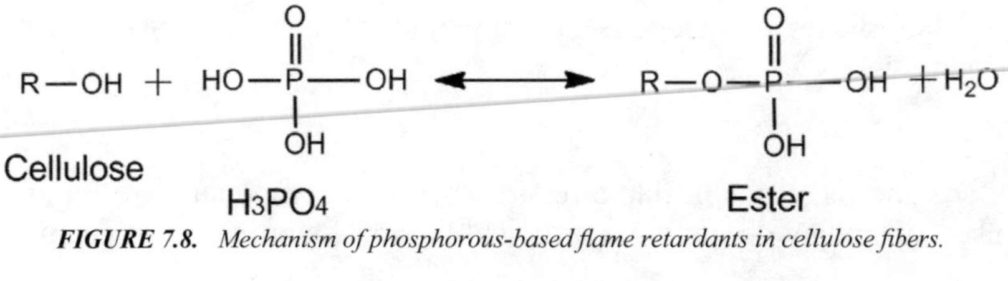

FIGURE 7.8. *Mechanism of phosphorous-based flame retardants in cellulose fibers.*

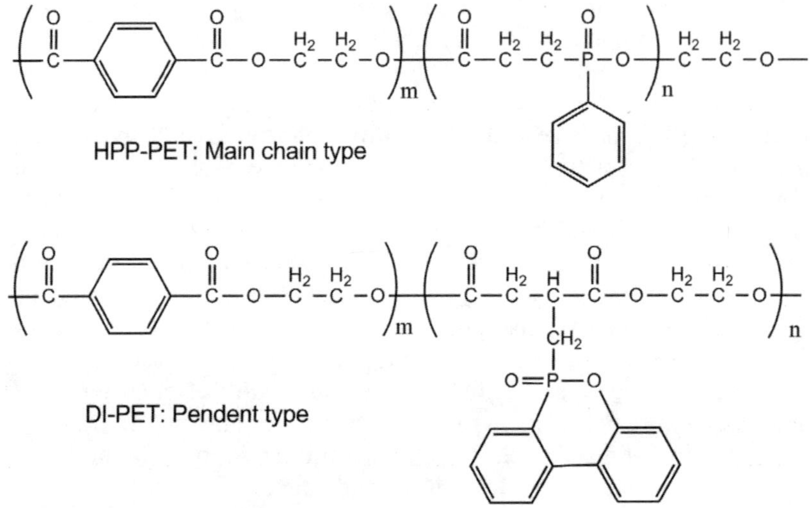

HPP-PET: Main chain type

DI-PET: Pendent type

FIGURE 7.9. *FR polyesters.*

developed and used to cause textile materials to be flame retardant (Green, 1996).

It is generally believed that the combustion of a polymer material is a free radical chain reaction (see the "Concept & Theory" box below). Halogenated compounds (e.g., the bromide compounds) decompose to release HBr [shown in Equation (7.4)], which competes with free radicals in the reaction shown in Figure 7.11. As a result, the much less reactive Br radicals replace the H, OH and O radicals [Equation (7.5)], thus cutting down the rate of free radical chain reaction and slowing down the release of energy, which helps extinguish the fire.

$$CH_4 + Br \rightarrow HBr + CH_3$$
$$H^* + HBr \rightarrow H_2 + Br^* \tag{7.4}$$

$$OH^* + HBr \rightarrow H_2O + Br^*$$
$$O^* + HBr \rightarrow OH^* + Br^* \tag{7.5}$$

The efficacy of halogenated compounds as flame retardant can be rated as:

$$I > Br > Cl > F$$

As the most potent flame retardant, iodine compounds are seldom used since they do not have sufficient thermal stability. Bromide com-

---

Concept & Theory: What Is the Free Radical Chain Reaction?

Chemically speaking, an atom is most stable in its ground state, where each electron in the outermost shell is paired with another that spins in the opposite direction. A free radical (or radical) is an atom or atom group with one or more highly reactive, unpaired electron(s) in its outermost shell. The formation of free radicals usually leads to a rapidly escalating chain reaction, like dominoes.

The combustion of polymer fibers is such a free radical chain reaction, generating large amounts of hydrogen (H*) and hydroxyl (OH*) free radicals as a result of the breaking down of chemical bonds in the polymer. These highly reactive radicals further fuel the combustion process. Methane can be taken as an example to describe the free radical chain reaction that happens in the combustion of polymer materials, as shown in Figure 7.10. It can be seen that the reaction of H* with oxygen (O_2) is an example of chain branching, in which the number of radicals (O* and OH*) is escalating; the reaction of CO being converted into CO_2 is a exothermic one (e.g., a chemical reaction that releases energy in the form of heat) that further enhances the temperature of the system (Green, 1996).

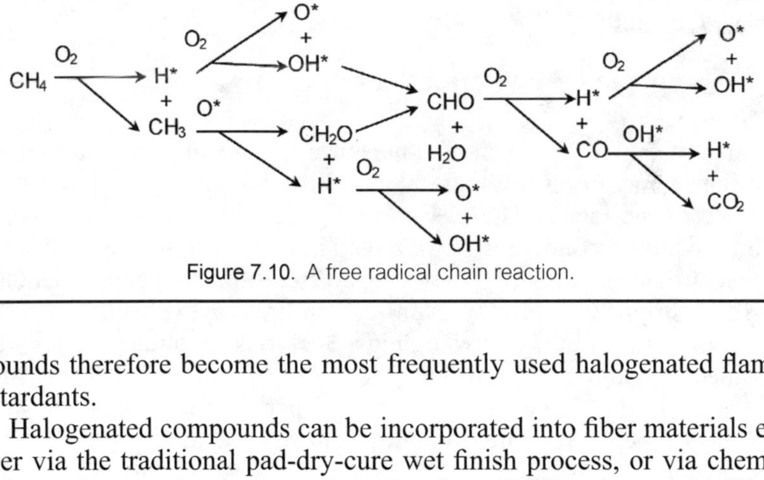

Figure 7.10. A free radical chain reaction.

---

pounds therefore become the most frequently used halogenated flame retardants.

Halogenated compounds can be incorporated into fiber materials either via the traditional pad-dry-cure wet finish process, or via chemical reactions to be permanently affixed to the fiber materials. They can also be incorporated into the main chain of a fiber material via copolymerization. Modacrylic fiber is a frequently used copolymerized flame resistant fiber. It is composed of copolymers of acrylonitrile and an FR component, often a halogen compound, such as vinyl chloride ($CH_2=CHCl$) or vinylidene chloride ($CH_2=CCl_2$), as shown in Figure 7.11. Modacrylic fibers do not burn and will self-extinguish after the flame source is removed. During the fire, the halogen components in the modacrylic promote formation of char, which acts as a flame barrier. Such an FR mechanism allows the modacrylic to be blended with

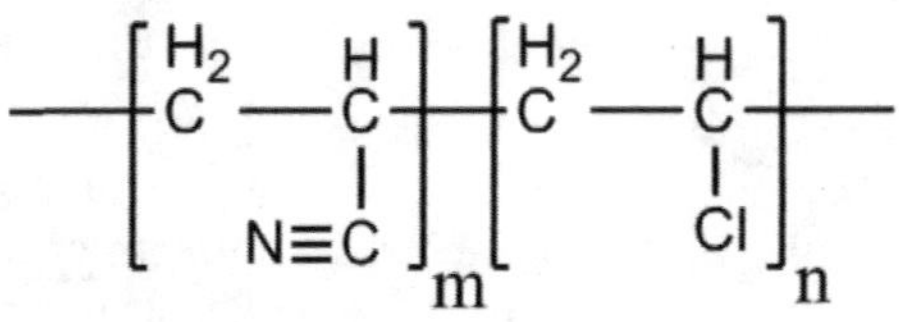

poly(acrylonitrile-co-vinyl chloride)

FIGURE 7.11. Modacrylics.

other cellulose fibers like cotton and rayon to enhance the comfort level of end products.

As a risk to health and life, fire hazards vary in severity with many factors, including the property and quantity of toxic fumes produced during the combustion. A recent concern is about the vapor-phase (or halogen-based) flame retardants in that the chemicals released in their vapor form during the fire may be toxic to humans and to the environment. As a result, there has been a tendency to shift from the halogen-based flame retardants to the phosphorous-based ones (Horrocks, Kandola, *et al.*, 2005).

7.3. ANTISTATIC TEXTILES

Electrostatic charge can be a nuisance for uses of textile products: the fabric may cling to the body and dirt may adhere to the charged surface of the fabric. The electrostatic discharges, or spark between the body and a conductor (e.g., a metal door knob, or the surface of an electronic instrument), may cause discomfort to people, damage to the instrument, and may even lead to fires or explosions if there are combustibles in the surroundings. Such risks should especially be avoided in healthcare facilities, where the patients, already in compromised health, have to rely on the proper functioning of the various electronic instruments. Naturally, antistatic textiles are even more needful in these places.

Electrostatic charges in textiles mostly originate from the contact between dissimilar surfaces that causes the transfer of charge between them. If one or both of the surfaces is low in electrical conductivity, the charge that has been transferred will remain on the surface after the two surfaces separate (Holme, McIntyre, *et al.*, 1998). Since most textile fibers are good insulators, they are poor electrical conductors. Repeated contacts (e.g., rubbing) may lead to a significant build-up of electrostatic charge.

Several factors may affect the electrostatic build-up. An increase in relative humidity or moisture content of the textile material will contribute to the increase of electrical conductivity of the textile material, and thus a decrease in static build-up. As water is a better conductor than the fiber material, the incorporation of water molecules into a fiber material helps dissipate the electrostatic charge. That is why textile materials are more prone to electrostatic build-up in a dry environment. Similarly, hydrophobic synthetic fibers usually are more vulnerable to electrostatic buildup than hydrophilic natural/regenerated fibers. The only exception is Polypropylene fiber, well known for its zero absorbency but still low electrostatic buildup as a result of the strength with which the electrons are held by atoms. Polypropylene fibers are non-polar in nature, indicating that the electrons are equally shared between different atoms and, as a result, can hardly be brought to the surface of the fiber.

In accordance with the mechanism of how the electrostatic charge is built up in and dissipated from the fiber material, a textile product can be rendered antistatic by several approaches, especially by (1) improving water absorbency of the fiber and (2) incorporating conductive materials or antistatic agents into the fiber.

Synthetic fibers can be used in blends with natural or hydrophilic fibers to improve their water absorbency. Hydrophilic finishes may also be utilized to improve the hydrophilicity of synthetic fibers. For example, polyester fibers can be treated with alkali (e.g., sodium hydroxide) to induce surface hydrolysis, which will result in the introduction of polar groups (e.g., hydroxyl and carboxyl groups) on the fiber surface. Improved water absorbency helps reduce static build-up on the fiber surface (at the cost of reduced fiber mechanical strength, though).

For synthetic fibers composed of copolymers (e.g., polyester and acrylic fibers), polar groups can be incorporated into the fibers by designing a copolymer to include a monomer-containing polar groups. For instance, copolymerization of acrylonitrile with a vinyl monomer containing such polar groups as hydroxyl, carboxyl, ester, amide or substituted amides (as shown in Figure 7.12) will lead to the formation of hydrophilic acrylic fibers that are antistatic (Bajaj, Gupta, *et al.*, 2000).

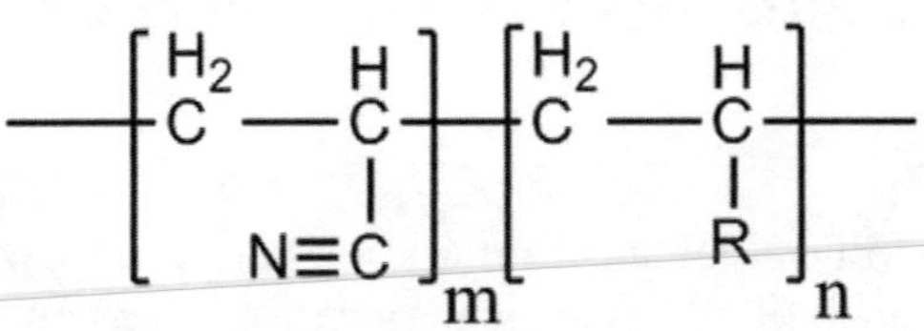

R=OH, COOH, COOR', CONH$_2$ or CONHR'

FIGURE 7.12. Antistatic acrylic fibers.

Electrical conductive materials or antistatic agents, usually small molecular compounds, have been used to render polymer fibers antistatic.

Carbon black, which is composed primarily of the element carbon in the form of clusters of fine particles, has been incorporated into acrylic fibers by mixing it into the fiber spinning solution to produce antistatic acrylic fibers, but this results in reduced mechanical strength of the product (Bajaj, Gupta et al., 2000). Metallic fibers can be blended with textile fibers to result in much improved electrical conductivity in the product. Steel is among the first metals used for this purpose. Steel fibers, usually constituting 1% by weight of the blended yarns, effectively reduce the static build-up in the end product (Holme, McIntyre, et al., 1998).

Metal oxides/salts (e.g., antimony oxide, tin oxide, titanium dioxide and copper sulfate) have also been used as additives to the fiber spinning solution to fabricate antistatic fibers. Similarly, these metal compound fillers may affect mechanical strength of the fiber product. Other ionic antistatic agents include quaternary ammonium compounds. Many of these ionic agents function to render the end product antibacterial and antistatic as well (see Section 7.2). Unfortunately, these metallic agents may become detached from the fibers during their end uses due to external mechanical forces, thus causing concerns about human and environmental health.

For medical textiles, especially disposable products (most often composed of meltblown polypropylene), antistatic agents in their aqueous solution can be sprayed onto the surface of the fabric, followed by heating to dry. Since the heating process reduces the mechanical strength of the product, an improved process is to spray the solution of the agent into the stream of the molten polymer ejected from the spinneret during fiber spinning, so that the water will evaporate and the agent will be deposited onto the fibers. A frequently used agent for such a purpose is a pH-adjusted alcohol phosphate salt, like potassium butyl phosphate ($C_4H_{12}KO_5P$). Since the end product is intended to be used only once or for a short time, durability of the treatment and product is of little consequence (Holme, McIntyre, et al., 1998).

7.4. SUMMARY

Humans need to be shielded from a large variety of hazards—from microorganisms, to bullets, to nuclear radiation. We can protect ourselves from these by a great many means, including going underground to hide in a concrete building, and uncomfortably staying there, worried or scared, until we deem we are out of danger. Protective textiles are important because they are often used for making articles for us to "wear", thus causing us to be protected and allowing us to live (or even work) almost as usual.

This book limits itself to protective textile products used for medical/ healthcare purposes, most often by hospitalized patients and medical/ healthcare personnel. The worst hazard for these people is microorganisms that cause infection and diseases, and the next worst is fire accidents. Accordingly, this chapter has given a detailed discussion about protective textiles for infection control (in Section 7.1) and those capable of retarding fire (in Section 7.2).

Electrostatic charges may either look harmless in normal situations or be a nuisance insofar as it may count against "comfort", but it is considered a hazard in healthcare facilities because people in these places (i.e., the hospitalized patients) are already in compromised health, which causes "comfort" to be more meaningful for them. Hence there is the discussion about textiles that are protective by reason of being "antistatic" (in Section 7.3).

Related to these three major types of hazards are the two major approaches to rendering a textile *protective:* (1) to cause the textile to physically be (or provide) a "barrier" to shield the hazard away and (2) to treat the textile with such finishes as to render the product antimicrobial, flame-retardant, or antistatic.

The physical barrier textiles will deter the penetration of microorganisms and provide a passive sort form of protection to the end users—that is, they physically block the passage through which the microorganisms may be transmitted. The respirator, a great example of such barriers, functions to protect wearers from the attack of diseases transmitted via air. Different types of respirators have been developed to provide different levels of protection. Some respirators are state enforced and recommended (of these, the N95 respirator is the best known).

Bacteria and viruses reach us not only by the air. Thus "waterproof" textiles have been developed. They are useful especially in healthcare facilities to protect the wearers (e.g., surgeons) from microorganisms transmitted via the liquid. Admirably, such products provide not only protection but also comfort by means of being "breathable".

While the various barrier textiles protect people physically from biological hazards, a wide range of antimicrobial agents have been incorporated into textiles to produce textile products capable of microorganism inhibition, considering that bacteria and viruses can be entrapped in textiles and further transferred to the outer environment via mechanical forces. These contaminated textiles, if not properly handled, may become a health threat, too. Antimicrobial agents for treating textiles include silver or metal compounds, quaternary ammonium compounds,

N-halamines, and chitosan. The concern about the currently available antimicrobial finishes is either their efficacy (e.g., that of chitosan) or their toxicity to human health and impact on the environment.

Fire is the second greatest hazard for people in healthcare facilities, which explains the extensive efforts and the many means used to develop textiles capable of working against fire. The simplest method is treating a textile with a *flame retardant,* a substance that is intrinsically flame "resistant", so that the textile product will be rendered prone either to self-extinguish the fire or to prevent the flame from spreading further.

Fire-related damages are to a large degree caused by flammable volatiles produced during the decomposition of the fiber before it starts to burn and by toxic fumes released during the combustion. Introduced in this chapter are the many measures to reduce such damages.

7.5. REFERENCES

Arai, T., G. Freddi, *et al.* (2001). Absorption of metal cations by modified B-mori silk and preparation of fabrics with an antimicrobial activity. *Journal of Applied Polymer Science* **80**(2): 297–303.

Arai, T., G. Freddi, *et al.* (2001). Acylation of silk and wool with acid anhydrides and preparation of water-repellent fibers. *Journal of Applied Polymer Science* **82**(11): 2832–2841.

ASTM (2008). D123-07 Standard terminology relating to textiles. West Conshohocken, PA: American Society for Testing and Materials.

Bajaj, P., A.P. Gupta, *et al.* (2000). Antistatic and hydrophilic synthetic fibers: A critique. *Journal of Macromolecular Science-Reviews in Macromolecular Chemistry and Physics* **C40**(2–3): 105–138.

Belkin, N.L. (1997). The evolution of the surgical mask: filtering efficiency versus effectiveness. *Infect. Control Hosp. Epidemiol.* **18**(1): 49–57.

Brown, R.C. (1993). Air filtration: an integrated approach to the theory and applications of fibrous filters. New York: Pergamon Press.

Burke, J.P. (2003). Infection control—A problem for patient safety. *New England Journal of Medicine* **348**(7): 651–656.

Cai, Z.S. and G. Sun. (2004). Antimicrobial finishing of acrilan fabrics with cetylpyridinium chloride. *Journal of Applied Polymer Science* **94**(1): 243–247.

Chen, C.C. and K. Willeke. (1992). Aerosol penetration through surgical masks. *American Journal of Infection Control* **20**(4): 177–184.

Derrick, J.L. and C.D. Gomersall. (2005). Protecting healthcare staff from severe acute respiratory syndrome: filtration capacity of multiple surgical masks. *Journal of Hospital Infection* **59**: 365–368.

El-Rafie, M.H., A.A. Mohamed, *et al.* (2010). Antimicrobial effect of silver nanoparticles produced by fungal process on cotton fabrics. *Carbohydrate Polymers* **80**(3): 779–782.

Franklin, T.J., G.A. Snow, *et al.* (2005). Biochemistry and molecular biology of antimicrobial drug action. New York: Springer.

Freddi, G., T. Arai, *et al.* (2001). Binding of metal cations to chemically modified wool and antimicrobial properties of the wool-metal complexes. *Journal of Applied Polymer Science* **82**(14): 3513–3519.

Gao, Y. and R. Cranston (2008). Recent advances in antimicrobial treatments of textiles. *Textile Research Journal* **78**(1): 60–72.

Ghosh, S., S. Yadav, *et al.* (2010). Antibacterial properties of cotton fabric treated with silver nanoparticles. *Journal of the Textile Institute* **101**(10): 917–924.

Gilman, J. W., C.L. Jackson, *et al.* (2000). Flammability properties of polymer—Layered-silicate nanocomposites. Polypropylene and polystyrene nanocomposites. *Chemistry of Materials* **12**(7): 1866–1873.

Green, J. (1996). Mechanisms for flame retardancy and smoke suppression—A review. *Journal of Fire Sciences* **14**(6): 426–442.

Gupta, D. and A. Haile (2007). Multifunctional properties of cotton fabric treated with chitosan and carboxymethyl chitosan. *Carbohydrate Polymers* **69**(1): 164–171.

Hatch, K.L. (1993). Textile science. Minneapolis/Saint Paul: West Pub.

Hinds, W.C. (1982). Aerosol technology: properties, behavior, and measurement of airborne particles. New York: J. Wiley.

Holme, I., J.E. McIntyre, *et al.* (1998). Electrostatic charging of textiles. *Textile Progress* **28**(1).

Holme, I., J.E. McIntyre, *et al.* (1998). Electrostatic charging of textiles: a critical appreciation of recent developments. Manchester, UK: Textile Institute.

Horrocks, A.R., B.K. Kandola, *et al.* (2005). Developments in flame retardant textiles— a review. *Polymer Degradation and Stability* **88**(1): 3–12.

Ignatova, M., N. Manolova, *et al.* (2009). Electrospun non-woven nanofibrous hybrid mats based on chitosan and PLA for wound-dressing applications. *Macromolecular Bioscience* **9**(1): 102–111.

Ignatova, M., N. Manolova, *et al.* (2007). Novel antibacterial fibers of quaternized chitosan and poly(vinyl pyrrolidone) prepared by electrospinning. *European Polymer Journal* **43**(4): 1112–1122.

Johnson, D.F., J.D. Druce, *et al.* (2009). A quantitative assessment of the efficacy of surgical and N95 masks to filter influenza virus in patients with acute influenza infection. *Clinical Infectious Diseases* **49**(2): 275–277.

Kim, C.H., J.W. Choi, *et al.* (1997). Synthesis of chitosan derivatives with quaternary ammonium salt and their antibacterial activity. *Polymer Bulletin* **38**(4): 387–393.

Kim, S.S., J.E. Park, *et al.* (2011). Properties and antimicrobial efficacy of cellulose fiber coated with silver nanoparticles and 3-mercaptopropyltrimethoxysilane (3-MPTMS). *Journal of Applied Polymer Science* **119**(4): 2261–2267.

Le Bras, M. (2005). Fire retardancy of polymers new applications of mineral fillers. Cambridge, UK: Royal Society of Chemistry.

Lee, H.J., S.Y. Yeo, *et al.* (2003). Antibacterial effect of nanosized silver colloidal solution on textile fabrics. *Journal of Materials Science* **38**(10): 2199–2204.

Li, S. (2003). Method of retaining antimicrobial properties on a halamine-treated textile substrate while simultaneously reducing deleterious odor and skin irritation effects. United States Patent 6,576,154

Lim, S.H. and S.M. Hudson. (2003). Review of chitosan and its derivatives as anti-microbial agents and their uses as textile chemicals. *Journal of Macromolecular Science-Polymer Reviews* **C43**(2): 223–269.

Lin, J., C. Winkelman, *et al.* (2001). Antimicrobial treatment of nylon. *Journal of Applied Polymer Science* **81**(4): 943–947.

Lin, J., C. Winkelmann, *et al.* (2002). Biocidal polyester. *Journal of Applied Polymer Science* **85**(1): 177–182.

Lu, G.Q., D.C. Wu, *et al.* (2007). Studies on the synthesis and antibacterial activities of polymeric quaternary ammonium salts from dimethylaminoethyl methacrylate. *Reactive & Functional Polymers* **67**(4): 355–366.

Madsen, P.O. and R.E. Madsen. (1967). A study of disposable surgical masks. *Am. J. Surg.* **114**(3): 431–5.

McDonnell, G. and A.D. Russell. (1999). Antiseptics and disinfectants: activity, action, and resistance. *Clinical Microbiology Reviews* **12**(1): 147–179.

Moyer, E.S. and M.S. Bergman. (2000). Electrostatic N-95 respirator filter media efficiency degradation resulting from intermittent sodium chloride aerosol exposure. *Appl Occup Environ Hyg* **15**(8): 600–8.

Mukhopadhyay, A. and V.K. Midha. (2008a). A review on designing the waterproof breathable fabrics, Part I: fundamental principles and designing aspects of breathable fabrics. *Journal of Industrial Textiles* **37**(3): 225–262.

Mukhopadhyay, A. and V.K. Midha. (2008b). A review on designing the waterproof breathable fabrics, Part II: construction and suitability of breathable fabrics for different uses. *Journal of Industrial Textiles* **38**(1): 17–41.

Nakashima, T., Y. Sakagami, *et al.* (2001). Antibacterial activity of cellulose fabrics modified with metallic salts. *Textile Research Journal* **71**(8): 688–694.

NIOSH. (1995). Respiratory Protective Devices. 42 CFR Part 84 Morgantown, West Virginia.

Price, D. (1999). Fire retardant polymeric materials '97—Preface. *Polymer Degradation and Stability* **64**(3): 351–352.

Qian, L. and G. Sun. (2004). Durable and regenerable antimicrobial textiles: Improving efficacy and durability of biocidal functions. *Journal of Applied Polymer Science* **91**(4): 2588–2593.

Qian, Y., K. Willeke, *et al.* (1998). Performance of N95 Respirators: Filtration Efficiency for Airborne Microbial and Inert Particles. *American Industrial Hygiene Association Journal* **59**: 128–132.

Reponen, T.A., Z. Wang, *et al.* (1999). Survival of mycobacteria on N95 personal respirators. *Infection Control and Hospital Epidemiology* **20**(4): 237–241.

Seong, H.S., H.S. Whang, *et al.* (2000). Synthesis of a quaternary ammonium derivative of chito-oligosaccharide as antimicrobial agent for cellulosic fibers. *Journal of Applied Polymer Science* **76**(14): 2009–2015.

Shin, Y., D.I. Yoo, *et al.* (2001). Molecular weight effect on antimicrobial activity of chitosan treated cotton fabrics. *Journal of Applied Polymer Science* **80**(13): 2495–2501.

Shin, Y., D.I. Yoo, *et al.* (1999). Antimicrobial finishing of polypropylene nonwoven fabric by treatment with chitosan oligomer. *Journal of Applied Polymer Science* **74**(12): 2911–2916.

Simpson, W.S. (1975). Resist treatment of wool with tannic acids. 1. Chemical aspects. *Textile Research Journal* **45**(11): 796–800.

Son, Y.A., B.S. Kim, *et al.* (2006). Imparting durable antimicrobial properties to cotton fabrics using quaternary ammonium salts through 4-aminobenzenesulfonic acid-chloro-triazine adduct. *European Polymer Journal* **42**(11): 3059–3067.

Son, Y.A. and G. Sun. (2003). Durable antimicrobial nylon 66 fabrics: Ionic interactions with quaternary ammonium salts. *Journal of Applied Polymer Science* **90**(8): 2194–2199.

Sun, G. and X.J. Xu (1998). Durable and regenerable antibacterial finishing of fabrics: Biocidal properties. *Textile Chemist and Colorist* **30**(6): 26–30.

Sun, Y.Y., T.Y. Chen, *et al.* (2001). Novel refreshable N-halamine polymeric biocides containing imidazolidin-4-one derivatives. *Journal of Polymer Science Part A-Polymer Chemistry* **39**(18): 3073–3084.

Vanturnhout, J., W.J. Hoeneveld, *et al.* (1981). Electret filters for high-efficiency and high-flow air cleaning. *IEEE Transactions on Industry Applications* **17**(2): 240–248.

Wang, C.S. (2001). Electrostatic forces in fibrous filters—a review. *Powder Technology* **118**(1-2): 166–170.

Weil, E.D. and S.V. Levchik. (2009). Flame retardants for plastics and textiles : practical applications. Cincinnati: Hanser Publications.

Yang, S.C. and J.P. Kim. (2007). Flame retardant polyesters. I. Phosphorous flame retardants. *Journal of Applied Polymer Science* **106**(5): 2870–2874.

Yeo, S.Y., H.J. Lee, *et al.* (2003). Preparation of nanocomposite fibers for permanent antibacterial effect. *Journal of Materials Science* **38**(10): 2143–2147.

Zhao, T. and G. Sun. (2007). Antimicrobial finishing of wool fabrics with quaternary aminopyridinium salts. *Journal of Applied Polymer Science* **103**(1): 482–486.

Zhu, J., F.M. Uhl, *et al.* (2001). Studies on the mechanism by which the formation of nanocomposites enhances thermal stability. *Chemistry of Materials* **13**(12): 4649–4654.

CHAPTER 8

Textiles for Wound Care

A wound is defined as "a disruption in the normal continuity of a body structure" (Shai and Maibach, 2005). Wounds can take many forms, such as acute trauma, chronic ulcers, superficial cuts, deep incisions, small abrasions or serious burns. Although different types of wound care products are used for different wounds to facilitate the healing process, they should meet a number of general expectations, including being able to: (1) prevent and/or control infection in the wound and/or the surrounding areas; (2) provide a suitable degree of moisture within the environment of the wound to favor the complex processes of wound healing; (3) improve comfort and protect the wound and its surroundings from mechanical trauma; (4) absorb secretions, if needed; and (5) accelerate wound healing, if possible.

Defined as prevention of wound complications and promotion of wound healing, *wound care* depends considerably on the use of wound care materials and means. In this chapter, a variety of fiber, textile materials and products that have been used for wound care will be introduced, beginning with a brief explanation of the process of wound healing. Wound dressings, wound care materials (products) most frequently used in first aid and nursing, will be the focus of this chapter. Another textile product for wound care, the pressure garment, will also be mentioned. Materials/products discussed in this chapter usually need to be changed regularly in their end applications. Those that permanently replace the damaged or wounded tissues are usually referred to as grafts or implantable materials/products. They will be discussed in the next chapter.

8.1. HUMAN SKIN AND SKIN WOUNDS

8.1.1. Human Skin

The skin is a large, important organ of the body, performing the three major functions of protection, thermoregulation and immunization (Irion, 2002).

The skin protects the body in several ways. Firstly, it acts as a physical barrier against a variety of trauma-causing objects and influences, ranging from the less harmful dust to the more harmful elements such as heat and ultraviolet light. Less often noticed, the skin prevents many microorganisms from entering the body by several means: (1) since it is *waterproof,* it protects the body from the penetration of the many microorganisms that live in the water; (2) the acidic surface of the skin helps to suppress the growth of some microorganisms; and (3) the presence of certain defense molecules such as defensins and collectins help to inhibit the growth of microorganisms. For these reasons, the skin functions as a vital part of the human host's defense mechanism.

Secondly, since the core temperature of the body is normally maintained in a very narrow range around 37°C, the skin, as the interface between the body core and the outer environment, is vitally important because it regulates the amount of heat being brought from the body core to the surface. This regulation is related to the blood flow rate, and the release and evaporation of water through sweat glands, which is responsible for the evaporative heat loss. Finally, when the integrity of the skin is broken, the elements of the immune system (such as T-cells, neutrophils and macrophages) will come into play to fight against infection on its behalf.

The human skin has a stratified structure composed of three layers (Figure 8.1), which are, from top to bottom, the epidermis (0.12 mm thick), the dermis (1.1 mm) and the subcutis (0.1 to several cm) (Agache and Humbert, 2004). The topmost layer of the epidermis is the stratum corneum (SC), composed of multiple layers of keratinized cells called corneocytes. The whole SC goes through constant renewal: normally, each day a new keratinized cell layer is produced by the viable epidermis underneath and appears on the deepest SC surface, and the top SC cell layer sheds from the body. Under the SC layer, there is the viable epidermis composed of about ten layers of cells called keratinocytes. The dermis (or cutis) is a thick skin layer that holds hair cells and sweat glands. The dermis is composed of connective tissues in the form of interconnected collagen fibers, elastin fibers and an interstitial substance rich in proteins and glycosaminoglycans (GAGs). All components of the dermis are synthesized by the fibroblasts (or fibrocytes)

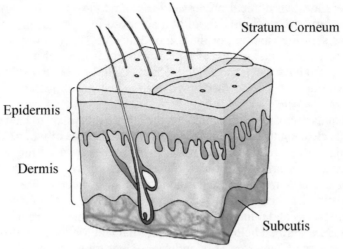

FIGURE 8.1. The structure of the human skin.

that are more plentiful in young tissues than in older ones. The bottom layer of the skin is usually referred to as subcutis (subcutaneous layer or hypodermis). Subcutis varies in thickness at different body sites. One component of subcutis is the interstitial tissue, which is a connective tissue that is similar to dermis in structure but much looser, and the other component is the subcutaneous adipose tissue (or subcutaneous body fat). Among the three skin layers, the epidermis is the only layer that can repair or regenerate itself spontaneously after being injured, while the dermis and subcutis tissues are not spontaneously regenerative.

8.1.2. Wound and Wound Healing

8.1.2.1. Acute Wound and Normal Wound Healing

Wound is the term commonly used to describe acute injury or acute mechanical trauma. Wounds vary in their severity: they may be confined to the epidermis (superficial), or be extended to some layers of the dermis (partial-thickness), or involve the complete thickness of the dermis (full-thickness) and even the subcutis tissues (Irion, 2002). Burn wounds, for example, are usually divided into three categories: the first degree burn is superficial and involves damage in the epidermis; the second degree burn involves burning damage all the way through the epidermis and further damage to the dermis; and the third degree burn refers to a burn wound through the dermis and damage to the subcutaneous tissues.

There are two clinical processes for wound closure (*healing*). The first, or primary, intention should be achieved by surgical procedures such as suturing, stapling or the use of adhesives, to result in *primary wound closure*. This process is typically used for surgical or traumatic wounds that have clean and smooth edges and little subcutaneous tissue loss. Appropriately performed, it will lead to faster healing than *secondary wound closure*.

Secondary closure or intention, on the other hand, refers to having the wounds close on their own, usually with the assistance of wound dressings that will be removed afterwards. This process is used for wounds not suitable for primary closure—for example, for wounds with tissue loss or necrosis, irregular edges and high microbial count. For secondary closure, the three phases of normal wound healing, in sequence, are: (1) hemostasis and inflammation; (2) proliferation; and (3) remodeling, which are described below (Irion, 2002; Shai and Maibach, 2005).

The phase of *hemostasis and inflammation* is triggered by the disruption of blood vessels, which go through immediate vasoconstriction in the first few minutes. Platelets start to aggregate along the inner surface of the injured vessels, causing the formation of a clot to prevent further leakage of blood from the injured vessels. Within an hour, a sequence of events of inflammation occurs, starting with a vasodilation induced by certain chemicals released from the injured tissues. The dilated vessels allow more plasma to leak through the vessel wall into the surrounding tissues, causing the injured sites to swell. Chemicals secreted and released into the wound are responsible for other signs of inflammation, such as redness, local warmth and pain. Just minutes after the wound occurs, an influx of white blood cells to the wound site will begin to act against pathogenic organisms; various growth factors will also be secreted to activate the wound healing process. This phase may also be accompanied by exudates, detachment of tissue debris and wound cleansing.

The phase of *proliferation* involves the most important events of wound healing, including re-epithelialization and granulation tissue formation, usually starting days after the wound occurs. Re-epithelialization is the process of resurfacing injured tissue via the migration and proliferation of keratinocytes from the free edges of the wound. Meanwhile, granulation tissue formation and wound contraction contribute to the filling of defects in the wounded site. The granulation tissue is named after its general appearance—a tissue containing a large number of tiny granules, which are actually newly formed young blood vessels. Other components of the granulation tissue are new cells and extracellular matrix (scaffolding materials outside of the cells) composed of immature collagen (type III).

Remodeling is the phase that coincides with the long-term response to the injury. It involves the continuous changes in the extracellular matrix: type III collagen is replaced by the more stable type I collagen, and the fibers of collagen are arranged in a more desired alignment. As a result of this remodeling process, strength of the healing wound is dramatically increased: two weeks after the wounding, the healing skin has a strength about 5% of its original strength, and reaches about 40% of its normal strength after a month. However, even after wound healing, it will not regain more than 80% of its original strength (Shai and Maibach, 2005).

8.1.2.2. Chronic Wound and Abnormal Wound Healing

Chronic wound, known also as chronic cutaneous ulcer, on the other hand, refers to any wound that has failed to heal within a reasonable length of time (e.g., 3–4 months) (Shai and Maibach, 2005). The process of normal wound healing is often interrupted in the case of a chronic wound. The chronic wound or ulcer usually involves localized damage in the epidermis, dermis, and possibly underlying tissues due to infections, pressure/shear, diabetes or venous stasis (Silver and Wang, 1992). Major medical, social and economic consequences can result from complications of skin ulcers. Pressure ulcers and diabetic foot ulcers are among the most frequently encountered chronic ulcers.

Pressure ulcers are skin ulcers caused by pressure, shear, friction or a combination of these (Cochrane, Rippon, *et al.*, 1999; EPUAP, 1999; Zhong, Xing, *et al.*, 2006). Compression of skin against bone may cause injury to underlying fat and muscle that precedes necrosis of dermis and epidermis (Silver and Wang, 1992). Pressure ulcers constitute a grave healthcare threat to hospitalized patients, especially those in geriatric care. Countries with a large and increasing geriatric population face significant cost increases for the treatment and care of patients with pressure ulcers (Cole and Nesbitt, 2004). Between 1990 and 2003, the overall estimate of the prevalence of pressure ulcers in patients in healthcare institutions across Canada was 26.0% (95% Confidence Interval, 25.2% to 26.8%) (Woodbury and Houghton, 2004).

Diabetic foot ulcers that lead to lower extremity amputation are another major health threat. Diabetics are susceptible to foot ulcers because of atherosclerosis, a condition in which fatty materials accumulate along the artery walls, thickening, hardening, and eventually blocking the arteries, and the resulting occlusive arterial disease and damages to the peripheral nervous system (Silver and Wang, 1992). Approximately 15% of diabetics develop foot ulcers; non-healing ulcers precede 84% of all lower extremity amputations in diabetic patients

(Reid, Martin, *et al.*, 2006). There have been pronounced increases in the number of patients with diabetic foot ulcers according to the statistics of the International Diabetes Federation (IDF) and World Health Organization (WHO) (Tecilazich, Dinh, *et al.*, 2011). In the US alone, an average of 6.5 million people suffers chronic skin wounds resulting from diabetic foot ulcers (Singer and Clark, 1999). It has been projected that two amputation surgeries are conducted every minute in the world, and 85% of the amputations are caused by skin ulcers, which costs 4 billion dollars in the US per year (Edmonds, 2009).

Abnormal healing occurs when a wound has failed to progress in a timely manner through the phases of normal wound healing. The chronicity or abnormality may manifest itself in any of the three phases. Many potential factors may contribute to a delayed wound healing process. For example, it may be caused by a disease or condition (e.g., AIDS, diabetes mellitus) that will further lead to the deficiency of some aspects of the immune system, or make it difficult for the necessary nutrients to reach the wound site (as a result of, say, problems in the circulation system and/or the digestive system). Infection, medications, and inappropriate wound care are among the other factors that evoke abnormal wound healing.

8.2. WOUND DRESSING AND WOUND DRESSING MATERIALS

An essential part of wound care, wound dressing (i.e., a wound care material or product) provides a barrier against environmental hazards and further mechanical injury/abrasion to the wound, and helps create conditions that are suitable for the wound healing process.

Wound dressings have been used by human beings for thousands of years. One of the earliest types of wound dressings was grease-soaked gauze bandages used by ancient Egyptians. Other materials used in ancient times include leaves, animal fat and honey. Dressings used in ancient times were prone to heavy contamination by microorganisms and could become sources of infection. It was not until the late 19th century that the importance of hygiene and aseptic practice was recognized as essential for medical procedures, including wound care (Queen, Orsted, *et al.*, 2004).

It used to be believed that, in the treatment of wounds or ulcers, they should ideally be left to dry out and exposed to the air. This practice favored the use of cotton gauze as wound dressing and was a tradition for many centuries. This type of dressing was structurally open and highly absorptive. It would, however, adhere to the wound bed and cause additional injury and pain during removal. To overcome this problem, gauze dressings were often impregnated with paraffin wax to reduce their adhesion (Shai and Maibach, 2005). In the 1960s, experiments on both animal models and human volunteers suggested that a moist environment was preferred for healing a wound or ulcer (Winter, 1962; Hinman, Maibach, *et al.*, 1963). It is generally accepted now that a proper degree of moisture in the wounded area provides a desirable biological environment for the complex processes of wound healing. As a result, occlusive dressings were introduced in the 1960s as a new generation of wound dressings. Since the 1980s, specific, advanced dressings have been developed for specific uses. To date, different types of wound dressing materials/products are available to treat a wide variety of wounds.

8.2.1. Design Considerations for Modern Dressings

Different types of wound dressings can have different properties and functions that suit specific types of wounds. Still, some of the functions are essential to any kind of dressings. Namely, wound dressings should all be able to (Shai and Maibach, 2005):

1. protect the wound from external sources of infection and prevent bacteria in the wound from contaminating the environment;
2. protect the wound and its neighboring tissues from mechanical abrasion and injury by acting as a cushion;
3. absorb and control exudates, if necessary; and
4. improve comfort for the patient.

In addition to these basic functions, there are others that must be taken into consideration for the design/choice of wound dressings (Irion, 2002; Mao and Russell, 2005; Shai and Maibach, 2005):

1. *Control of moisture content* in the wound bed is important for wound healing. A moderately moist environment is necessary for cellular interactions and favors metabolic activities of the cells and tissues, and thus promotes healing in the wound bed. However, an excessively moisturized wound would complicate the treatment and slow down the healing process, for it may cause skin breakdown and/or maceration and infection. Content of moisture in the wound bed is influenced by the choices of dressing materials and their structures.
2. Gas (e.g., oxygen) *permeability* is another performance indicator for dressings. Oxygen plays important roles in the several phases of wound healing. In the initial stage, a deficiency of oxygen (hypoxia) in the wound area may, as a rule, stimulate formation and growth of new blood vessels, and stimulate the growth of fibroblasts, which is

essential to the production of the new tissue. However, this rule may not necessarily apply in the long-term remodeling of wound tissue, because hypoxia may also impair immunity and collagen synthesis. In the case of chronic ulcers, it is more obvious that hypoxia impedes and delays wound healing. Hypoxia is often related to the use of occlusive dressings.

3. Local *pH value* affects the wound healing process, too. An acidic environment is beneficial because it inhibits the growth of bacteria. It has been demonstrated that wound fluid is more acidic under occlusive hydrocolloid dressings than under permeable polyurethane dressings (Varghese, Balin, *et al.*, 1986).

4. Dressing materials of *low adherence* are desirable because they will not adhere to the wound bed to cause pain or trauma during dressing changes.

5. *Infection control* is critical in wound care because the wounded area is the most vulnerable to infection. Antibacterial drugs are useful in controlling infection, but systemic administration of these may cause undesirable side effects, such as renal and liver toxicity (Stadelmann, Digenis, *et al.*, 1998; Suzuki, Tanihara, *et al.*, 1998), not to mention that an oral administration of antibiotics provides an insufficient dosage to the wounded tissues, where the antibiotics are the most needed (Stadelmann, Digenis, *et al.*, 1998). An effective means to remedy this shortcoming is topical administration (Jacob, Cierny, *et al.*, 1993; Stadelmann, Digenis, *et al.*, 1998; Fallon, Shafer, *et al.*, 1999), where the drugs are used in minimal amounts at the site of infection, and efforts are made to ensure that the drugs function efficiently at the site. The new generation of wound dressings involves incorporation of the antibacterial agents onto/into the dressing material. These dressings provide a sustained release of drugs into the wounded site, where infection control is critical to wound healing.

6. Newly developed functional wound dressings have been given new, *advanced functions.* For example, some bioactive molecules (e.g., growth factors) have been found to be significant to wound healing because they play active roles in the production of new cells and tissues. Since patients who have diseases such as diabetes may suffer from a deficiency in those essential growth factors, they may experience impaired wound healing. To overcome this problem, functional wound dressings can be designed to be loaded with growth factors that can be released into the wound tissues in a controlled manner to promote wound healing. One type of such functional wound dressings is composed of electrospun nanofibers loaded with growth factors (also see Chapter 3).

8.2.2. Classification of Modern Wound Dressings

A wide spectrum of wound dressings have been developed and produced for the treatment of different types of wounds. In line with the water vapor transmission rate of the dressings (i.e., occlusiveness), they can generally be divided into two categories: non-occlusive and micro-environmental (occlusive and semi-occlusive) dressings (Irion, 2002).

Non-occlusive dressings, mostly based on woven cotton gauze (Figure 8.2), allow water vapor and fluid to freely transmit into and out of the wound. These dressings are used when fluid/mass transmission is necessary for wound healing. For example, they are used for acute wounds closed already with primary intention, so as to absorb the large amounts of body fluid and bleeding. Non-occlusive dressings can be pre-moistened with normal saline or antiseptic solution to treat infected wounds. They are also used in wounds that contain large amounts of necrotic (i.e., dead) tissues and that need rapid medical removal of dead or damaged tissues from a wound to promote wound healing. However, use of non-occlusive dressings is limited by their high rate of fluid transmission, which may lead to desiccation of the wound bed and consequently cause the dressing to adhere to it. To deal with this problem, some gauze dressings are designed to be non-adhering by coating the dressing surface with Vaseline or petrolatum. Nevertheless, the problem remains when exudates are absorbed into the interstices between yarns/

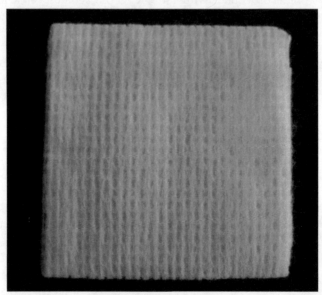

FIGURE 8.2. *A gauze pad.*

fibers and then dry. New tissues may grow through these interstices and cause adherence. In addition, abrasion between tissues and the dressing may cause small pieces of fiber materials to detach from the dressing and fall into the wound bed, which may induce wound contamination and inflammation. This is why gauze dressings need to be frequently changed.

Micro-environmental dressings, on the other hand, have important advantages for wound healing: they maintain wound moisture, which is critical for the healing of most wounds (except infected ones), and they require less changes and handling. The major objective to be achieved in designing such a dressing material is to ensure an optimized micro-environment for wound healing. Different types of micro-environmental dressings are listed below (Irion, 2002; Shai and Maibach, 2005; Hess, 2008). Some of the dressings are not made of fibers or textiles; they are described here so as to make the list fairly complete.

8.2.2.1. Semi-permeable (Semi-Occlusive) Film Dressings

Semi-permeable film dressings are made of polyurethane thin films that are permeable to moisture vapor and gases, but impermeable to fluid and bacteria. They maintain a moist environment in the wound bed, but have low absorbency, and are therefore not suitable for wounds with moderate to high level of exudates. They are usually used for superficial wounds or wounds with a low level of exudates. Since most of these film dressings are coated with adhesives, they may also be used as a secondary dressing (i.e., not in direct contact with the wound) to hold a more absorbent one (i.e., primary dressing, which is in direct contact with the wound). The most frequently used adhesive for these film dressings is soft silicone, which is hydrophobic and inert, so that it does not stick to a moist wound but adheres only to the surrounding dry skin.

8.2.2.2. Semi-permeable (Semi-Occlusive) Foam Dressings

Foam dressings are usually made of polyurethane, a material known for its ability to be processed into foam. A small amount of foaming agent (e.g., distilled water) is usually added into the reaction mixture during the synthesizing of the polyurethane (Oh, Kim, *et al.*, 2011). The water will react with one of the reacting agents (isocyanate) to create a gas (i.e., carbon dioxide), which then produces and expands the numerous void cells in the foam.

Foam dressings are also permeable to water vapor and gases, although their permeability may be smaller than film dressings. They have high absorption, the level of which may be dependent on the thick-

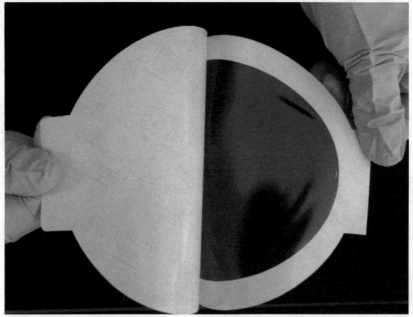

FIGURE 8.3. *A semi-permeable film dressing.*

ness of the dressing materials. These dressings are therefore not suitable for wounds with a low level of exudates, as it may cause an over drying effect on such wounds. A foam dressing usually has a hydrophilic side that is to be in contact with the wound and absorb the exudates, as well as a hydrophobic side that blocks the excessive loss of moisture from the wound bed to the outer environment. The wound-contacting layer is soft, and made to be either adherent or non-adherent (Figure 8.4). It functions also as a physical cushion to protect the wound bed, and acts as a thermal insulator to maintain an appropriate temperature in the wound bed. A number of additives are added into the foam dressings to enhance their functions. For example, charcoal can be incorporated to absorb odor, while silver can be incorporated to provide antibacterial functions.

8.2.2.3. Hydrocolloid Dressings

Hydrocolloid dressings are occlusive, containing hydrocolloid hydrophilic particles (e.g., sodium carboxymethyl cellulose, gelatin and pectin) that will swell to form a gel after absorbing fluid(s). Hydrocolloid dressings are either in the form of a sheet or are spreadable. A sheet-form dressing is composed of a hydrocolloid lining that is to be in

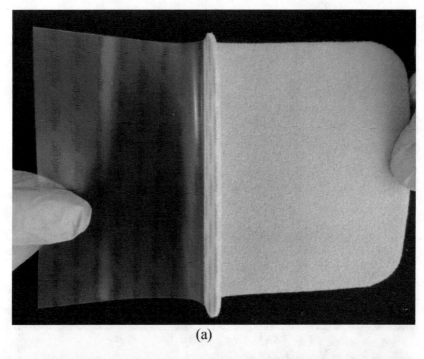

(a)

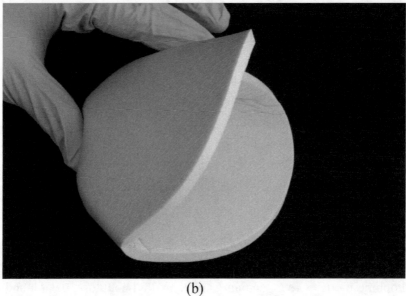

(b)

FIGURE 8.4. *Semi-permeable foam dressings: (a) an adhesive foam dressing; (b) a non-adhesive heel dressing (thick foam).*

176

contact with the wound and an outer hydrophobic coating that is impermeable to gases, water and bacteria. The sheet dressings usually adhere to the skin. The spreadable dressings, on the other hand, can be in the forms of pastes, granules or spiral-cut sheets. A secondary dressing may be necessary to hold these spreadable dressings in place. Hydrocolloid dressings are suitable for mild to moderate exuding ulcers, burn wounds and donor sites. They can be left on the wound for 5 days or more before being changed, thus causing less disturbance or trauma to the newly formed tissues of the wound. However, they are not suitable for moderately- to heavily-exuding wounds, as they can be overwhelmed within a few days. Hydrocolloid dressings may also leave a residue in the wound, possibly with an odor.

8.2.2.4. Hydrogel Dressings

Hydrogels are a water-swollen three-dimensional (3D) network composed of physically or chemically cross-linked hydrophilic polymers (Peppas, Huang, *et al.*, 2000). As previously discussed, for example, hydrogel is the gel formed by superabsorbent polymers (found also in diapers) after absorbing a large amount of fluid during their end uses (see Chapter 6). Hydrophilic polymers that have been used to produce

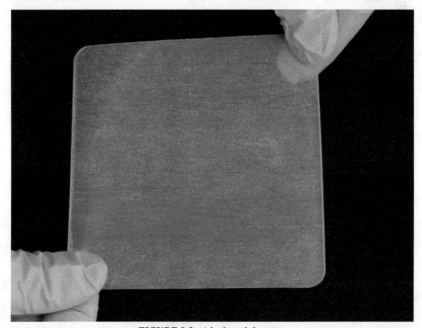

FIGURE 8.5. *A hydrogel dressing.*

hydrogels for wound care include carboxymethyl cellulose (CMC) and polyethylene oxide. Mechanisms of formation of hydrogels for wound care are similar to what have already been discussed (in Chapter 6) and will not be described here. Because of their high water content, they may not be able to absorb large amounts of exudates. Instead, hydrogel dressings are primarily used for hydrating dry wounds. They are rather soothing on the wound, and are non-adherent, causing minimal disturbance to the wound bed upon removal. They are also available in the form of sheets, spreadable gel, or hydrogel-impregnated gauze.

8.2.2.5. Alginate and Hydrofiber Dressings

Alginate dressings are made of biocompatible and biodegradable alginate fibers composed of an anionic polysaccharide (Figure 8.6) derived from brown seaweed. Alginate fibers are able to absorb large amounts of exudates and swell to form a hydrophilic gel to conform to the wound bed and act as a hemostat. The formed soft gel also maintains a moist healing environment. An alginate dressing can absorb exudates of up to 20 times its own weight (Hess, 2008). As a result, alginate dressings are suitable for wounds with moderate to high levels of exudates, especially for filling such irregularly-shaped wounds as cavities. They are not for wounds with low levels of exudates because they may dehydrate and adhere to the wound. Alginate dressings are available as sheets of nonwoven mats, ropes (containing strands of alginate fibers) or gels. The latter two forms of dressings are usually used for filling cavity wounds. An alginate dressing usually requires a secondary dressing to hold it in place.

Alginate can be formed into fibers via wet spinning. Commercial alginate fibers for wound care usually consist of metal (e.g., calcium, sodium, zinc and silver) salts of alginic acid. Calcium alginates are most frequently used because calcium cations are believed to have a hemostatic effect on wounds. Zinc and silver ions can contribute to infection control of the wound. Sodium ions, on the other hand, enhance solubility of the alginate, and consequently the swelling/absorption capacity of the dressing materials. A dressing composed of two different types of metal-salt alginate fibers (e.g., sodium and calcium) can be developed to benefit from a combination of functions.

Alginate fibers can be processed into nonwoven dressing sheets via different methods. Staple alginate fibers can be turned into a nonwoven mat by wet-laying and hydro-entangling (spunlacing). A carded and lapped web of alginate fibers can be compression-bonded or needle-punched to form a dressing mat. Spun-laying is another method adopted in the production of alginate dressings (Mao and Russell, 2005).

Alginate

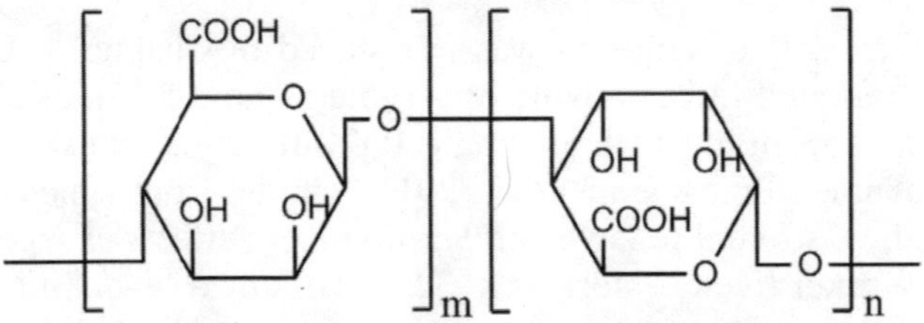

COOH

OH   OH

OH   OH

COOH

FIGURE 8.6. Chemical structure of alginate (alginic acid).

Hydrofiber dressings are composed of sodium carboxymethyl cellulose (CMC) fibers. They are similar to alginate dressings in that they swell to form a gel after absorbing exudates from the wound. Hydrofibers can be mechanically bonded to form nonwoven dressing sheets. CMC is also used in hydrocolloid dressings in the form of particles. However, CMC in the hydrofiber form is believed to have the advantage of complete removal from the wound upon changes. Hydrocolloid dressings, on the other hand, may leave a gelatinous mass on the surface of the wound, which may need extra care.

In addition to the above mentioned wound dressings that have been widely accepted for clinical applications, there are other wound dressings that are still in the stage of research or development, or are only commercialized on a relatively small scale.

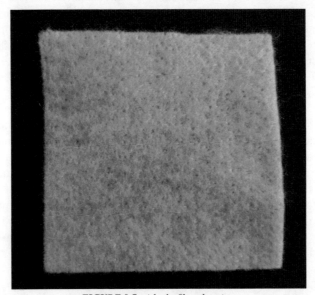

FIGURE 8.7. A hydrofiber dressing.

8.2.2.6. Chitosan Dressings

The chemistry of chitosan was introduced in Chapter 3. Chitosan has been reported to be capable of serving as both a hemostat and an antibacterial agent, thus stimulating cell proliferation and wound healing (Jayakumar, Prabaharan, *et al.*, 2011). Chitin, from which chitosan is derived, was found to have similar biological effects except that the effect is weaker (Ueno, Mori, *et al.*, 2001). Quite a few chitin- or chitosan-based dressings are commercialized to date. They are in the form of nonwovens (e.g., Beschitin®), microfibrils derived from a microalga (e.g., Syvek-Patch®), or freeze-dried sponges (e.g., Chitipack S®). There are also chitosan-based dressings in the form of powders (e.g., Chitodine®), wet-spun fibers (e.g., Chitopack C®), and nonwovens (e.g., Chitosan Skin®) (Muzzarelli, 2009).

8.2.2.7. Collagen Dressings

Collagen is the most abundantly-occurring protein of a fibrous form. It is biocompatible and biodegradable, thus suitable for wound care. Collagen is a naturally-occurring protein in the human body, and when used as a dressing material, is believed to stimulate cell growth and new tissue development, and therefore promote wound healing. Commercialized collagen dressings may be in the form of gel/powder (e.g., Cellerate RX®) or sheets (e.g., Puracol®). Collagen can be used in dressing products in combination with other materials, including oxidized regenerated cellulose (e.g., Promogran®) and alginate (e.g., Fibracol® Plus). Collagen dressings can deal with wounds with low to heavy exudates, depending on the form of the dressings.

8.2.2.8. Nanofibrous Dressings

Nanofibrous structures have the advantages of good absorption and a high level of comfort and are therefore frequently applied in wound care products. However, this type of dressing material is still in the stage of research and development in laboratories, due to limitations such as small yield rate and difficulties encountered in manufacturing (e.g., electrospinning). A more detailed discussion about these materials can be found in Chapter 3.

8.2.3. Modification and Functionalization of Modern Wound Dressings

Extensive research and development work has been conducted to enhance the performance of various wound dressings. Some of the important outcomes are introduced as follows.

8.2.3.1. Incorporation of Bioactive Agents into Wound Dressings

Activated charcoal (or activated carbon) is known for its high porosity, surface area and capacity of adsorption. It is therefore incorporated into the dressing materials so that they will be endowed with the antibacterial and anti-odor functions. Activated charcoal particles are usually bound to a semi-permeable dressing material to contribute to infection control by physically absorbing exudates and bacteria from the wound bed into the dressing materials (Frost, Jackson, *et al.*, 1980). Alternatively, a charcoal cloth can be prepared from carbonizing (i.e., heating without supply of oxygen) and activating (i.e., being treated with oxygen to render a highly porous structure) a knitted viscose fabric, and be sandwiched between two face fabrics (e.g., spun-bonded viscose fabrics) to form a wound dressing. These dressings also absorb and filter the malodorous chemicals released from the wound bed to reduce odor from the wound.

Silver is another frequently used antibacterial agent for wound dressings. Silver compounds (e.g., silver sulphadiazine) in the form of cream have for decades been used as a topical treatment for burns and chronic wounds. However, this topical treatment requires frequent applications to keep its efficacy. To overcome this shortcoming, new dressing materials/products have been developed to provide sustained, long-term release of silver into the wound by incorporating the silver compound into the dressings. For example, sodium CMC hydrofiber dressings impregnated with silver ions (e.g., Aquacel AG®) have been designed to provide both high absorption of exudates and infection control. Silver compounds can also be incorporated into polyurethane foam (e.g., Contreet foam®) or hydrocolloid (e.g., Contreet hydrocolloid®) dressings, from which silver ions are released upon contact with wound fluid (Lansdown, Jensen, *et al.*, 2003). Another design involves nanocrystalline silver-coated, high-density polyethylene mesh that is bound to a rayon/polyester dressing core which regulates the moisture level in the wound (e.g., Acticoat®). The silver nanocrystals provide large surface area for the antibacterial activity (Dowsett, 2003). In addition to these commercialized products, extensive research work has been performed for the development of silver-loaded nanofibrous mats that are potentially useful for wound care (see Chapter 3 for details). However, there have been concerns about silver used in wound care, in that it may stain the wound or the surrounding skin, and cause toxicity or sensitization.

There are also dressings that combine both activated charcoal and silver to provide odor and infection control in the wounds. For example, a charcoal cloth produced by carbonizing and activating a knitted viscose rayon fabric is enclosed in a sleeve of spun-bonded nonwoven nylon fabric, resulting in such a dressing (e.g., Actisorb®) (Furr, Russell, *et al.*, 1994).

Other antibacterial agents that have been incorporated into wound dressings include Chlorhexidine (e.g., Bactigras®), iodine (Inadine®) and honey (Mesitran®). Other bioactive agents or molecules that can be incorporated into wound dressings include extracellular matrix proteins (e.g., Xelma®) and growth factors that promote cell differentiation and wound healing. Most of these efforts are still in the laboratory stage (more detailed information can be found in Chapter 3).

8.2.3.2. Making and Using Composite Dressings

A composite wound dressing usually consists of two or more of the dressing materials discussed in the previous section. For example, a multi-layer dressing composed of a hydrophobic wound contact layer (e.g., polypropylene) and a highly absorbent inner layer (e.g., cellulose, hydrogel) may be free from adherence of the dressing to the wound while maintaining its permeability/non-occlusiveness, and is therefore suitable for acute or infected wounds. A waterproof and bacteria-resistant outer layer can also be incorporated into such dressings. A hydrofiber/alginate fiber layer (wound contact layer) combined with a foam layer has also been adopted in the design of composite dressings, which conform well to the wound bed and are rather absorptive.

8.2.4. Secondary Dressings

Secondary dressings are usually not applied in direct contact with the wound bed. They are used in combination with primary dressings (as described in previous sections) to provide extra functions (e.g., to hold the primary dressings in place and to provide additional absorption, compression, cushion, warmth and/or comfort as required). They include absorptive pads, adhesive bandages, surgical tapes and bandage rolls. Some of the secondary dressings are discussed in this section.

8.2.4.1. Absorptive Pads

Absorptive pads are usually multilayer dressings composed of highly absorptive layers of cellulose fibers. They can be used as secondary dressings over most primary dressings to provide extra absorption of exudates. The typical construction of such a pad includes

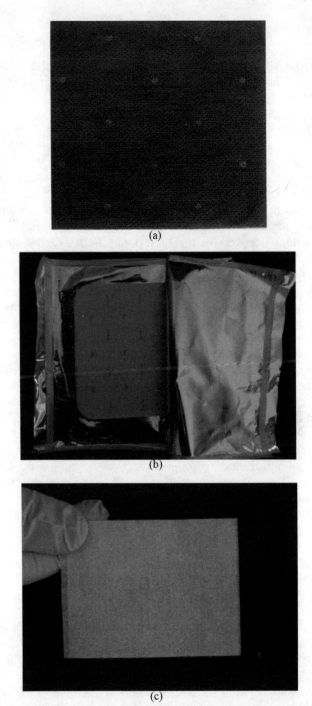

(a)

(b)

(c)

FIGURE 8.8. *Antibacterial agent-incorporated dressings: (a) A silver-coated multi-layer dressing, (b) A Silver-incorporated foam dressing, (c) A gauze impregnated with an antibacterial agent (0.5% chlorhexidine acetate BP).*

183

soft nonwoven top/back layers, with cellulose fluff fillers inside for absorbency. The edges of the pad are sealed to prevent lint leakage from the pad.

8.2.4.2. Tapes

Tapes are simple forms of secondary dressings that can be used to hold primary dressings in place for smaller wounds. Four types of tapes are currently available: silk tapes, plastic tapes, paper tapes and foam tapes (Irion, 2002). Silk tapes (e.g., Durapore®) are silk-like tapes with strong adhesion to the skin. They are made of acetate cellulose fibers in a tightly-woven plain weave (i.e., taffeta). Plastic tapes (e.g., Transpore®) are made of perforated plastic films (e.g., PET) that are waterproof and breathable, or composed of viscose or polyester nonwovens. Silk and plastic tapes are coated with a layer of acrylic adhesive that adheres them to the skin (Mao and Russell, 2005). These two tapes are highly adhesive, and therefore require cautious handling to avoid trauma during changing. They may not be suitable for fragile skin (e.g., that of the young and elderly). Paper tapes (e.g., Micropore®) are made of viscose nonwoven fabrics coated with an acrylic adhesive. They are less adhesive than the previous two types of tapes and can be occasionally applied on fragile skin. A foam tape (e.g., Microfoam®) is usually composed of an elastic foam coated with an acrylic adhesive. The foam tape is the least adhesive among the four types, and is therefore used on skins at risk. Among the four types of tapes, silk and paper tapes are permeable to both liquid and vapor water, while the plastic and foam tapes are semi-permeable—that is, permeable to gas and water vapor but impermeable to liquid water.

8.2.4.3. Bandage Rolls

Bandage rolls come in various widths. They can be in the form of woven fabrics, e.g., cotton gauze (in either loose plain weave or leno weave). Elastic fibers (e.g., rubber) can be blended into the yarns to provide higher elasticity and compression of the bandages. Knitted (usually warp-knitted) bandages are also available to provide more elasticity. These bandage rolls may come in the form of flat sheets or tubular net fabrics. The latter type can be used for such parts of the body as digits, hand, foot and head, to allow easy application and unimpaired movement of the joints. These tubular bandages are composed of cellulose/ elastic fiber (e.g., rubber or lycra) blends in the knit structure.

Special designs for bandages based on their textile structure can be represented by the *cohesive elastic retention bandages*. They are ban-

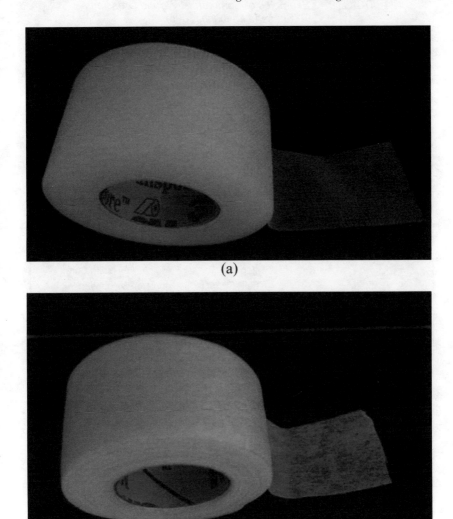

FIGURE 8.9. *Surgical tapes: (a) a roll of plastic tape; (b) a roll of paper tape.*

dages that will adhere to themselves and do not adhere to the skin, hair or clothing. They can be used on fragile skin that may be traumatized by other bandages with stronger adhesion properties. These bandages are usually made of cellulose fibers (i.e., cotton or viscose). The yarns to form the fabric are highly twisted (also known as crepe-twisted), in both S and Z twists; they are also starched before weaving to maintain their stability during processing. These highly-twisted yarns with dif-

TABLE 8.1. *Examples of Commercial Wound Dressings*
(Shai and Maibach, 2005).

Categories		Brand Name	Manufacturer
Primary Dressings	Film Dressings	Bioclusive®	Johnson & Johnson
		Blisterfilm®	Kendall
		Carrafilm®	Carrington Laboratories
		Cutifilm®	Smith & Nephew
		Opsite®	Smith & Nephew
		Polyskin®	Kendall
		Tegaderm®	3M Health care
	Foam Dressings	Allevyn®	Smith & Nephew
		Biatain®	Coloplast
		Carrasmart foam®	Carrington Laboratories
		Curafoam®	Kendall
		Flexzan®	UDL Laboratories
		Lyofoan®	Seton Healthcare
		Mepilex®	Mölnlycke Health Care
		Tielle®	Johnson & Johnson
	Hydrocolloid Dressings	Comfeel®	Coloplast
		Duoderm®	Convatec
		Granuflex®	Convatec
		Tegasorb®	3M Health care
	Hydrogel Dressings	Geliperm®	Geistlich
		Granugel®	Convatec
		Intrasite®	Smith & Nephew
		Oxyzyme®	Insense
		Vigilon®	Bard
	Alginate & Hydrofiber Dressings	Algisite® M	Smith & Nephew
		Aquacel®	Convatec
		Kaltocarb®	Convatec
		Kaltostat®	Convatec
		Tegagel®	3M Health Care
		Sorbsan®	UDL Laboratories
	Chitin/Chitosan Dressings	Beschitin®	Unitika
		Chitipack S®	Eisai
		Chitodine®	IMS
		Chitopack C®	Eisai
		Chitosan Skin®	Hainan Xinlong non-wovens
		Syvek-Patch®	Marine Polymer Technologies
	Collagen Dressings	Cellerate RX®	Hymed Group
		Fibracol® Plus	Johnson & Johnson
		Promogran®	Johnson & Johnson
		Puracol®	Medline Industries

(continued)

186

*TABLE 8.1. (continued) Examples of Commercial Wound Dressings
(Shai and Maibach, 2005).*

Categories		Brand Name	Manufacturer
Functional Dressings	Silver-containing Dressings	Acticoat®	Smith & Nephew
		Aquacel AG®	Convatec
		Contreet®	Coloplast
		Mepilex AG®	Mölnlycke Health Care
	Dressings with activated charcoal	Carbonet®	Smith & Nephew
		Kaltocarb®	Convatec
		Clinisorb®	CliniMed
	Dressings containing both silver & charcoal	Actosorb®	Johnson & Johnson
	Dressings with other bioactive compounds	Bactigras®	Smith & Nephew
		Inadine®	Johnson & Johnson
		Mesitran®	Theo Manufacturing BV
		Xelma®	Mölnlycke Health Care
Secondary Dressings	Composite Dressings	Alldress®	Mölnlycke Health Care
		Thinsite®	Swiss-American Products
	Absorptive Pads	Curity®	Kendall
		DuPad®	Derma Sciences
	Tapes	Durapore®	3M Health Care
		Hypafix®	Smith & Nephew
		Mepitac®	Mölnlycke Health Care
		Microfoam®	3M Health Care
		Transpore®	3M Health Care
	Bandage Rolls	Elastocrepe®	Smith & Nephew
		Quinaband®	Mölnlycke Health Care
		Tensopress®	Smith & Nephew

ferent twists (S or Z twist) are laid alternatively in the warp direction on a weaving loom for the construction of a plain weave fabric. A crepe effect (i.e., an irregular fabric surface) is finally achieved by a degumming process to remove the starch and release the highly-twisted yarns from their set condition, resulting in the contrary pull of the two crepe-twisted yarns and the shrinking of the fabric to form a crinkly fabric surface. Such a special fabric surface morphology enables the fabrics to adhere to each other but not to other surfaces. As a result, such dressing materials impose less disturbance to the skin, but may be subjected to dislocation after application. These bandages can be further coated with a layer of adhesive to enhance their security on the wound.

8.3. PRESSURE GARMENT

The normal and intact skin maintains an appropriate pressure against its underlying tissues. For a patient with a severe burn injury, if a considerable amount of skin (in partial or full thickness) is gone, the skin is no longer able to apply the normal pressure to the underlying tissues. As a result, a thick and stiff scarring, known also as hypertrophic scarring, may form at the site of the injury. Such scarring leads to aesthetic impairment and difficulty in movement if a scar is located near a joint. It is estimated that the prevalence of hypertrophic scarring after severe burns can range from 32–67% (Esselman, Thombs, *et al.*, 2006). To reduce or prevent scarring, the pressure garment is usually worn by the patient to put a substitute pressure on the damaged skin and its underlying tissues. This garment should be worn almost 24 hours a day and the whole therapy may last for 1 year or until the scar matures (Ripper, Renneberg, *et al.*, 2009).

Pressure garments are tightly fit garments, gloves, masks, sleeves, and stockings that can be worn to cover part of the human body and to exert pressure on a compromised skin that has healed from a burn injury (i.e., the wound is closed and able to sustain pressure). A pressure garment is expected to apply an appropriate amount of pressure (i.e., no less than 24 mm Hg) (Yildiz, 2007) on the injured skin. To meet the requirement of high elasticity and elastic recovery, pressure garments are usually made of nylon fibers or nylon/lycra blends. In structure, the fabric can either be a weft or warp knit. Two types of pressure garments are available: the *ready-to-use* and the *custom-made.* The ready-to-use (or *off-the-shelf*) garments are usually available in a variety of styles and sizes, although they may need adjustment if they do not fit perfectly; they provide immediate treatment, especially when a custom-made garment is under construction (Macintyre and Baird, 2006). A medical-grade elastomer sheet or pad can usually be used as an insert or lining under a pressure garment (i.e., to be in direct contact with the skin), particularly over such fragile areas as joints.

Comfort is a critical issue for the development of pressure garments, as it is both physical discomfort (e.g., pain, itching, increased perspiration, blistering, ulceration or skeletal and dental deformity) and emotional distress (e.g., shame and embarrassment to wear a visible garment) that have combined to prevent burn patients from adherence to the pressure garment therapy (Macintyre and Baird, 2006; Ripper, Renneberg, *et al.*, 2009).

8.4. SUMMARY

This chapter is devoted to a discussion of skin wound care materials (wound dressings). It started with the basics of "skin" and provided details on "wound care" for wound "healing" before addressing the dressing materials proper. Such a sequence is expected to benefit learning.

The human skin is a special organ because it is the most vulnerable to getting wounded. In addition to the fact that it is the most frequent organ to receive wounds is the fact that it receives many different types of wounds, owing to the human capacity for violence and reckless behavior. This is the first reason why we need so many different types of wound care materials to assist in the healing of wounds.

Many different types of wound care products are needed because wounds themselves differ in causes, sizes, and severity; wound care materials that suitable in one case may not be suitable in another. This chapter has therefore specified the many types and forms of wound care materials and products used for the care of various kinds of wounds, and has justified such uses by adequately discussing their function mechanisms.

Since this book may be read also by product development professionals, this chapter has covered in great detail the many specific functions that wound dressings are expected to perform—namely, what must be taken into consideration in the development and design of wound dressings—and has included instances of successful stories in such development work.

This chapter is largely to serve practical purposes, to be read most likely by those who make decisions about what to use. Thus it gives fairly full lists (even "brands") of wound care products. For such purposes, this chapter tells what to use, what not to use, and adequately explains WHY (e.g., how "permeability" of the dressing material influences maintenance of moisture, which can be critical to wound healing, and why the highly absorptive alginate dressings are suitable for some wounds and not for others).

Discussed towards the end, "pressure garment" is not typically a wound dressing (but, rather, a means to give comfort or "last aid" to the skin that has recovered from serious wounding). It is discussed here because this may be the relatively best place for such a discussion.

8.5. REFERENCES

Agache, P.G. and P. Humbert. (2004). Measuring the skin: non-invasive investigations, physiology, normal constants. New York: Springer.

Cochrane, C., M.G. Rippon, *et al.* (1999). Application of an *in vitro* model to evaluate bioadhesion of fibroblasts and epithelial cells to two different dressings. *Biomaterials* **20**(13): 1237–1244.

Cole, L. and C. Nesbitt. (2004). A three year multiphase pressure ulcer prevalence/incidence study in a regional referral hospital. *Ostomy Wound Manage* **50**(11): 32–40.

Dowsett, C. (2003). An overview of Acticoat dressing in wound management. *Br. J. Nurs.* **12**(19 Suppl): S44-9.

Edmonds, M. (2009). The treatment of diabetic foot infections: focus on ertapenem. *Vascular Health and Risk Management* 5.

EPUAP. (1999). European pressure ulcer advisory panel guidelines on treatment of pressure ulcers. *EPUAP Review* **1**: 31–33.

Esselman, P.C., B.D. Thombs, *et al.* (2006). Burn rehabilitation—State of the science. *American Journal of Physical Medicine & Rehabilitation* **85**(4): 383–413.

Fallon, M.T., W. Shafer, *et al.* (1999). Use of cefazolin microspheres to treat localized methicillin-resistant Staphylococcus aureus infections in rats. *Journal of Surgical Research* **86**(1): 97–102.

Frost, M.R., S.W. Jackson, *et al.* (1980). Adsorption of bacteria onto activated charcoal cloth an effect of potential importance in the treatment of infected wounds. *Microbios Letters* **13**(51-52): 135–140.

Furr, J.R., A.D. Russell, *et al.* (1994). Antibacterial activity of actisorb-plus, actisorb and silver-nitrate. *Journal of Hospital Infection* **27**(3): 201–208.

Hess, C.T. (2008). Skin & wound care. Philadelphia: Wolters Kluwer Health/Lippincott Williams & Wilkins.

Hinman, C.D., H. Maibach, *et al.* (1963). Effect of air exposure and occlusion on experimental human skin wounds. *Nature* **200**(490): 377-8.

Irion, G. (2002). Comprehensive wound management. Thorofare, NJ: SLACK.

Jacob, E., G. Cierny, *et al.* (1993). Evaluation of biodegradable cefazolin sodium microspheres for the prevention of infection in rabbits with experimental open tibial fractures stabilized with internal-fixation. *Journal of Orthopaedic Research* **11**(3): 404–411.

Jayakumar, R., M. Prabaharan, *et al.* (2011). Biomaterials based on chitin and chitosan in wound dressing applications. *Biotechnology Advances* **29**(3): 322–337.

Lansdown, A.B., K. Jensen, *et al.* (2003). Contreet Foam and Contreet Hydrocolloid: an insight into two new silver-containing dressings. *J. Wound Care* **12**(6): 205–10.

Macintyre, L. and M. Baird. (2006). Pressure garments for use in the treatment of hypertrophic scars—a review of the problems associated with their use. *Burns* **32**(1): 10–15.

Mao, N. and S.J. Russell. (2005). *Nonwoven Wound Dressings.* Manchester, UK: The Textile Institute.

Muzzarelli, R.A.A. (2009). Chitins and chitosans for the repair of wounded skin, nerve, cartilage and bone. *Carbohydrate Polymers* **76**(2): 167–182.

Oh, S.T., W.R. Kim, *et al.* (2011). The preparation of polyurethane foam combined with pH-sensitive alginate/bentonite hydrogel for wound dressings. *Fibers and Polymers* **12**(2): 159–165.

Peppas, N.A., Y. Huang, *et al.* (2000). Physicochemical, foundations and structural design of hydrogels in medicine and biology. *Annual Review of Biomedical Engineering* **2**: 9–29.

Queen, D., H. Orsted, *et al.* (2004). A dressing history. *Int. Wound J.* **1**(1): 59–77.

Reid, K.S., B.D. Martin, *et al.* (2006). Diabetic foot complications in a northern Canadian Aboriginal community. *Foot Ankle Int.* **27**(12): 1065–73.

Ripper, S., B. Renneberg, *et al.* (2009). Adherence to pressure garment therapy in adult burn patients. *Burns* **35**(5): 657–664.

Shai, A. and H.I. Maibach. (2005). Wound healing and ulcers of the skin. Berlin: Springer.

Silver, F.H. and M.C. Wang. (1992). A review of the etiology and treatment of skin ulcers with wound dressings—comparison of the effects of occlusive and nonocclusive dressings. *Journal of Long-Term Effects of Medical Implants* **2**(4): 267–288.

Singer, A.J. and R.A. Clark. (1999). Cutaneous wound healing. *N. Engl. J. Med.* **341**(10): 738–46.

Stadelmann, W.K., A.G. Digenis, *et al.* (1998). Impediments to wound healing. *American Journal of Surgery* **176**(2A): 39s–47s.

Suzuki, Y., M. Tanihara, *et al.* (1998). A new drug delivery system with controlled release of antibiotic only in the presence of infection. *Journal of Biomedical Materials Research* **42**(1): 112–116.

Tecilazich, F., T. Dinh, *et al.* (2011). Treating diabetic ulcers. *Expert Opin. Pharmacother.* **12**(4): 593–606.

Ueno, H., T. Mori, *et al.* (2001). Topical formulations and wound healing applications of chitosan. *Advanced Drug Delivery Reviews* **52**(2): 105–115.

Varghese, M.C., A.K. Balin, *et al.* (1986). Local environment of chronic wounds under synthetic dressings. *Archives of Dermatology* **122**(1): 52–57.

Winter, G.D. (1962). Formation of scab and rate of epithelization of superficial wounds in skin of young domestic pig. *Nature* **193**(4812): 293-&.

Woodbury, M.G. and P.E. Houghton. (2004). Prevalence of pressure ulcers in Canadian healthcare settings. *Ostomy Wound Manage* **50**(10): 22–38.

Yildiz, N. (2007). A novel technique to determine pressure in pressure garments for hypertrophic burn scars and comfort properties. *Burns* **33**(1): 59–64.

Zhong, W., M.M.Q. Xing, *et al.* (2006). Textiles and human skin, microclimate, cutaneous reactions: An overview. *Cutaneous and Ocular Toxicology* **25**(1): 23–39.

CHAPTER 9

Biotextiles

BIOTEXTILES is a type of biomaterial, which is defined as "a nonviable material used in the fabrication of a medical device and intended to react with biological systems" (Williams, 1987). Similarly, a biotextile can be defined as "a structure composed of textile fibers and designed for use in a specific biological environment, where its performance depends on its interactions with cells and biological fluids as measured in terms of biocompatibility and biostability (Martin and Burg, 2003). A wide variety of biotextile devices and materials has been used in the treatment of disease or injury, or as substitutes for damaged or diseased human tissues/organs. As indicated in its definition, biocompatibility and biostability are two critical criteria for the design and development of biotextile products and materials (see Chapter 5).

This chapter covers a series of implantable biotextiles, including sutures, vascular grafts, ligament prostheses and hernia repair mesh grafts. The extracorporeal biotextiles (e.g., artificial kidney)—devices that perform their functions outside of the human body but still react with human tissues (e.g., blood)—will also be discussed in this chapter.

9.1. SUTURES

The most frequently used biotextile, especially in the process of surgery, sutures help close the wound, a function that will last for a relatively long time until the natural healing process is restored to provide a sufficient level of wound strength. The use of sutures dates thousands of years. Natural materials, including flax, hair, cotton, silk and catgut, had been used for this purpose in the many centuries before the invention and commercialization of synthetic sutures in the 1940s. Suture materials can be evaluated according to the following (Bennett, 1988):

1. Physical properties
   a. *physical configuration*—whether the material is of a single-strand/monofilament or multi-strand/multifilament structure
   b. *diameter* (or caliber)
   c. *capillarity*—the capacity of a suture to adsorb or imbibe fluid
   d. *fluid absorption ability*—the capacity to absorb fluid into the fiber material
   e. *tensile strength*
   f. *knot strength*—the force necessary to cause a knot to slip
   g. *elasticity*—the ability to regain its original form and length after being stretched
   h. *plasticity*—the ability to retain its new, deformed length and form after being stretched
   i. *memory*—the capacity to return to its original shape upon deformation.

Appropriate physical properties of sutures are related to their performance. Capillary and fluid absorption may influence a suture's tendency to take up and retain water-borne bacteria, which can induce infection. A multifilament suture can take up more fluid and bacteria than a monofilament suture that is made of the same polymer material. To maintain its strength during the wound healing process, or to avoid the risk of early degradation of the suture before the wound heals, a bioabsorbable suture should have predictable degradation and absorption (usually accompanied by a reduction of mechanical strength). A suture should also be flexible to allow easy bending and stretching to accommodate wound edema (which is an accumulation of an excessive amount of watery fluid in cells, tissues, or body cavities) and to recoil to its original length after the wound contracts. Memory can be related to elasticity and plasticity of a suture. A suture material (e.g., nylon) with high memory tends to untie from a knot to result in decreased knot security, whereas a suture material (e.g., silk) with low memory usually has a high knot security.

2. *Handling properties* dictate a suture's pliability, knottability and surface/frictional features. Pliability is the measure of how easily the suture can be handled by a surgeon in a surgical operation, especially how flexible it is to bending. Braided sutures are usually more pliable than monofilament sutures. Knottability is important because a suture should be tied easily to form a secure and minimized knot. Surface/frictional properties (e.g., coefficient of friction) indicate how easily the suture will slip through the tissue and be knotted.

TABLE 9.1. Types of Sutures.

	Natural Sutures	Synthetic Sutures
Absorbable	Catgut	Polyglycolic acid, Polyglactin, Polydioxanone
Non-absorbable	Silk	Polyamide (Nylon), Polyester (Dacron), Polypropylene, Polytetrafluoroethylene (PTFE)

3. *Tissue response (or tissue reaction)* is, on the other hand, undesirable because it impedes wound healing and may cause infection and discomfort. Generally, higher tissue response is associated with lower biocompatibility of the suture material, and a larger quantity of foreign material implanted. Therefore, a desirable suture should demonstrate low tissue response. To minimize tissue response, a suture should have high biocompatibility and consist of the least possible amount of foreign material. Tissue response to absorbable sutures is usually more obvious than to nonabsorbable sutures, and such response will persist until the suture is absorbed. A more detailed discussion about tissue responses, material biocompatibility and bioresorbability has been provided in Chapter 5.

Sutures can be grouped into two categories according to their source of raw materials: natural sutures and synthetic sutures. Sutures also vary in their capacity to retain a long-term physical integrity in the body, and can therefore be differentiated into absorbable and non-absorbable sutures. The various types of sutures are summarized in Table 9.1.

The following are types of sutures that better known and more often used.

9.1.1. Absorbable Sutures

Catgut, known also as surgical gut, is derived from the small intestines of sheep or cattle. The major component of catgut is strands of highly purified collagen, a fibrous protein. Catgut as a traditional suture material has now been largely replaced by synthetic sutures because of several disadvantages. Catgut may contain such contaminants as muscle fibers or mucoproteins, which may cause tissue reaction problems. Catgut can be treated with chromium salt, in a procedure similar to the tanning of leather. The resulted chromic gut is stronger and more resistant to degradation after implantation. Catgut sutures generally are low in mechanical strength. Plain gut starts to degrade 12 hours after implantation, and it will retain significant strength for only 5–7 days, whereas chromic gut may last twice as long (Meyer and Antonini, 1989). Both plain and chromic gut sutures completely lose their tensile strength in 2 to 3 weeks. The complete absorption of a gut suture is unpredictable and may last about 12 weeks. Catgut degrades via digestion of proteins by enzymes (proteolysis) (Bennett, 1988; Moy, Waldman, et al., 1992). These sutures also have poor handle and knot security: the knots may harden and traumatize adjacent tissues in the presence of body fluid (Levin, 1980). Catgut is known to cause high degrees of tissue reaction (the highest among currently available sutures) and impede wound healing.

   Polyglycolic acid (PGA) (Figure 3.8) suture was the first synthetic absorbable suture (i.e., Dexon®), introduced in 1970. PGA sutures usually contain braided filaments produced via solvent spinning and heat stretching. A highly crystalline material, a PGA suture has better mechanical properties than a catgut suture. It retains 60% of its original breaking strength at day 7 (Morgan, 1969) and 20% of its original strength by day 28 (Herrmann, Kelly, et al., 1970). It is completely dissolved within 90–120 days (Craig, Williams, et al., 1975). PGA is broken down in the body via hydrolysis (i.e., having its long polymer chain disintegrated as a result of the attack of water) in the presence of body fluid.

   The original PGA suture (i.e., Dexon® S) has a rough surface, making it difficult to handle and secure a knot. The rough surface also increases drag force to the tissue when the suture is pulled through. The next generation of PGA suture (i.e., Dexon® plus) adopts a surface coating to lubricate the suture surface, so that the suture can slip through the tissue more smoothly and allow easier handling and knotting. The coating is soluble in an aqueous environment and is eliminated within a few days, resulting in an uncoated suture with the rough surface to retain good knot security (Rodeheaver, Foresman, et al., 1987).

   Absorbable PGA sutures are useful for procedures inside the body, as no removal procedure is required. However, they are not often used for cutaneous surgery in which the sutures can later be removed, because the braided multifilament sutures may allow the penetration of bacteria into the wound by capillary action. Besides, the degradation and absorption rate of the suture is unpredictable if it is not totally buried and is in contact with body fluid (Bennett, 1988).

   Polyglactin 910 suture (i.e., Vicryl®) was introduced in 1974 as another synthetic and bioresorbable suture. It contains a copolymer of 90% glycolide and 10% lactide, known as *poly(lactic-co-glycolic acid)*, or PLGA, as shown in Figure 9.1. The structure and properties of Polyglactin 910 suture are similar to those of the PGA suture. Vicryl® is also available in the form of braided filaments produced from solvent spin-

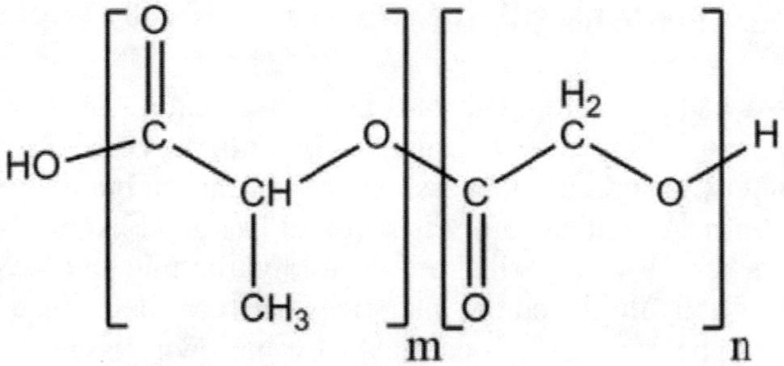

FIGURE 3.2. *PLGA (for Polyglactin 910, m: n = 10:90).*

ning. Vicryl® retains 8% of its strength by day 28. Complete absorption of Vicryl® takes less time (60–90 days) than that of Dexon®, because the polylactide blocks render the submicroscopic polymer chains apart and therefore make the copolymer more vulnerable to hydrolytic degradation (Craig, Williams, *et al.*, 1975). Coated Vicryl® was also developed to improve the suture's passage through tissue and its knotting properties. Tissue response, handling qualities and physical properties of coated Vicryl® are very similar to those of Dexon® plus. Also, Vicryl® suture is more suitable for procedures inside the body than cutaneous surgery.

Polydioxanone suture (e.g., PDS®) is composed of a polymer synthesized from monomer paradioxanone. It is manufactured as a monofilament suture, and therefore has a lesser affinity for bacteria. PDS® retains 58% of its tensile strength by day 28 after implantation and is completely absorbed in 180 days (Ray, Doddi, *et al.*, 1981). Unlike other synthetic absorbable sutures, PDS® has a slow degradation profile because of its slow hydrolysis, enabling it to be used for situations where a longer period of time is required for the wounded skin to regain considerable strength. The PDS suture, as well as its degradation products, impose minimal tissue response, although the monofilament suture is stiffer than multifilament sutures, thus negatively affecting its handle and knotting properties (Moy, Waldman, *et al.*, 1992).

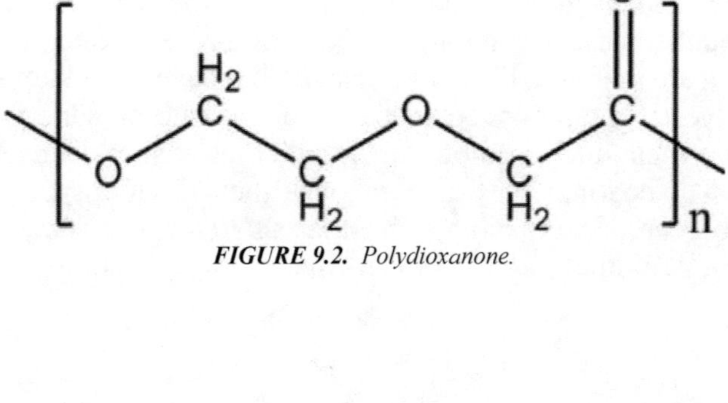

FIGURE 9.2. *Polydioxanone.*

9.1.2. Non-absorbable Sutures

Silk is a natural protein (fibroin) fiber. Silk sutures are categorized as a non-absorbable suture because it takes almost two years for it to be completely absorbed. They are available either in braided or monofilament form. A braided suture is soft and has good handle and knotting properties. However, silk sutures are hydrophilic and swell in the presence of body fluid, and the interstices between filaments in braided sutures may be covered or penetrated by ingrowth tissues, therefore causing pain during suture removal. A monofilament silk suture, on the other hand, does not allow tissue penetration and ingrowth, thus imposing less pain during removal (Bennett, 1988). The silk suture is weaker than other synthetic sutures, and it is generally believed that it induces a higher level of tissue response than most other sutures except catgut (Postlethwait, Willigan, *et al.*, 1975). However, a recent report suggests that the higher level of tissue response may be caused by the residual sericin (glue-like proteins) on the silk fiber surface, while the core silk fibroin fibers exhibit comparable biocompatibility with other commonly used biomaterials (Altman, Diaz, *et al.*, 2003).

Polyamide (Nylon) suture was the first synthetic suture, introduced in 1940. It is slowly absorbable, classified as a non-absorbable suture. It loses its strength by hydrolysis at a rate of 15–20% each year. The nylon suture comes in either monofilament (e.g., Ethilon® and Dermalon®) or braided (e.g., Surgilon® and Nurolon®) forms. The braided sutures are more pliable and have better handling properties, but are more costly than monofilament sutures. Nylon sutures have high mechanical strength, high elasticity, and low cost. They are also inert, and therefore impose minimal tissue responses. However, nylon has low knot security because of its tendency to return to original state (memory), and thus an increased number of knot throws is needed to hold a stitch in place. An increase in the size or number of the knots, on the other hand, may lead to increased tissue responses (Meyer and Antonini, 1989).

Polyester sutures are made from polyethylene teraphthalate (PET), which is melt spun, stretched and braided into a multifilament strand. It has lower tissue response than silk sutures. They can be uncoated (e.g., Mersilene® and Dacron®) or coated (e.g., Ethibond®). Uncoated sutures have a rougher surface and may produce drag when pulled through the tissue, and are therefore difficult to handle but have good knot security. Other polyester sutures are coated with polybutilate, silicone or Teflon® to increase their surface smoothness, but at the cost of decreased knot security. The coatings may also enhance their tissue response. There have also been concerns about the coating's cracking after knots are tied (Moy, Waldman, *et al.*, 1992). Since polyester sutures maintain their high mechanical strength indefinitely after implantation, they can be used to fix implanted prosthetic materials (Meyer and Antonini, 1989).

Polypropylene is a linear hydrocarbon polymer. Polypropylene suture (e.g., Surgilene® and Prolene®) is a flexible monofilament in form, with an above average strength among sutures made of different materials. Polypropylene is also highly inert, and thus causes very low tissue response or adherence to the tissue. A distinctive characteristic of polypropylene sutures is that they have an extremely smooth surface and exert a minimal drag force when pulled through the tissue. The force required to remove the suture has been reported to be about one-third to two-thirds that of nylon and one-fourth to one-half that of silk (Freeman, Homsy, *et al.*, 1970). As a result, polypropylene can be a good choice for cutaneous procedures because, during its removal, it can be a "pull-out" suture with little disturbance to the tissue. The smooth surface, on the other hand, may cause low knot security, as the knots tend to slip easily. Polypropylene suture is known for its good plasticity. It stretches and deforms to accommodate wound swelling to avoid cutting through the tissue.

PTFE is the most inert polymer of all, and therefore PTFE sutures (e.g., Cytoplast®) induce minimal tissue response. Expanded PTFE (ePTFE) is used to produce monofilament sutures (e.g., Gore-Tex® suture) known for their high porosity. High porosity may reduce the mechanical strength of the sutures, but give them a unique compression capacity. This feature allows a needle-to-suture diameter ratio of nearly 1, which contributes to reduced suture hole blood leakage as compared to other sutures without compressive ability. In addition, the PTFE sutures also impose minimal drag to the tissue during the implantation and removal procedures (Gayle, Wheeler *et al.*, 1988; Ratner, 2004).

Sutures made from other materials are also known, but are not used as widely as the above mentioned:

1. Surgical cotton is a natural cellulose fiber; a cotton suture can be handled easily but is physically weak. It loses half of its strength in 6–9 months.

2. Polyethylene (e.g., Dermalene®) sutures are similar to polypropylene but have less tensile strength and knot security. It also slowly loses strength and eventually breaks down (Meyer and Antonini, 1989).

3. Polybutester (e.g., Novafil®) is a non-absorbable suture material occurring in monofilament form. It has high elasticity and memory, similar to a rubber band (Moy, Waldman, *et al.*, 1992).

4. Stainless steel is the strongest and least tissue reactive among all

TABLE 9.2. Relative Tensile Strength of Commonly Used Suture Materials
(Bennett, 1988).

Relative Tensile Strength	Nonabsorbable Sutures	Absorbable Sutures
High	Steel	
	Polyester	Polyglycolic acid
↑	Nylon (monofilament)	Polyglactin 910
	Nylon (braided)	
	Polypropylene	Polydioxanone
	Silk	
Low		Catgut

suture materials. However, it is stiff and may break at sites of bending, twisting and knotting. Handling and knotting of steel sutures
are difficult, but the knots are secure. They are usually used for bone
fixation (Meyer and Antonini, 1989).

Among the wide variety of sutures available today, not one of them
possess performance attributes that would suit all types of end uses. The
two major properties (strength and tissue reactivity) of the sutures are
compared in Tables 9.2 and 9.3. In addition to the performance of a suture, its choice also depends on criteria such as cost and type of surgery.

9.2. VASCULAR GRAFTS

Blood vessels are an essential part of the circulation system that
transport blood along with nutrients throughout the human body. Injured or diseased vessels may affect this critical transport process, causing cell death and tissue necrosis. When these happen to major arteries
such as the coronary arteries, the results may be severe and even lethal.

TABLE 9.3. Relative Tissue Reactivity of Commonly Used Suture Materials
(Bennett, 1988).

Relative Tissue Reactivity	Nonabsorbable Sutures	Absorbable Sutures
High		Catgut
	Silk, cotton	
↑	Coated polyester	Polyglactin 910
	Uncoated polyester	Polyglycolic acid
	Nylon	
	Polypropylene	
Low	Steel	

Product Development Question 9.1

The knot-tying process leads to residual force and distortion of the tissue. The knots may obstruct blood perfusion through capillary vessels and hinder wound healing. They are also the source of significant tissue response. Is there any way to minimize knotting or remove the knot during the use of sutures?

Suggested answer: When it is possible, a surgeon may choose to use a suture that will result in the smallest possible knots (e.g., a suture that is small in diameter) or/and require the smallest possible number of knots (e.g., a suture with better knot security). A newly developed barbed suture may provide a solution to this problem: such a suture is designed to be self-anchoring and knotless. A first trial of a non-absorbable barbed suture was conducted when a nylon barbed suture was applied in a flexor tendon repair, which proved to be an innovation that led to reduced tissue response (McKenzie, 1967). However, the non-absorbable suture needs to be removed afterwards. To date, most of the barbed sutures are made from absorbable materials such as polydioxane, so that no removal procedure is needed. A bi-directional barbed suture (Figure 9.3) contains barbs in a spiral pattern around the circumference of the suture, with the barbs divided into two groups facing each other in opposing directions (Dattilo, King, *et al.*, 2002). Clinical trials have suggested that the use of knotless barbed sutures can facilitate surgical wound closure (Einarsson, Chavan, *et al.*, 2011).

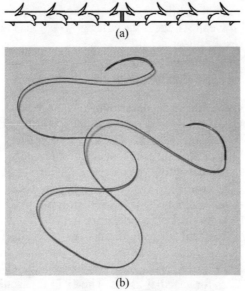

(a)

(b)

Figure 9.3. Bi-directional barbed suture: (a) a Sketch of a Bi-directional barbed suture, (b) Bi-directional barbed suture. The device is composed of delayed-absorbable polydioxanone (PDO), cut with barbs that change direction at the mid-point of the double-armed suture. [Reprinted with permission from (Siedhoff, Yunker *et al.*, 2011). Copyright (2011) Elsevier].

Cardiovascular disease has become the leading cause of death in developed countries. In 2004, coronary atherosclerosis, a condition in which fatty material accumulates along the walls of arteries, was reported to be responsible for 1.2 million hospital stays and result in over $44 billion in expense in the U.S. Peripheral arterial disease was reported to affect about 8 million Americans and be responsible for significant mortality. Treatment of coronary artery and peripheral vascular diseases often involves replacement of the diseased vessels with vascular grafts (Roger, Go, *et al.*, 2011).

Clinically speaking, the best replacements for the bypass of coronary artery and peripheral diseases are autologous veins or arteries from the patient. However, many patients do not have suitable vessels for implantation because of vascular diseases or previous treatments (Piccone, 1987). Implantation of vascular grafts from manmade materials thus became an alternative treatment, representing an annual market of approximately $200 million worldwide (Ku and Allen, 2006). An ideal vascular graft should be inert to cause minimum tissue response. It is also expected to provide mechanical properties (e.g., strength and elasticity) similar to host blood vessels so that it will be sufficiently compliant but not lead to overexpansion or bursting. It should possess a long-term mechanical stability in the human body to prevent graft leakage and abrasion wear. An ideal vascular graft is expected to serve the patient for the rest of his or her life.

9.2.1. Materials and Structures for Vascular Grafts

Vascular grafts with a textile structure have been used clinically since the 1950s. Polyamide fibers were used to fabricate the first vascular graft in 1956, but were soon replaced. A wide variety of grafts with different materials or structures are now commercially available. The majority of the vascular grafts, however, is made of polyethylene teraphthalate (PET/Dacron®), expanded polytetrafluoroethylene (ePTFE/ Gore-Tex®), or polyurethane (PU)-based polymers (Zilla, Bezuidenhout, *et al.*, 2007). All of the materials are hydrophobic and inert. PET fibers have high mechanical strength and can be easily fabricated into either woven or knit fabrics. The first PET vascular graft was introduced in 1957. PTFE is a relatively weak material, used usually in the form of membranes for vascular grafts. The ePTFE vascular grafts were first used in 1969. PU vascular grafts constitute a younger generation, and are known for two advantages over PET and ePTFE: elasticity and ease of handling. PU vascular grafts are available in fibrous or foamy forms. These different structures for vascular grafts will be explained as follows (Pourdeyhimi and Text, 1987).

9.2.1.1. Woven Vascular Grafts

Vascular grafts are in a woven structure, mostly plain wovens. They can be fabricated as seamless tubes on a shuttle loom. Bifurcated grafts are more complicated in structure and are often produced on a jacquard loom. Woven grafts are dimensionally stable, high in bursting strength, and low in their tendency to fatigue. They can be woven tightly to minimize water/blood leakage. However, they are very difficult to handle and suture, and tend to fray at the edges.

The woven vascular grafts can either have a smooth-walled or velour surface. The velour grafts are fabricated by introducing an extra end to the base fabric, as shown in Figure 9.4. It can produce floats on one or both sides of the graft surface. The velour yarns are less frequently interlaced with warp yarns than the ground warp yarns. They can be textured (i.e., yarns being endowed with significantly enhanced apparent volume, by the introduction of coils or loops into the fibers, via physical, chemical and/or heat treatments). The introduction of velour yarns makes the grafts softer, and allows reduction of the fabric tightness without adversely affecting their permeability. The velour structure allows greater yarn mobility, making the graft more compliant and easier to handle. It is suggested that velour woven grafts may have better healability than those that are smooth-walled.

9.2.1.2. Weft Knitted Vascular Grafts

Plain (jersey, stockinette) knits are some of the most frequently used structures for weft knitted vascular grafts. Weft knits are known for their high elasticity, especially in the course, or radial, direction. Such a characteristic is compliant with the behavior of the host artery. The weft knitted grafts have greater yarn mobility than the woven grafts,

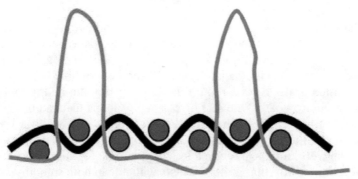

FIGURE 9.4. *The velour woven structure.*

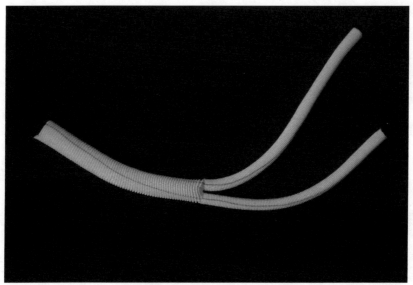

FIGURE 9.5. *A bifurcated vascular graft.*

making it easier for surgeons to handle and suture. On the other hand, the worst problem of weft knitted grafts has been traced to their high elasticity: it renders them vulnerable to leakage. Pre-coating treatment, as a result, is usually required before their implantation. In the early years of development, weft knitted grafts (or vascular grafts in another structure, if necessary) were subjected to the process of pre-clotting, in which a vascular graft was impregnated by the patient's blood to close the interstices of the graft through the clot formation. Such a practice has now largely been replaced by pre-coating grafts with other biocompatible polymers, like collagen and gelatin, not only to reduce leakage, but also enhance biocompatibility of the grafts (see also Section 9.3.3 for more detailed information).

The weft knit structure suffers for another problem: its cut-edge can curl up to make it difficult to suture. It can also have poor elastic recovery after implantation and exposure to cyclic loading, leading to graft enlargement in the radial direction. Another possible failure of the weft knitted grafts can be rupture because of running and unraveling of the structure; that is, the loss of a group of loops that can propagate throughout the length of the graft. A run usually starts with a breaking yarn. All these can lead to serious problems after implantation, and make the weft knitted structure a less popular one for vascular grafts.

Weft knitted vascular grafts are also available in both smooth-walled and velour surface forms. Velour grafts can be produced by using two (or more) sets of yarns in the fabrication and giving each set of yarns different loop heights (i.e., one set of yarns form the elongated or velour loops while the other form the ground loops). The velour loops usually face the inside of the tube. Velour grafts are easier to suture and handle than smooth-walled grafts, have higher degrees of healability, but do not run as easily.

9.2.1.3. Warp Knitted Vascular Grafts

The mechanical properties of warp knitted fabrics are somewhere between those of the woven fabrics and weft knitted fabrics, making the fabrics versatile in the design to resemble either woven or weft knitted fabrics. The most frequently used warp knitted structures for vascular grafts are the locknit and reverse locknit. Locknit (Figure 9.6) is also the most popular warp knitted structure, accounting for 70–80% of total output for all end uses. These structures are dimensionally stable and show a higher compliance in the course direction (i.e., radial direction of the tube) than in the wale direction (i.e., the longitudinal direction of the tube). Their compliance is higher than that of the woven grafts but lower than that of the weft knitted grafts. Locknit fabrics have smooth and soft handle. They are less likely to snag, split and curl than weft knitted fabrics, thus reducing the problems of running, unraveling, and curling up. Reversed locknit fabrics have a lower elasticity than locknit but do not curl (Spencer, 2001). The warp knitted grafts do not fray at the edge like woven grafts.

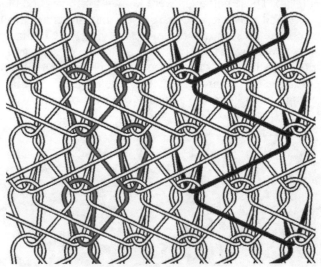

FIGURE 9.6. *A locknit structure.*

Warp knitted vascular grafts can have either a smooth-walled or velour surface. The velour grafts are produced by feeding an extra set of
textured yarns under a low tension and at a higher rate than the ground
yarns. As a result, the textured yarns are more exposed to the surface to
create the velour structure. The velour surface may further improve the
handle and healability of the grafts.

9.2.1.4. Membrane Vascular Grafts

Membrane grafts (e.g., Gore-Tex®, Impra® and Vitagraft®) are made
from expanded polytetrafluoroethylene (ePTFE). They are produced
from a PTFE film, which is stretched to produce a micro-porous structure, with an average pore size of 30 μm (Ku and Allen, 2006). PTFE is
the most chemically inert of all polymer materials, with minimal tissue
response as a result. However, these grafts are relatively non-compliant,
and have low mechanical strengths. They are mostly applied in small-
caliber vascular replacement. Dual-layer ePTFE grafts can be designed
to provide a tube with a high-porosity outer layer and low-porosity inner layer (Zilla, Bezuidenhout, et al., 2007).

9.2.1.5. PU Vascular Grafts

Vascular grafts made of PU-based polymers are relatively new and
still under extensive research and development. The most frequently
used polymers are poly(ether urethane) (PEU) and poly(carbonate urethane)s (PCUs). These polymers were known for their good blood biocompatibility and elasticity. PU-based vascular grafts are available in
a variety of structures: in one example (Corvita®), PCU filaments are
wound onto a rotating mandrel to form a multilayer tube, and a kitted
polyester (PET) structure is used as an external reinforcement to stabilize the graft. The PET reinforcement is bonded to the PCU tube through
a low melting point (30–50°C) adhesive of low-molecular weight PCU

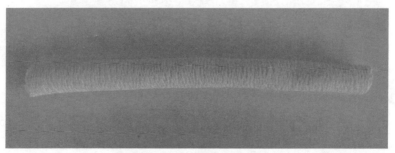

FIGURE 9.7. An ePTFE vascular graft.

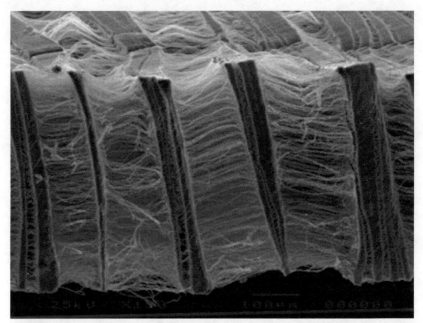

FIGURE 9.8. *Scanning electron micrograph of a cross-section through a high porosity ePTFE vascular graft [Reprinted with permission from (Zilla, Bezuidenhout, et al., 2007). Copyright (2007) Elsevier].*

(Wilson, MacGregor, *et al.*, 1993). Other PU-based vascular grafts may be fabricated via a phase-separation technique into a porous structure (Liu and Kodama, 1992): PU solution can be injected into a tubular mold, frozen at low temperature, and the solvents are dissolved out using water to form a porous tube (e.g., Pulse-Tec®, made of PEU). PU-based vascular grafts are usually developed for small-diameter (e.g., about 6 mm) vascular grafts (Zhang, Xie, *et al.*, 2010).

9.2.2. Problems of Current Vascular Grafts

Currently, vascular grafts suffer a number of limitations that need to be amended, circumvented, or resolved in future research and development. These problems are discussed in this section and some of the efforts to tackle them are explained in the next section.

9.2.2.1. Patency

Patency refers to the condition of being open and unobstructed. Patency is essential for the normal functioning of a vascular graft. Loss of patency is the leading cause of failure of vascular grafts. The life

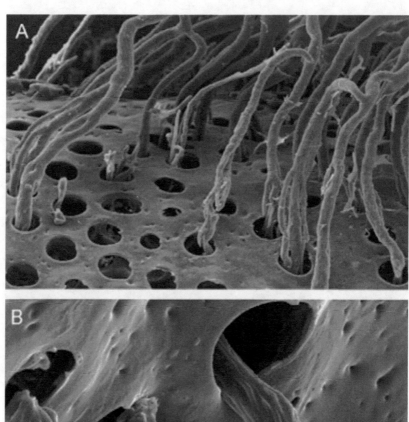

FIGURE 9.9. *A porous PU graft showing vessel ingrowth into its pores [Reprinted with permission from Zilla, Bezuidenhout, et al., 2007. Copyright (2007) Elsevier].*

span of vascular grafts is usually reported in the form of graft patency rate over a year. There has been no reported significant difference in patency rate between polyester and ePTFE grafts. Small-diameter vascular grafts, however, are more vulnerable to obstruction than grafts with larger diameters. Both polyester and ePTFE grafts perform well in large-diameter, high-flow and low-resistance sites. For example, grafts used for a bypass joining the abdominal aorta and the femoral arteries (aortofemoral bypass) have 5 to 10 year patency rates of 90% (Ratner, 2004). On the other hand, small-caliber grafts (< 6 mm) have much lower performance, with a 3-year patency below 25% (Dahl, Kypson, *et al.*, 2011). When a vascular graft is implanted into the human body, a series of events take place to affect its patency, including thrombosis in the early stage and tissue ingrowth in the next couple of years (Ku and Allen, 2006).

Thrombosis refers to the formation of thrombus, a fibrin clot that forms in a blood vessel or chamber of the heart. Thrombosis negatively affects the patency of a blood vessel, and may eventually lead to obstruction and failure of an implanted vascular graft. The mechanism of biomaterial-related thrombosis is not fully clear. To current knowledge, it involves a series of complicated reactions that will further result in platelet adhesion and formation of a clot. Blood flow dynamics play an important role in the growth of thrombi. The mismatch in mechanical (e.g., compliance) and surface properties (porosity and smoothness) between grafts and host vessels is believed to lead to cell damages and turbulent flows, which contribute to thrombosis (Gorbet and Sefton, 2004). As a result, it is an important task to develop vascular grafts that are less thrombogenic (i.e., more blood compatible).

Platelets and thrombin quickly accumulate on the inner surface of a graft within 24 hours after implantation. After that, cells may migrate from the host artery into the graft and proliferate, and a large amount of extracellular substance may be synthesized and deposited inside the vessel, leading to significant occlusion.

9.2.2.2. Dilation

Dilation is the enlargement of the grafted vessel diameter after implantation. The implanted vascular graft is subjected to both static pressure and cyclic pulsating load so that permanent deformation (i.e., enlargement of the diameter, or dilation) to some extent is unavoidable. It is suggested that dilation of a graft at an early stage after implantation is primarily caused by the fabric structure. Weft knitted fabrics are especially vulnerable to such dilation, because their constituent loops can be easily straightened. Warp knitted grafts are more stable than weft knitted grafts, while woven structures are most resistant to structural deformation. On the other hand, the dilation of a graft late in its service life may be induced by material fatigue, or the permanent deformation or breakage of fibers or polymer chains caused by cyclic load (Pourdey-himi and Wagner, 1986).

9.2.2.3. Other Mechanical Failure

Other mechanical failure of vascular grafts may include surface abrasion caused by interactions between the grafts and neighboring tissues, as well as suture-line deterioration. Sutures are usually needed during an implant operation to join a vascular graft to the host vessels. A suture line represents an area of stress concentration caused by the mismatch in compliance between a host vessel and a graft: a host artery has higher compliance than a graft. The interactions between the implants (sutures and grafts) and body fluid may further weaken the materials to induce suture-line deterioration failure and blood leakage. The suture-line deterioration may manifest in one or more of the following ways. The suture may lose its strength with time due to fatigue and degenerative reactions in the presence of body fluids and enzymes, and finally fracture. Another possible failure can be graft yarn slippage (which is common for woven grafts, especially at the fabric edges) or breakage (more common in knitted grafts) at the suture line. Finally, a suture may tear from a host vessel wall, caused either by a diseased host vessel or strength of suture/graft materials larger than that of the host vessel (Pourdeyhimi, Harrison, et al., 1986).

These problems often lead to failure of a vascular graft during its service. They constitute grave threats to the stability and life span of vascular grafts, and have engendered extensive research and development work to improve the performance and stability of vascular grafts, especially the small-diameter ones. Some of the important efforts are discussed in the next section.

9.2.3. Modification Processes for Vascular Grafts

Freshly taken from a knitting machine or weaving loom, the tubular fabrics for vascular grafts usually need further treatment before they can be used. Processes for such treatment include compaction, crimping and sterilization (Pourdeyhimi, Harrison et al., 1986).

Compaction is adopted to reduce the porosity of vascular grafts to avoid leakage during their end uses. This procedure is especially important for knitted grafts. During their fabrication processes, fabrics are usually subjected to tension, which causes degrees of structural elongation or deformation in fabrics, yarns, fibers and even polymer chains. Either thermal (i.e., dry or wet heat that cause shrinking) or chemical (swelling agents or solvents, or a combination of the two) means can be used to reverse such deformation. However, both chemical and thermal treatments may reduce the mechanical strength of the grafts. In addition, there are concerns about whether a chemical treatment may affect biocompatibility and toxicity of the materials to be implanted.

Crimping (i.e., the creation of curls or pleats on the surface of a graft) is used to increase the bulkiness of the graft surface so as to enhance a graft's resistance to compression. Compression exerted on a graft by neighboring tissues, especially bones or joints, may bend the graft and cause occlusion. To achieve the goal of crimping, a mold designed according to the desired configuration is coupled to a heat-setting to operate together. Such a process will significantly improve a vascular graft's compression resistance. However, it is suggested that a graft surface thus crimped may increase the likelihood of thrombosis and occlusion as compared to a non-crimped graft (Herring, Dilley, *et al.*, 1980). An alternative design to solve the problem is to fabricate an externally supported vascular graft: a polypropylene monofilament is wrapped and heat-fused onto the outer surface of the graft and, as a result, the graft will be given a smooth inner surface that allows smooth flow of the blood to improve the patency, and a bulky outer surface to enhance the compression resistance (Kenney, Sauvage, *et al.*, 1982).

Sterilization, a treatment to follow manufacturing, is essential for the grafts to be free from bacteria so as to reduce the risk of infection. γ-irradiation is the most popular treatment adopted by graft manufacturers, while thermal (dry or wet heat) or chemical sterilization is preferred in hospitals when re-sterilization is needed.

In addition to the above commonly used treatments, other modifications have been developed and used to improve performance of vascular grafts. The most frequently employed modification process is surface immobilization of bio-molecules to reduce infection and/or thrombosis of the grafts. A variety of treatments have been used to modify the surface of vascular grafts so as to control infection and suppress platelet and/or protein adhesion.

Cases of vascular graft-related infection are more frequently attributed to the surgery than to the grafts themselves (Pourdeyhimi, Harrison, *et al.*, 1986). Whatever the cause, they may cause serious problems. A vascular graft can be given a capacity for *infection control* with a coating of anti-bacterial agent(s), including silver compounds (Clark and Margraf, 1974) and/or antibiotics (e.g., rifampicin) (Selan, Artini, *et al.*, 2010).

Anti-thrombosis is another major target in the treatment of vascular grafts. Collagen or gelatin is among the first bio-molecules used to treat vascular grafts for improved blood compatibility (reduced thrombosis). Collagen is a natural polymer found in human connective tissues; gelatin is a denatured collagen. Both of them are known for being biocompatible and bioresorbable. However, it is vital that the agents for use, especially collagen, be absolutely clean and pure, for contaminants may cause abnormal inflammatory responses (Yamamoto, Noishiki, *et al.*, 1993). Vascular grafts are usually impregnated with these proteins not only to aid clotting and reduce graft leakage after implantation, but also to improve their biocompatibility. Poly(ethylene glycol) (PEG) is another frequently used polymer to treat vascular grafts, because it has been found to be able to reduce platelet adhesion and non-specific protein adhesion, and thereby alleviates immune and inflammatory responses (Dimitrievska, Maire, *et al.*, 2011). Heparin (Figure 9.10) is a highly-sulfated glycosaminoglycan known as an anticoagulant. Heparin-treated vascular grafts have received much attention recently. Heparin can be immobilized onto graft materials via a variety of methods, which, in the sequence of increasing binding stability, are impregnation, ionic interactions and covalent binding (Wendel and Ziemer, 1999). However, results of research work towards improvement on the *in vivo* biocompatibility of vascular grafts by means of heparin treatment remain mixed and unproven (Levy and Hartman, 1996; Gorbet and Sefton, 2004).

There have been many approaches to the improvement of the overall biocompatibility of vascular grafts, including the use of antibodies (Fitch, Rollins, *et al.*, 1999), inhibitors (Murkin, 1997) and growth factors (Heidenhain, Veeravoorn, *et al.*, 2011). Still one more effort is the introduction of viable cells into the vascular graft, an effort typically found in the field of tissue engineering and regenerative medicine, as will be discussed in greater detail in the next chapter.

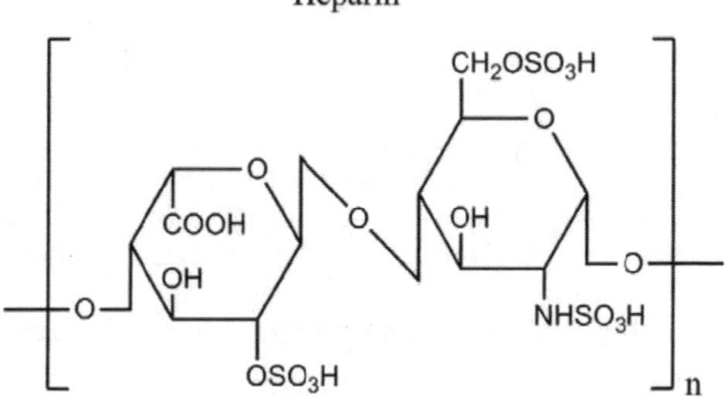

Heparin

FIGURE 9.10. *Heparin.*

9.3. LIGAMENT PROSTHESIS

Ligaments are strong and highly elastic strips of tissue that connect one bone to another. There are four main stabilizing ligaments at the knee joint (Figure 9.11): anterior cruciate ligament (ACL), posterior cruciate ligament (PCL), medial collateral ligament (MCL) and lateral collateral ligament (LCL). Among them, ACL is the one that connects the femur bone to the tibia bone and controls the extent to which the tibia can move in relation to the femur. ACL is the most frequently injured ligament and can be torn at a force of about 3.3 times the body weight (Noyes and Grood, 1976). ACL injuries are usually associated with sports that require sudden hyperextension or rotation forces, such as basketball, soccer, football and skiing. An injured ACL has poor intrinsic healing potential and needs surgical intervention. It is estimated that in the United States about 95,000 new ACL injuries occur each year, and more than 50,000 ACL reconstructions are performed annually (Frank and Jackson, 1997).

Three types of treatment are available. *Autograft* involves taking tendon (i.e., a fibrous cord or band that connects a muscle with its bony attachment) tissues (Dirckx, 2001) from the patient to have his ACL reconstructed. Tissues for this purpose are harvested from the hamstring (i.e., a tendon bounding the space behind the knee) (Dirckx, 2001) or patella (i.e., knee cap) tendons (Spindler, Magnussen, *et al.*, 2011). Autograft is generally believed to be the best treatment because there is no issue of host responses. However, it has the drawback of additional injury and pain in the harvesting site, and can be limited by the availability or adequacy of healthy tissues from the patient. The next option is *allograft,* in which graft tissues are obtained from a donor's cadaver. Allografts, however, are associated with such concerns as host responses, mechanical properties and risk of disease transmission (Nutton, McLean, *et al.*, 1999). The last option for treating ACL injuries is the use of a *ligament prosthesis.* Synthetic materials such as PET, PTFE and carbon fibers have been used to produce ligament prostheses. A performing ligament prosthesis is expected to have a high tensile strength, a high elongation and recovery, and a stiffness that matches that of the host ACL, which are requirements on which the choice of ligament prosthesis materials is based, as discussed in the following.

PTFE ligament prostheses are fabricated from braided filaments of expanded PTFE (a porous material comprising about 75% air by volume), containing approximately 180 strands (Indelicato, Pascale, *et al.*, 1989). Short-term clinical outcomes have shown that the grafts have excellent biocompatibility, easy handling and reduced healing time (Vogel, 1992). However, reports about problems related to PTFE ligament

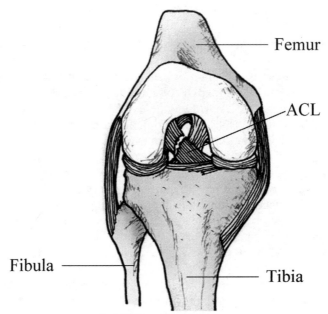

FIGURE 9.11. *ACL at the knee joint.*

prostheses increased in the 1990s. The problems include graft breakage and weakening, as well as inflammation. As a result, the graft was withdrawn from the market in 1993 (Muren, Dahlstedt, *et al.*, 2005).

Carbon fibers are used as ligament prostheses in the form of braided bundles. They have high mechanical strength and good biocompatibility, and have been reported to support tissue proliferation (Osborne, Telfer, *et al.*, 1984). However, the drawback of carbon fibers used as ligament prostheses is their high fragility and brittleness, which will result in relatively low resistance to abrasion and strain failure (Blazewicz, Wajler, *et al.*, 1996).

PET is a popular material for ligament prostheses, given its good biological and mechanical properties (Seitz, Marlovits, *et al.*, 1998). It is also available in the form of braided filament strands. A clinical follow up study suggested that the long-term (1–8.3 years) stability of PET ligament prostheses is acceptable, with over 80% good and excellent results (subjective patients' evaluation). The rest, however, may fail within a short time due to different causes (e.g., inflammation, ruptures and infection), or lead to complaints like pain, swelling and lack of motion (Krudwig, 2002).

Ultrahigh molecular weight polyethylene (UHMWPE) is a relatively new material for ligament prostheses. Therefore, clinical data for its performance are limited. In a 14-year prospective study on a small number of patients (16), the UHMWPE braided ligament prosthesis was found to function in a way similar to an autograft. Such a UHMWPE braided ACL prosthesis contains more than 4000 filaments, and has a high tensile strength (9000N) (Purchase, Mason, *et al.*, 2007).

Other fiber materials that have been used to produce ligament prostheses include polypropylene (Kdolsky, Gibbons, *et al.*, 1997), aramid fibers (Dauner, Planck, *et al.*, 1990), and carbon/PET fiber composites (Campbell and Rae, 1995). Despite decades of research and development work in the area, there has been no perfect graft for ACL reconstruction. There are problems to be solved. Long-term stability is still the major concern. Mechanical problems include creep (permanent deformation as a result of applied stress), fatigue caused by cyclic loads, and wear fragments as a result of abrasion damage. Clinical symptoms that follow may be pain, swelling and inflammation, which can lead to the failure of a graft, too. There is also concern about the weak link where a ligament prosthesis is surgically fixed to a bone, usually via staples or screws. Failures at these sites may be ascribed to the implantation procedures (Krudwig, 2002). With such problems looming so large, usefulness of the ligament prosthesis for ligament reconstruction has been a controversial issue. Efforts to bring about significant improvement, however, have not been slackened nor suspended. Among these, tissue engineering seems to be promising, as will be discussed in the next chapter.

9.4. HERNIA REPAIR MESH GRAFTS

A hernia usually refers to the protrusion of a part of or a structure through the tissues normally containing it (Dirckx, 2001). Hernias can occur in a number of locations in the body, but is most commonly found in the abdomen, where a bag forms by the lining of the abdominal cavity and protrudes through the fascia (i.e., the connective tissue surrounding the muscle in the abdominal wall). Abdominal hernias may occur at a weak area or a scar (e.g., due to a previous abdominal surgery) in the abdominal wall, and cause pain or lead to life-threatening complications. Inguinal hernia (i.e., a hernia in the groin) is the most common, and affects about 16% of adult men (Cheek, Black, *et al.*, 1998). It is reported that over 700,000 cases of inguinal hernia surgery are performed per year in the US and Europe (Grant and Collaboration, 2002).

Typical hernia repair procedures usually involve mesh grafts to be placed and sutured onto the weak spot to prevent hernia recurrence. An ideal mesh graft will provide both appropriate mechanical strength and flexibility, as well as a scaffold for tissue incorporation and infection resistance (Parker, Ayubi, *et al.*, 2008). Both absorbable (e.g., polyglactin, collagen) and non-absorbable (e.g., polypropylene, polyester) materials have been used, as explained below.

Polypropylene (PP) is the most popular non-absorbable material for hernia mesh grafts. PP is hydrophobic and chemically inert. However, it is relatively low in flexibility. As a result, PP mesh grafts (e.g., Marlex®, Prolene®) for hernia repair are usually constructed in a warp knitted structure to favor elasticity (Jiang, Miao, *et al.*, 2005). They are fabricated from either monofilament or multifilament strands. Tissue responses to PP meshes may vary, depending on properties and structures of the material. It is generally believed that lighter-weight and more porous PP meshes perform better in terms of biocompatibility and handling, although the optimal density and porosity remains unknown (Earle and Mark, 2008). Still, PP mesh grafts for hernia repair bring concerns about adhesion between the graft and host tissue, which may lead to chronic pain and complications like intestinal obstruction (Bellon, Rodriguez, *et al.*, 2007).

Polyethylene terephthalate (PET) is another nonabsorbable synthetic material frequently used for implants. It has been reported to provide adequate strength, good elasticity, moderate tissue response and minimal risk of infection (Hamy, Pessaux, *et al.*, 2003). PET mesh grafts (e.g., Surgimesh®, Mersilene®) are usually in a knitted structure, made from either monofilament or multifilament strands. However, there are also concerns about adhesion between the graft and host tissue and consequent complications (Marchal, Brunaud, *et al.*, 1999). Their degradation over time, especially in an infected environment, may be a potential problem (Earle and Mark, 2008).

Polytetrafluoroethylene (ePTFE) is the most inert polymer. ePTFE mesh grafts (e.g., Gore® Dualmesh®) have the important advantage of inducing minimal graft-tissue adhesion, as compared to other nonabsorbable mesh grafts (Earle and Mark, 2008). It is suggested that the ePTFE mesh graft can be a good alternative to the PP mesh graft because of its several features: minimal tissue response, stability in the presence of body fluid, and softness (owing to its smooth surface) that will diminish adhesion (Athanasakis, Saridaki, *et al.*, 2000).

Partially absorbable mesh grafts is a product developed to reduce polymer density (and consequently tissue response) but maintain handling properties and long-term material strength. They can be fabricated by mixing a nonabsorbale polymer (e.g., PP) with an absorbable polymer (e.g., polyglactin). A composite mesh containing both PP and polyglactin multifilament (e.g., Vypro®) has been found to impose less tissue response than pure PP mesh (Rosch, Junge, *et al.*, 2003), although the pure PP mesh has a higher strength than the composite one (Earle and Mark, 2008).

Collagen is the most frequently used material for absorbable mesh grafts, known also as *biologic prosthetics,* the application of which is limited because of their much higher cost. Collagen mesh grafts (e.g., Surgisis®, Permacol®) are designed to provide a scaffold for native cells to grow and to produce connective tissues to replace the defected ones. The design is conceptually similar to tissue engineering approaches (as discussed in the next chapter) and shares objectives—that is, to minimize tissue response and promote healing. However, comparative studies *in vivo* have found no significant difference between absorbable and nonabsorbable mesh grafts in terms of healing time, post-surgical complications or recurrence (Sadat, Markar, *et al.*, 2010).

Various types of treatment have been developed to enhance performance of the mesh grafts by endowing them with antibacterial and antiadhesion functions, or to impart better biocompatibility. For example, grafts can be impregnated with silver carbonate and chlorhexidine diacetate to render the graft antibacterial (as is Dualmesh® Plus). An absorbable omega-3 fatty acid derived from fish oil was coated onto a PP mesh (C-Qur™) to avoid immune response, with the coating to be about 70% absorbed in 120 days and all the protein removed (Earle and Mark, 2008). Another absorbable carbohydrate, oat beta glucan, was coated onto a PP mesh, and the coated graft was found (according to the 2-year follow-up study) to have significantly reduced severe pain as compared to an uncoated graft (Champault and Barrat, 2005).

Despite large amounts of research and development work on hernia repair mesh grafts, an ideal graft for such repair has not yet been found. Future efforts should aim to improve the overall properties of such grafts, including appropriate mechanical strength and elasticity, ease of handling, minimal tissue response, diminished adhesion and recurrence.

9.5. EXTRACORPOREAL DEVICES: ARTIFICIAL KIDNEY

A human being's life depends on the normal function of all his or her organs. Some of them are involved in the complicated processes of filtration of the waste, detoxification, metabolism, and transfer or exchange of mass and nutrients to the other parts of the body. Acute failure of any of these organs will lead to serious disturbance to the entire system of life, and is often fatal. Accordingly, extracorporeal devices and/or systems of devices have been developed either as substitutes for the failing organs or as a means of temporary aid to the patient whose organs are failing him. Fibrous materials are suitable for applications involving filtration and transport because they have larger surface areas and highly porous structures. Medical filters made from porous hollow fibers have important applications in providing long-term or temporary extracorporeal supports for such failed human organs as the kidney, liver, lungs and pancreas.

In this section, the artificial kidney, or hemodialyzer, which has been widely adopted in clinics for renal support, will be discussed. Other extracorporeal devices (e.g., artificial liver) that involve living cells will be discussed in the next chapter.

The kidney serves to filter waste products out of the human body and regulate levels of electrolytes (ionizable substances in solutions, e.g., NaCl) that are essential for the normal functioning of the body (e.g., maintaining a stable pH level and regulating a normal blood pressure). The kidney is also responsible for secreting certain hormones. A person can live with one healthy kidney. However, if both kidneys fail, toxins and fluids can accumulate in the body to cause malfunction of the blood. If untreated, these conditions may lead to serious illnesses and even death.

According to statistics provided by the US National Kidney Foundation (www.kidney.org), more than 26 million American adults (about 13% of the adult population) suffer from chronic kidney disease; more than 526,000 Americans are being treated for kidney failure, including over 367,000 patients who are receiving dialysis treatment and 158,000 receiving kidney transplants. The artificial kidney, or hemodialyzer, is the first synthetic device that has been used to perform the major functions of a human organ, and as a therapy is the only successful long-term ex vivo (i.e., out of the body) organ substitution to date (Humes, Fissell, *et al.*, 2006).

9.5.1. Hemodialyzer

The hemodialyzer has been used clinically as an artificial renal support since 1923 (Clark, 2000). It provides two basic functions expected of the human kidney: hemodialysis and ultrafiltration. A hemodialyzer usually consists of two compartments divided by a semi-permeable membrane. The semi-permeable membrane will allow small molecules such as water and electrolytes to freely pass through. Red and white blood cells and fat and protein molecules will be prevented from passing through the membrane owing to their larger sizes, and be left behind in the blood compartment. As a result, only body waste will be filtered out of the human blood.

The membrane used in a clinical dialyzer is made from cellulose or synthetic polymers, and consists of bundles of about 10,000 hollow fibers, the internal diameter of which is around 200 μm (Klein, Ward, *et al.*, 1987). It allows blood to flow, a few ounces at a time, through the lumen of hollow fibers. Concentrations of the various electrolytes in the blood must be maintained within narrow limits if serious harm to the patient is to be avoided. To that end, the extracapillary space of the dialyzer is filled with a dialysate bath, a mineral solution; its concentrations of sodium, potassium, chloride, and other electrolytes are made to approximate normal levels in the human blood serum. As a result, concentrations of these particles will in the course of dialysis become nearly equal on both sides of the membrane, and the undesirable waste products in the blood will be filtered out owing to the constant supply of fresh solution to keep levels of the waste low in the dialysate bath.

The other function of the artificial kidney, ultrafiltration, is the removal of excess water from the body of the patient by the pressure difference between the lumen and extracapillary space. In the case where the patient has gained more than the recommended amount of fluid since the last dialysis, a negative pressure (suction) can be applied to the dialysate.

In the case described above, blood is taken from the artery of a patient by a system of tubes to the artificial kidney for dialysis and ultrafiltration, and will eventually be returned by another tube to the patient's vein (Noordwijk, 2001). For a patient to undergo dialysis for 15 years, his blood will have to have contact with approximately 4,000 m^2 of foreign surface (Stamatialis, Papenburg, *et al.*, 2008).

9.5.2. Materials for Hemodialyzer

As noted from the above description, the semi-permeable filtering membrane or cellophane is the key element for the hemodialyzer. Early-stage hemodialyzers contain cellophane tubing or stacked cellophane sheets (Clark, 2000), and are nowadays looked upon with disfavor for their instability and poor efficiency. New, more efficient hemodialyzers are based on the function of hollow–fiber bioreactors (Figure 9.12). A bioreactor consists of a large number of small fibers made from semipermeable membranes, functioning collectively through a cylindrical shell/jacket (Sueoka and Takakura, 1991; Clark, 2000; Tzanakakis, Hess, *et al.*, 2000). The intratubular space of such a fiber is called the lumen or capillary space, and the space at the outside is called the extracapillary space. They constitute the two compartments across which filtration takes place. Two types of polymers are exploited in building hollow fiber bioreactors: cellulose-based polymers and synthetic polymers (Woffindin and Hoenich, 1995).

Cellulose-based polymers are the first used materials for hollow fiber membranes. It is now clear that free hydroxyl groups (–OH) give poor blood compatibility (Bowry, 2002), and this explains why modified cellulosic materials have come to be used. Quite a few cellulose-based polymers have been used for hemodialyzers, including cellulose acetate, cellulose triacetate and cuprammonium rayon (Cuprophan). Cuprammonium rayon is produced by dissolving cellulose into an ammonium solution of copper hydroxide. The copper-ammonia-cellulose complex is then extruded into an acid bath to yield the fibers. Cuprammonium rayon is often referred to as unmodified cellulose and regarded as bio-incompatible (Boure and Vanholder, 2004). Other modified cellulose-based polymers can be produced by replacing part (cellulose acetate) or almost all three (cellulose triacetate) of the hydroxyl groups (–OH) in the six-membered rings with acetyl groups (–OCOCH$_3$). Although it is suggested that free hydroxyl groups contribute to poor blood compatibility, *in vivo* data show that there has been no correlation made between the number of hydroxyl groups replaced and the improvement in blood biocompatibility of the material—that is, the cellulose triacetate membrane does not necessarily have better blood compatibility than the cellulose acetate membrane, indicating not all hydroxyl groups behave in the same manner (Hoenich, Woffindin, *et al.*, 1995).

Synthetic polymers for synthetic hollow fiber membranes can be polysulfone, polyamide, and polyacrylonitrile, among which polysulfone is the most frequently used. These synthetic hollow fiber membranes are made from hydrophobic polymers and are designed to have

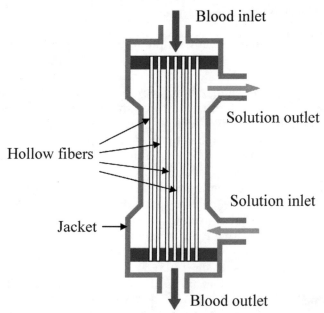

FIGURE 9.12. *A typical hollow fiber dialyzer.*

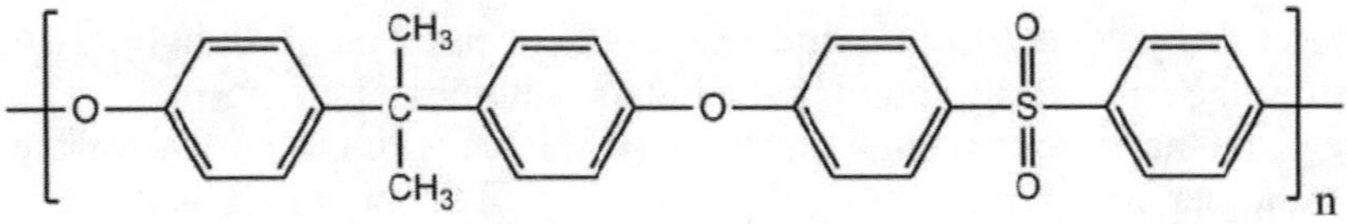

FIGURE 9.13. *Polysulfone.*

larger pore sizes and higher water permeability than cellulose-based membranes. They are therefore referred to as "high-flux" membranes as compared to traditional "low-flux" cellulose-based membranes.

Polysulfone polymers (Figure 9.13) were introduced in the 1960s. Polysulfone membranes have good thermal and chemical stability, and outstanding mechanical and film-forming properties, which cause them to be the most popular synthetic polymer used for hemodialyzers. Comparative studies suggest that there is no significant difference between polysulfone and modified cellulose-based dialyzers in terms of blood compatibility (Hoenich, Woffindin, *et al.*, 1995; Jaber, Alonso, *et al.*, 2009). However, these two types of dialyzers do differ in their efficiency of clearance or removal of drugs, and in their capacity to maintain the normal level of plasma lipids: clearance rates of drugs, such as Ranitidine (Tsuruoka, Sugimoto, *et al.*, 2000) and ofloxacin (Thalhammer, Kletzmayr, *et al.*, 1998), were found to be significantly higher with polysulfone dialyzers than with modified cellulose-based dialyzers, and patients using polysulfone dialyzers were found to be better off in terms of plasma lipid levels than using modified cellulose-based dialyzers (Kovacic and Roguljic, 2003).

9.5.3. Problems and Solutions: Modification for Hemodialyzers

Hemodialysis as a therapy has no doubt changed the lives of patients with kidney failure. However, existing hemodialysis devices (particularly the hollow fiber membranes) are still reported to have an annual mortality rate of over 20%. Therefore it is essential to tackle the various shortcomings of these devices to effect performance improvement (Humes, Fissell, *et al.*, 2006).

Biocompatibility is the most important criterion for any polymer material to be used in direct contact with living organisms. In the case of hollow fiber bioreactors for hemodialysis, blood compatibility is essential because it helps avoid thrombus, or blood coagulation. Also, since some of the small molecular weight toxins may adhere quickly to the albumin in the course of hemodialysis, making it difficult for them to be removed through diffusion, it is desirable that a hollow fiber bioreactor is anti-fouling, a property much dependent on the device's compatibility with blood. To that end, a modification is made to hollow fiber bioreactors by using a novel material: polymers based on phospholipids, a substance plentifully found in the human cell membrane.

2-methacryloyloxyethyl phosphorylcholine (MPC) is a methacrylate monomer with a phospholipid polar group. Its copolymers have been used for the modification of hollow fiber membranes. MPC polymers are used as an additive for polysulfone membranes, and have proved able to effectively reduce protein adsorption and platelet adhesion, improving blood compatibility as a result (Ishihara, Fukumoto, *et al.*, 1999; Ishihara, Fukumoto, *et al.*, 1999). Cellulose acetate hollow fiber membranes are also modified with MPC polymers by means of blending or surface coating (Ye, Watanabe, *et al.*, 2005; 2006). These membranes manifest better permeability, hemocompatibility and cytocompatibility, and therefore can be used for the purpose of hemopurification and in the construction of liver assist bioreactors.

Synthetic membranes are hydrophobic, making them vulnerable to adsorption of proteins, which affect their permeability and clearance efficiency. As a result, there has been a trend to enhance the hydrophilicity of synthetic membranes. Polymers or monomers have also been used to modify the surface of hollow fiber membranes. Polyvinylpyrrolidone (PVP), a hydrophilic polymer, can be covalently conjugated with polysulfone membranes to improve their hydrophilicity. For polysulfone membranes, this modification procedure has been related to a much smaller number of adhering platelets and lower level of plasma protein adsorption, as compared to those that have not undergone such modification (Higuchi, Shirano, *et al.*, 2002). PVP can also be used as an additive to polyethersulfone membranes to improve their hydrophilicity and blood compatibility (Torrestiana-Sanchez, Ortiz-Basurto, *et al.*, 1999; Wang, Yu, *et al.*, 2009). Poly(ethylene glycol) (PEG) is a hydrophilic polymer, very compatible with peptides and proteins, and nontoxic in the body. Polysulfone membranes with surface-grafted PEG have been reported to have better hydrophilicity and blood compatibility (Song, Sheng, *et al.*, 2000). Poly(acrylic acid) is believed to be able to improve surface performance of polysulfone membranes (Ulbricht and Riedel, 1998). There is evidence that single strand DNA immobilized onto polysulfone membranes with UV-irradiation helps reduce protein adsorption onto, and increase blood compatibility of, the membranes (Zhao, Liu, *et al.*, 2003).

The use of physical methods, such as low-temperature plasma treatment, has been reported for the purpose of hydrophilic surface modification of polysulfone and polyacrylonitrile membranes (Ulbricht and Belfort, 1996; Song, Sheng *et al.*, 2000; Steen, Hymas, *et al.*, 2001). For instance, treatment with water plasma and helium plasma will drastically increase the surface hydrophilicity of polysulfone membranes and reduce their protein retention (Ulbricht and Belfort, 1996). It is believed that the low-temperature water plasma treatment will result in permanent hydrophilic surface modification: the plasma-treated polysulfone membranes will remain wettable for over 16 months after the treatment (Steen, Hymas, *et al.*, 2001).

Traditional hemodialyzers have been performing, with degrees of success, two critical functions on behalf of the human kidney in cases when it has failed to function naturally: dialysis and ultrafiltration. Traditional hemodialyzers have not been able to fulfill other important functions, such as excretion of hormones essential for the normal functioning of organs of the human body. In addition, current efforts to modify hollow fiber materials have not fully solved the critical problem of blood biocompatibility. Fortunately, new efforts have been added from the field of tissue engineering, with promising approaches to the solution of their shared problems. See the next chapter.

9.6. SUMMARY

This chapter provides a discussion of the various textiles that are used *biologically*, i.e., used either as a material to be implanted into the human flesh (as is the case of sutures and vascular grafts) or into a medical device (e.g., artificial kidney) to be in contact with human tissues (e.g., blood). In both cases these textiles encounter, or even interact with, human cells and/or human biological fluids—hence the name "biotextiles". Such use predetermines the many prerequisites for the textiles, especially that the material and device to be implanted must biologically suit the physiological environment in the human body, and be able to stay there for a relatively long period of time. These two properties, respectively known as biocompatibility and biostability, the two fundamental properties of any biomaterial or biological device, are highlighted throughout the chapter.

Biological qualities are multidimensional—they are physically, chemically, or even psychologically determined and measured. Thus we are concerned about the physical and chemical features. We also have to attend to a psychological dimension of physical comfort, namely, the patients' complaint about "pain".

Discussion in this chapter is arranged to follow these lines:

1. The discussion of materials and devices is performance-oriented. Since performance is the combined consequence of the various properties, the discussion of performance is a discussion of properties. For instance, a most important performance of a vascular graft

is to better serve the patient for the rest of his life. Therefore, the material must have high mechanical strength, and be chemically inert, which are properties necessary for biostability.

2. This discussion of properties includes both desirable properties and undesirable ones, so that we know what material is compatible with its end use. For instance, the performance of sutures depends on physical properties such as elasticity and knot strength, which are closely related to their handling properties, such as pliability and knottability. These properties indicate how easily the suture can be handled by the surgeon, and depend on the extent to which the use of sutures causes *tissue response,* an obviously undesirable property of suture materials. A clarification of both desirable and undesirable properties favors wise choice of materials.

3. This discussion of properties is important because it is related to specific structures or materials (sometimes with product brands) and devices. For instance, in the discussion of vascular grafts to be implanted into the body as replacement of the diseased blood vessels, many structures have been identified and clarified: the membrane, warp knitted, weft knitted, and woven structures. For the same purpose, many materials have been listed for sutures: catgut, polyamide (Nylon), polydioxanone, polyester, polyglactin 910, polyglycolic acid (PGA), polypropylene, PTFE, and silk. Discussions of materials are often aided with tables, where they can be directly related to properties.

4. Since performance is often a function of fabrication and modification processes, such processes have been combined into the discussion. Generally, they are discussed for three purposes, i.e., to represent them as means of: (a) solving problems originating in materials and/ or manifested in devices, such as the high elasticity-related leakage problem suffered by weft knitted grafts, which has its solution in the process of pre-coating; (b) performance improvement, e.g., by the process of "crimping" there will be significant improvement in the compression resistance of a vascular graft; and (c) adding new functions, as instanced by adding a coating of anti-bacterial agent(s) to the surface of a vascular graft so as to render it capable of "infection control".

By highlighting performance, related aspects have been addressed in two directions: (1) materials to constitute the bio-textile and the bio-textile as a material to constitute the various biological devices— presented in such a way that each material is correlated to its properties; (2) the various fabrication and modification processes—presented in such a way that they are correlated to the problems they are intended to tackle and the performance improvement they bring about as a result.

9.7. REFERENCES

Altman, G.H., F. Diaz, *et al.* (2003). Silk-based biomaterials. *Biomaterials* **24**(3): 401–416.

Athanasakis, E., Z. Saridaki, *et al.* (2000). Surgical repair of inguinal hernia: Tension free technique with prosthetic materials (Gore-Tex Mycro Mesh expanded polytetrafluoroethylene). *American Surgeon* **66**(8): 728–731.

Bellon, J.M., M. Rodriguez, *et al.* (2007). Peritoneal effects of prosthetic meshes used to repair abdominal wall defects: monitoring adhesions by sequential laparoscopy. *Journal of Laparoendoscopic & Advanced Surgical Techniques* **17**(2): 160–166.

Bennett, R.G. (1988). Continuing medical-education—selection of wound closure materials. *Journal of the American Academy of Dermatology* **18**(4): 619–640.

Blazewicz, S., C. Wajler, *et al.* (1996). Static and dynamic fatigue properties of carbon ligament prosthesis. *Journal of Biomedical Materials Research* **32**(2): 215–219.

Boure, T. and R. Vanholder (2004). Which dialyser membrane to choose? *Nephrology Dialysis Transplantation* **19**(2): 293–296.

Bowry, S.K. (2002). Dialysis membranes today. *International Journal of Artificial Organs* **25**(5): 447–460.

Campbell, A.C. and P.S. Rae. (1995). Anterior cruciate reconstruction with the ABC carbon and polyester prosthetic ligament. *Annals of the Royal College of Surgeons of England* **77**(5): 349–350.

Champault, G. and C. Barrat. (2005). Inguinal hernia repair with beta glucan-coated mesh: results at two-year follow up. *Hernia* **9**(2): 125–30.

Cheek, C.M., N.A. Black, *et al.* (1998). Groin hernia surgery: a systematic review. *Annals of the Royal College of Surgeons of England* **80**: S1–S80.

Clark, R.E. and H.W. Margraf (1974). Antibacterial vascular grafts with improved thromboresistance. *Archives of Surgery* **109**(2): 159–162.

Clark, W.R. (2000). Hemodialyzer membranes and configurations: a historical perspective. *Seminars in Dialysis* **13**(5): 309–311.

Craig, P.H., J.A. Williams, *et al.* (1975). Biologic comparison of Polyglactin-910 and polyglycolic acid synthetic absorbable sutures. *Surgery Gynecology & Obstetrics* **141**(1): 1–10.

Dahl, S.L.M., A.P. Kypson, *et al.* (2011). Readily available tissue-engineered vascular grafts. *Science Translational Medicine* **3**(68): 11.

Dattilo, P.P., M.W. King, *et al.* (2002). Medical textiles: application of an absorbable barbed bidirectional surgical suture. *Journal of Textile and Apparel, Technology and Management* **2**(2).

Dauner, M., H. Planck, *et al.* (1990). Para-aramid fiber for artificial ligament. Amsterdam: Elsevier Science Publ.

Dimitrievska, S., M. Maire, *et al.* (2011). Low thrombogenicity coating of nonwoven PET fiber structures for vascular grafts. *Macromolecular Bioscience* **11**(4): 493–502.

Dirckx, J.H. (2001). Stedman's concise medical dictionary for the health professions: illustrated, 4th Edition. Baltimore: Lippincott Williams & Wilkins.

Earle, D.B. and L.A. Mark (2008). Prosthetic material in inguinal hernia repair: how do I choose? Surgical Clinics of North America **88**(1): 179–201.

Einarsson, J.I., N.R. Chavan, *et al.* (2011). Use of bidirectional barbed suture in laparoscopic myomectomy: evaluation of perioperative outcomes, safety, and efficacy. *Journal of Minimally Invasive Gynecology* **18**(1): 92–95.

Fitch, J.C.K., S. Rollins, *et al.* (1999). Pharmacology and biological efficacy of a recombinant, humanized, single-chain antibody C5 complement inhibitor in patients undergoing coronary artery bypass graft surgery with cardiopulmonary bypass. *Circulation* **100**(25): 2499–2506.

Frank, C.B. and D.W. Jackson (1997). The science of reconstruction of the anterior cruciate ligament. *J. Bone Joint Surg. Am.* **79**(10): 1556–76.

Freeman, B.S., C.A. Homsy, *et al.* (1970). An analysis of suture withdrawal stress. *Surgery Gynecology and Obstetrics with International Abstracts of Surgery* **131**(3): 441-7.

Gayle, R.G., J.R. Wheeler, *et al.* (1988). Evaluation of the expanded polytetrafluoroethylene (ePTFE) suture in peripheral vascular-surgery using ePTFE prosthetic vascular grafts. *Journal of Cardiovascular Surgery* **29**(5): 556–559.

Gorbet, M.B. and M.V. Sefton (2004). Biomaterial-associated thrombosis: roles of coagulation factors, complement, platelets and leukocytes. *Biomaterials* **25**(26): 5681–5703.

Grant, A.M. and E.H.T. Collaboration (2002). Repair of groin hernia with synthetic mesh—meta-analysis of randomized controlled trials. *Annals of Surgery* **235**(3): 322–332.

Hamy, A., P. Pessaux, *et al.* (2003). Surgical treatment of large incisional hernias by an intraperitoneal Dacron mesh and an aponeurotic graft. *Journal of the American College of Surgeons* **196**(4): 531–534.

Heidenhain, C., A. Veeravoorn, *et al.*, (2011). Fibroblast and vascular endothelial growth factor coating of decellularized vascular grafts stimulates undesired giant cells and graft encapsulation in a rat model. *Artificial Organs* **35**(1): E1–E10.

Herring, M., R. Dilley, *et al.* (1980). The effects of crimping on the healing of prosthetic arterial grafts. *Journal of Cardiovascular Surgery* **21**(5): 596–603.

Herrmann, J.B., R.J. Kelly, *et al.* (1970). Polyglycolic acid sutures—laboratory and clinical evaluation of a new absorbable suture material. *Archives of Surgery* **100**(4): 486-&.

Higuchi, A., K. Shirano, *et al.* (2002). Chemically modified polysulfone hollow fibers with vinylpyrrolidone having improved blood compatibility. *Biomaterials* **23**(13): 2659–2666.

Hoenich, N.A., C. Woffindin, *et al.* (1995). Biocompatibility of membranes used in the treatment of renal-failure. *Biomaterials* **16**(8): 587–592.

Humes, H.D., W.H. Fissell, *et al.* (2006). The future of hemodialysis membranes. *Kidney International* **69**(7): 1115–1119.

Indelicato, P.A., M.S. Pascale, *et al.* (1989). Early experience with the Gore-Tex polytetrafluoroethylene anterior cruciate ligament prosthesis. *American Journal of Sports Medicine* 17(1): 55–62.

Ishihara, K., K. Fukumoto, *et al.* (1999). Modification of polysulfone with phospholipid polymer for improvement of the blood compatibility. Part 1. Surface characterization. *Biomaterials* 20(17): 1545–1551.

Ishihara, K., K. Fukumoto, *et al.* (1999). Modification of polysulfone with phospholipid polymer for improvement of the blood compatibility. Part 2. Protein adsorption and platelet adhesion. *Biomaterials* 20(17): 1553–1559.

Jaber, B.L., A. Alonso, *et al.* (2009). Biocompatible hemodialysis membranes for acute renal failure (Review). *Cochrane Database of Systematic Reviews* (3).

Jiang, G.M., X.H. Miao, *et al.* (2005). Process of warp knitting mesh for hernia repair and its mechanical properties. *Fibres & Textiles in Eastern Europe* 13(3): 44–46.

Kdolsky, R.K., D.F. Gibbons, *et al.* (1997). Braided polypropylene augmentation device in reconstructive surgery of the anterior cruciate ligament: Long-term clinical performance of 594 patients and short-term arthroscopic results, failure analysis by scanning electron microscopy, and synovial histomorphology. *Journal of Orthopaedic Research* 15(1): 1–10.

Kenney, D.A., L.R. Sauvage, *et al.* (1982). Comparison of noncrimped, externally supported (exs) and crimped, nonsupported dacron prostheses for axillofemoral and above-knee femoro-popliteal bypass. *Surgery* 92(6): 931–946.

Klein, E., R.A. Ward, *et al.* (1987). Membrane processes: dialysis and electrodialysis. *In:* Handbook of separation process technology, pp. 954–981. R.W. Rousseau (ed.). New York: Wiley.

Kovacic, V. and L. Roguljic. (2003). A comparison of low-flux cellulose acetate and polysulfone dialyzers: impact on plasma lipid concentration in chronic hemodialysis patients. *Dialysis & Transplantation* 32(9): 552–560.

Krudwig, W.K. (2002). Anterior cruciate ligament reconstruction using an alloplastic ligament of polyethylene terephthalate (PET-Trevira((R))-hochfest). Follow-up study. *Bio-Medical Materials and Engineering* 12(1): 59–67.

Ku, D.N. and R.C. Allen (2006). Chapter 65: Vascular Grafts. *In:* Tissue engineering and artificial organs. J.D. Bronzino (ed.). Boca Raton, CRC/Taylor & Francis.

Levin, M.P. (1980). Periodontal suture materials and surgical dressings. *Dental Clinics of North America* 24(4): 767–781.

Levy, M. and A.R. Hartman (1996). Heparin-coated bypass circuits in cardiopulmonary bypass: Improved biocompatibility or not. *International Journal of Cardiology* 53: S81–S87.

Liu, S.Q. and M. Kodama (1992). Porous polyurethane vascular prostheses with variable compliances. *Journal of Biomedical Materials Research* 26(11): 1489–1502.

Marchal, F., L. Brunaud, *et al.* (1999). Treatment of incisional hernias by placement of an intraperitoneal prosthesis: a series of 128 patients. *Hernia* 3: 141–147.

Martin, J. and K.J.L. Burg (2003). Textiles and biomedical devices. *AATCC Review* 3(11): 41–44.

McKenzie, A.R. (1967). An experimental multiple barbed suture for the long flexor tendons of the palm and fingers. Preliminary report. *J. Bone Joint Surg. Br.* **49**(3): 440–7.

Meyer, R.D. and C.J. Antonini. (1989). A review of suture materials, Part I. *Compendium* **10**(5): 260-2, 264–5.

Meyer, R.D. and C.J. Antonini. (1989). A review of suture materials, Part II. *Compendium* **10**(6): 360-2, 364, 366–8.

Morgan, M.N. (1969). New synthetic absorbable suture material. *British Medical Journal* **2**(5652): 308.

Moy, R.L., B. Waldman, *et al.* (1992). A review of sutures and suturing techniques. *Journal of Dermatologic Surgery and Oncology* **18**(9): 785–795.

Muren, O., L. Dahlstedt, *et al.* (2005). Gross osteolytic tibia tunnel widening with the use of Gore-Tex anterior cruciate ligament prosthesis—A radiological, arthrometric and clinical evaluation of 17 patients 13–15 years after surgery. *Acta Orthopaedica* **76**(2): 270–274.

Murkin, J.M. (1997). Cardiopulmonary bypass and the inflammatory response: A role for serine protease inhibitors? *Journal of Cardiothoracic and Vascular Anesthesia* **11**(2): 19–23.

Noordwijk, J.V. (2001). Dialysing for life: the development of the artificial kidney. Boston: Kluwer Academic Publishers.

Noyes, F.R. and E.S. Grood. (1976). The strength of the anterior cruciate ligament in humans and Rhesus monkeys. *J. Bone Joint Surg. Am.* **58**(8): 1074–82.

Nutton, R.W., I. McLean, *et al.* (1999). Tendon allografts in knee ligament surgery. *J. of the Royal Coll. Surg. Edinb.* **44**(4): 236–40.

Osborne, A.H., R.C. Telfer, *et al.* (1984). Recent experience with carbon fibre. *Journal of the Royal Naval Medical Service* **70**(2): 66–9.

Parker, D.M., F.S. Ayubi, *et al.* (2008). Abdominal wall hernia repair: a comparison of Permacol® and Surgisis® grafts in a rat hernia model. *Hernia* **12**(4): 373–378.

Piccone, V. (1987). Alternative techniques in coronary artery reconstruction. New York: McGraw-Hill.

Postlethwait, R.W., D.A. Willigan, *et al.* (1975). Human tissue reaction to sutures. *Annals of Surgery* **181**(2): 144–150.

Pourdeyhimi, B., P.W. Harrison, *et al.* (1986). Vascular grafts: textile structures and their performance: a critical appreciation of recent developments. Manchester, Engl.: Textile Institute.

Pourdeyhimi, B. and C. Text. (1987). A review of structural and material properties of vascular grafts. *Journal of Biomaterials Applications* **2**(2): 163–204.

Pourdeyhimi, B. and D. Wagner (1986). On the correlation between the failure of vascular grafts and their structural and material properties—a critical analysis. *Journal of Biomedical Materials Research* **20**(3): 375–409.

Purchase, R., R. Mason, *et al.* (2007). Fourteen-year prospective results of a high-density polyethylene prosthetic anterior cruciate ligament reconstruction. *Journal of Long-Term Effects of Medical Implants* **17**(1): 13–19.

Ratner, B.D. (2004). *Biomaterials science: an introduction to materials in medicine.* Boston: Elsevier Academic Press.

Ray, J.A., N. Doddi, *et al.* (1981). Polydioxanone (PDS), a novel mono-filament synthetic absorbable suture. *Surgery Gynecology & Obstetrics* **153**(4): 497–507.

Rodeheaver, G.T., P.A. Foresman, *et al.* (1987). A temporary nontoxic lubricant for a synthetic absorbable suture. *Surgery Gynecology & Obstetrics* **164**(1): 17–21.

Roger, V.L., A.S. Go, *et al.* (2011). Heart disease and stroke statistics-2011 update: a report from the American Heart Association. *Circulation* **123**(4): E18–E209.

Rosch, R., K. Junge, *et al.* (2003). Vypro II (R) mesh in hernia repair: Impact of polyglactin on long-term incorporation in rats. *European Surgical Research* **35**(5): 445–450.

Sadat, U., S.R. Markar, *et al.* (2010). Partially or completely absorbable versus nonabsorbable mesh repair for inguinal hernia: a systematic review and meta-analysis. *Surgical Laparoscopy Endoscopy & Percutaneous Techniques* **20**(4): 213–219.

Seitz, H., S. Marlovits, *et al.* (1998). Biocompatibility of polyethylene terephthalate (Trevira (R) hochfest) augmentation device in repair of the anterior cruciate ligament. *Biomaterials* **19**(1-3): 189–196.

Selan, L., M. Artini, *et al.* (2010). Comparison of anti-bacterial prophylactic properties of two different vascular grafts: action of anti-bacterial graft coating and systemic antibiotic treatment. *International Journal of Immunopathology and Pharmacology* **23**(1): 383–386.

Siedhoff, M.T., A.C. Yunker, *et al.* (2011). Decreased incidence of vaginal cuff dehiscence after laparoscopic closure with bidirectional barbed suture. *Journal of Minimally Invasive Gynecology* **18**(2): 218–223.

Song, Y.Q., J. Sheng, *et al.* (2000). Surface modification of polysulfone membranes by low-temperature plasma-graft poly(ethylene glycol) onto polysulfone membranes. *Journal of Applied Polymer Science* **78**(5): 979–985.

Spencer, D.J. (2001). Knitting technology: a comprehensive handbook and practical guide. Cambridge, England: Woodhead Publishing.

Spindler, K.P., R.A. Magnussen, *et al.* (2011). Does autograft choice determine intermediate-term outcome of ACL reconstruction? *Knee Surgery Sports Traumatology Arthroscopy* **19**(3): 462–472.

Stamatialis, D.F., B.J. Papenburg, *et al.* (2008). Medical applications of membranes: drug delivery, artificial organs and tissue engineering. *Journal of Membrane Science* **308**(1–2): 1–34.

Steen, M.L., L. Hymas, *et al.* (2001). Low temperature plasma treatment of asymmetric polysulfone membranes for permanent hydrophilic surface modification. *Journal of Membrane Science* **188**(1): 97–114.

Sueoka, A. and K. Takakura. (1991). Hollow fiber membrane application for blood treatment. *Polymer Journal* **23**(5): 561–571.

Thalhammer, F., J. Kletzmayr, *et al.* (1998). Ofloxacin clearance during hemodialysis: a comparison of polysulfone and cellulose acetate hemodialyzers. *American Journal of Kidney Diseases* **32**(4): 642–645.

Torrestiana-Sanchez, B., R.I. Ortiz-Basurto, *et al.* (1999). Effect of nonsolvents on properties of spinning solutions and polyethersulfone hollow fiber ultrafiltration membranes. *Journal of Membrane Science* **152**(1): 19–28.

Tsuruoka, S., K.I. Sugimoto, *et al.* (2000). Ranitidine clearance during hemodialysis with high-flux membrane: comparison of polysulfone and cellulose acetate hemo-dialyzers. *European Journal of Clinical Pharmacology* **56**(8): 581–583.

Tzanakakis, E.S., D.J. Hess, *et al.* (2000). Extracorporeal tissue engineered liver-assist devices. *Annual Review of Biomedical Engineering* **2**: 607–632.

Ulbricht, M. and G. Belfort. (1996). Surface modification of ultrafiltration membranes by low temperature plasma 2. Graft polymerization onto polyacrylonitrile and poly-sulfone. *Journal of Membrane Science* **111**(2): 193–215.

Ulbricht, M. and M. Riedel. (1998). Ultrafiltration membrane surfaces with grafted polymer 'tentacles': preparation, characterization and application for covalent pro-tein binding. *Biomaterials* **19**(14): 1229–1237.

Vogel, U.B. (1992). Clinical experiences with the Gore-Tex 5-Ptfe cruciate-ligament prosthesis—greater-than-4-year follow-up. *Helvetica Chirurgica Acta* **58**(6): 943–947.

Wang, H.T., T. Yu, *et al.* (2009). Improvement of hydrophilicity and blood compat-ibility on polyethersulfone membrane by adding polyvinylpyrrolidone. *Fibers and Polymers* **10**(1): 1–5.

Wendel, H.P. and G. Ziemer (1999). Coating-techniques to improve the hemocompat-ibility of artificial devices used for extracorporeal circulation. *European Journal of Cardio-Thoracic Surgery* **16**(3): 342–350.

Williams, D.F. (1987). Blood compatibility. Boca Raton, Fla.: CRC Press.

Wilson, G.J., D.C. MacGregor, *et al.* (1993). A compliant Corethane/Dacron composite vascular prosthesis. Comparison with 4-mm ePTFE grafts in a canine model. *ASAIO journal* (American Society for Artificial Internal Organs) **39**(3): M526–31.

Woffindin, C. and N.A. Hoenich (1995). Hemodialyzer performance—a review of the trends over the past two decades. *Artificial Organs* **19**(11): 1113–1119.

Yamamoto, K., Y. Noishiki, *et al.* (1993). Unusual inflammatory responses around a collagen-impregnated vascular prosthesis. *Artificial Organs* **17**(12): 1010–1016.

Ye, S.H., J. Watanabe, *et al.* (2005). Design of functional hollow fiber membranes mod-ified with phospholipid polymers for application in total hemopurification system. *Biomaterials* **26**(24): 5032–5041.

Ye, S.H., J. Watanabe, *et al.* (2006). High functional hollow fiber membrane modi-fied with phospholipid polymers for a liver assist bioreactor. *Biomaterials* **27**(9): 1955–1962.

Zhang, Z., X.Y. Xie, *et al.* (2010). Five types of polyurethane vascular grafts in dogs: the importance of structural design and material selection. *Journal of Biomaterials Science-Polymer Edition* **21**(8-9): 1239–1264.

Zhao, C.S., X.D. Liu, *et al.* (2003). Surface characterization of polysulfone membranes modified by DNA immobilization. *Journal of Membrane Science* **214**(2): 179–189.

Zilla, P., D. Bezuidenhout, *et al.* (2007). Prosthetic vascular grafts: wrong models, wrong questions and no healing. *Biomaterials* **28**(34): 5009–5027.

CHAPTER 10

Tissue Engineering

THE injury or disease of a tissue or organ (e.g., skin, blood vessel, ligament and bone) is a grievous and costly event in health care, affecting millions of people worldwide annually. Only a few types of tissues can be spontaneously regenerated (i.e., restoring the normal structure and function) when injured. These are epithelial tissues (e.g., epidermis), bone tissues and smooth muscle tissues (i.e., one of the muscles of the internal organs, having no striations). Even for the regenerative tissue like bone, it is difficult or impossible to have large defects repaired/restored. Those that do not have the capacity to regenerate themselves need surgical intervention, of which the latest means is *tissue engineering* for the purpose of tissue regeneration.

According to records of United Network for Organ Sharing (UNOS at www.unos.org), as of today, over 114,000 people in the United States are on the waiting list for organ transplantation. In 2011, 28,535 transplants were performed, involving both deceased and living donors. The severe shortage of donors has been a devastating problem for patients who are waiting for matching organs/tissues. Many of them may die before they get what they need. On the other hand, immune repression and disease transmission between patients and donors also increase the difficulties of transplantation. Artificial implants have been used as an alternative means to replace the functions of damaged or failed tissues/ organs, either temporarily when a patient is waiting for a transplant, or as a long-term solution. To date, however, human tissues or organs that can be replaced by artificial devices (as discussed already in Chapter 9 and continued in Chapter 10) are limited, not to mention that almost all prosthetic devices are associated with problems of biocompatibility and/or biostability.

Currently regarded as the most promising approach to treating damaged or failed human tissues/organs, *tissue engineering* refers to "an interdisciplinary field that applies the principles of engineering and the life sciences toward the development of biological substitutes that restore, maintain, or improve tissue function" (Langer and Vacanti, 1993). In a tissue engineering process, appropriate living cells are seeded on a matrix or scaffold and then guided to develop into a new and functional living tissue. Grafts as a result of such regeneration are known as *bioengineered* grafts, which will be able to function as substitutes for injured or diseased skin, vascular, bone, or other tissues. Generally speaking, tissue engineering is based on the tripod of scaffold (i.e., environment for the living of cells), regulator(s) (such as growth factors) and cells (such as stem cells).

Viable cells taken from the patient's body or other sources are essential for most tissue engineering approaches. These cells are expected to cause minimal immunological responses, and to rapidly expand/differentiate to produce the volume of tissue necessary to replace the lost ones. Stem cells are frequently used sources of cells for tissue engineering because of their capacity for proliferation and differentiation into one or more types of specialized cells. There are two types of stem cells according to their sources: embryonic and adult tissue stem cells. Embryonic stem cells (ESCs) are derived from developing embryos five to eight days after fertilization. ESCs are capable of unlimited expansion and differentiation into almost any line of cells. However, ESCs are difficult and costly to obtain, and the use of human ESCs is subjected to strict ethical constraints. On the other hand, adult tissue stem cells can be derived from epithelial tissues (e.g., epidermis, intestinal epithelium), blood, bone marrow (e.g., mesenchymal stem cells [MSC]), etc. They are limited in their capacity of differentiation, but are easier to obtain for tissue engineering purposes (Lanza, Langer, *et al.*, 2007).

A *scaffold* is a 3-dimensional (3D) porous solid biomaterial that has been developed to perform some or all of the following functions: (1) provide an environment that is both suitable for the cells to live and will also promote cell adhesion and proliferation; (2) allow transport of gas, nutrients and regulators that are necessary for the cells to perform their functions and to proliferate; (3) biodegrade in a controllable manner; and (4) cause minimal host responses. Depending on the specific tissue/ organ to be regenerated, different biomaterials can be used for such a scaffold. They include naturally-occurring biomaterials, synthetic materials, or hybrid materials, in the format of nanofibrous structures, gels, ceramics or composites (Lanza, Langer, *et al.*, 2007), as discussed in greater details in the following sections.

A *regulator* usually refers to a type of biomolecule that may promote the growth and/or guide the differentiation of the cells in question. The most well-known regulators are the various growth factors. They are incorporated into the scaffolding materials via different methods, including physical mixing, chemical conjugation, and nano-encapsulation. They are expected to be released in a controlled and sustained manner during their application.

There have been two basic approaches to tissue engineering: *in vitro* and *in vivo*. The latter approach refers to therapies in which bioengineered grafts are implanted and allowed to mature inside the human body for the repair or regeneration of damaged or diseased tissues. On the other hand, the *in vitro* (or *ex vivo*) approach depends on therapies in which the bioengineered grafts are cultured outside the human body to achieve appropriate functions before implantation (Lanza, Langer, *et al.*, 2007).

Theoretically, the approach of tissue engineering can be applied to repair and regenerate any injured or diseased tissue or organ in the human body, which is exactly the ultimate goal of research in this area. To date, however, only a few types of bioengineered grafts have been successfully adopted in hospitals to help patients who have had their tissues/organs lost or injured. Extensive research and development efforts are being made to expand the scope of research and application. This chapter will briefly relate these efforts, covering tissue engineering approaches to the regeneration of several major human organs, including skin, blood vessels, and some bioartificial extracorporeal devices. Readers who are interested in a particular topic may find information from literature listed at the end of the chapter.

10.1. BIOENGINEERED SKIN GRAFTS

The earliest application of tissue engineering involved the use of a 2-dimensional, or flat, biomaterial as a template to regenerate damaged skin and stimulate wound healing. Bioengineered skin grafts have been used in treatment for patients with severe skin damage that cannot heal spontaneously, even with the application of wound dressings. It is estimated that there are 35.2 million cases of significant skin loss in the U.S. each year, and 7 million of these wounds turn chronic (Clark, Ghosh, *et al.*, 2007). Among causes of significant skin loss, thermal injury is the most common, accounting for about one million hospital emergency visits annually. Chronic ulcerations caused by diabetes mellitus and pressure are another major cause of severe skin damages. For example, every year about 2 million Americans suffer from chronic diabetic ulcers, and about 82 thousand of them eventually have to receive amputation (Ehrenreich and Ruszczak, 2006).

There are several options for treating severe skin loss. The *autograft therapy* involves taking skin from an intact site of the patient himself/ herself and having it transplanted into the damaged location. Such an approach avoids any issue of host response, but the patient has to be subjected to extra pain and skin loss. *Allograft therapy,* on the other hand, depends on skin tissues transplanted from a donor to a patient. Such a practice may encounter problems of host response and transmitted disease. The tissue engineering therapy based on the use of bioengineered skin graft may avoid the disadvantages associated with autograft and allograft therapies, especially the need for skin tissues removed from the patient or the dependence on a donor source from which to harvest skin cells. Instead, a biocompatible and biodegradable porous scaffold (usually in a sheet form) is used to support cell proliferation and tissue regeneration, and to facilitate wound healing. Since the first clinical application of skin tissue engineering in the early 1980s, over 200,000 people have received therapy with bioengineered skin grafts (Lanza, Langer, *et al.*, 2007).

The epidermis is one of the few types of tissues that are capable of spontaneous regeneration. However, in cases where large areas of the epidermis are damaged, such spontaneous regeneration is unlikely. The underlying dermis is hardly able to regenerate itself. Once the dermis is damaged, there will form, in its absence, scar tissue, which is inelastic and weaker than the normal dermis tissue, and may as a result limit movement, and cause discomfort and/or cosmetic problems. Therein arises the need to replace both damaged epidermis and dermis tissues. For burn patients, it is generally believed that an early excision of the burned skin and the covering of the excised area with a skin graft are important to increase its rate of survival (Caldwell, Wallace, *et al.*, 1996). Currently there are several types of bioengineered skin grafts available, as discussed below.

Autologous epidermal cell sheet (e.g., Epicel®) is also referred to as cultured epithelial autograft (CEA). In a therapy when it is applied, skin tissues of punch biopsy size (e.g., 1 cm^2) are taken from the donor sites and cultured in appropriate conditions, and cells are allowed to proliferate and spread until the tissues are mature enough to be transplanted. One of the advantages of this approach is that only a small amount of donor tissue is needed and there is little pain associated with the tissue harvesting. Tissues taken from different donors may vary in their capacity for proliferation. Usually, the younger the donor is, the higher the proliferation capacity will be. By starting with 1 cm^2 of a newborn's skin, for example, the overall expansion of the epithelium by the end of 14–21 days will be about 1500-fold, resulting in a graft of 1500 cm^2 (Green, Kehinde, *et al.*, 1979). However, disadvantages of the CEA include: (1) the time factor—it takes a couple of weeks for the graft to be ready, and not all patients can afford to wait; (2) the grafts are expensive; (3) the grafts are very fragile after implantation; and (4) there have been concerns about the low rates of engraftment (i.e., with an average of only 51% of successful initial engraftment, and about 60% of delayed loss as a percentage of initial engraftment) (Sheridan and Tompkins, 1995).

Acellular matrix skin graft (e.g., Integra®, Alloderm®) provides a matrix without cells to facilitate wound healing. It usually consists of dermal replacement layer(s) in the form of a porous matrix containing cross-linked fibers of collagen and glycosaminoglycan (GAG). The acellular matrix can be derived from skins of either animals or deceased human donors by removing the epidermis layer and cells (e.g., fibroblasts) in the remaining dermal layer without altering the extracellular matrix structure (Wainwright, 1995). Such a dermal replacement serves as a scaffold for the infiltration of cells (e.g., fibroblasts) and tissues (e.g., capillaries). During the healing process, the infiltrated fibroblasts produce and deposit collagen to replace the biodegraded collagen/GAG of the acellular skin graft, leading to the formation of a new dermal layer (Fette, 2005). These acellular matrix skin grafts are usually supplied with a silicone outer layer that temporarily closes the wound to protect the wound bed from infection as well as heat/fluid loss. This silicone layer is removed after the formation of the new dermal layer, often in 14–21 days. An epidermal graft is then transplanted to complete the process. The advantage of the therapy involving acellular matrix skin grafts is that the products can be used immediately for patients. Such grafts have also been reported to prevent post-burn scar formation and joint movement limitation (Yim, Cho, *et al.*, 2010). However, there have been concerns that the acellular matrix dermal grafts do not lead to true dermal regeneration, due to: (1) limitation in the cells' infiltration into the grafts; (2) limits in the type of fibroblast growing in the grafts; and (3) the ability of the cells to degrade the grafted matrix while producing a new matrix (Lanza, Langer *et al.*, 2007). In addition, two procedures, i.e., dermal regeneration and epidermal transplant, and prolonged treating time are needed for the recovery.

Allogenic dermal substrate (e.g., Dermagraft®, Matriderm®) is a product developed to overcome some of the problems associated with acellular matrix dermal grafts discussed in the above. To that end, human neonatal fibroblasts derived from newborn foreskins are grown on biodegradable meshes and allowed to proliferate into the degrading temporary matrix and to synthesize a new matrix in the interstices of the mesh. It is reported that cells harvested from a single donor foreskin are able to provide enough seeds to produce as much as 250,000 square feet of finished dermal substrates, which will reconstruct a dermal base over which the patient's own epidermis can migrate to heal the wound (Edmonds, Foster, et al., 1997). However, early products of such skin substitutes (e.g., Dermagraft®, in which polyglactin was used for the matrix) encountered problems of short life span of implanted fibroblasts (which were found to die in a few weeks after implantation). It is thus reasonable to believe that this product functioned only as a delivery vehicle for growth factors and ECM produced by the fibroblasts while they were alive (Kamolz, Lumenta, et al., 2008). A recent dermal substitute (Matriderm®) adopts a matrix containing native bovine type I, II and V collagen fibre template coated with elastin. This grafted matrix will convert into native host collagen in a few weeks (Kamolz, Haslik, et al., 2007). Although results of initial clinical use of this new product are promising, its effectiveness needs further proof.

Human skin equivalent (HSE, e.g., Orcel®, Apligraf®), also known as bi-layered bioengineered skin substitute, consists of both epidermal and dermal substitutes. A HSE is a bi-layered composite containing (1) a collagen matrix seeded with dermal cells (fibroblasts), and (2) an overlying epidermal cell (keratinocytes) sheet. The total production time is about 17 to 20 days, during which: (1) fibroblasts and keratinocytes with a high capacity for proliferation are isolated from allogeneic human neonatal foreskin and allowed to grow and proliferate; (2) a solution of purified bovine type I collagen is mixed with the fibroblasts and the mixture is turned into a gel, where the fibroblasts cause the collagen matrix to contract so as to form a dermal equivalent in about 4–6 days; (3) the subsequent epidermalization involves seeding keratinocytes on top of the dermal equivalent and culturing for 2 days so that they will cover the dermal equivalent; and (4) the bi-layered graft is ready when the epidermis layer is mature (Eaglstein and Falanga, 1997). HSE has been used to treat patients with venous leg ulcers and diabetic foot ulcers, bringing about degrees of success in clinical application (Curran and Plosker, 2002). However, HSE also faces the problem of short life span of donor cells (which die in 4–8 weeks after implantation). In addition, the product is expensive ($30 per square cm) (Clark, Ghosh, et al., 2007).

For three decades, various types of bioengineered skin grafts have been used clinically to treat patients with skin injuries and diseases. Such a graft usually contains a biocompatible and biodegradable matrix to support cell proliferation *in vitro* or *in vivo*. For grafts involving allogenic cells, antigen-presenting cells (i.e., cells that may provoke host responses) should be avoided so as to elude tissue reaction. Nevertheless, despite the intensive research and development work already carried out in the related fields, an ideal graft or therapy for skin regeneration is not yet known, due to problems already mentioned above. A future breakthrough in this field may be the result of a better knowledge of how biopolymers interact with cells/tissues and how these interactions affect the activities and functions of cells and tissues.

10.2. BIOENGINEERED VASCULAR GRAFTS

As mentioned in Chapter 9, thrombosis is the leading cause of the failure of synthetic vascular grafts. For the native blood vessel, its inner surface is covered by endothelial cells (EC) that perform a variety of physiologic functions, among which the most important is to resist thrombosis. EC has limited capacity for regeneration. Compared with EC of native blood vessels, the function of EC in a synthetic vascular graft is less than 10% of physiologic levels (Walles, Gorler, *et al.*, 2004). As a result, persistent efforts have been made to develop bioengineered vascular grafts involving viable cells. To date, some bioengineered vascular grafts have been tested in clinical trials, but there is not yet a commercial product. A discussion of bioengineered vascular grafts involves three aspects: (1) cells, (2) scaffolds, and (3) regulators.

10.2.1. Cells

Playing vital roles in native vessels, the endothelial cell was the first viable cell to be seeded onto a bioengineered synthetic vascular graft (Herring, Gardner, *et al.*, 1978). Results of clinical trials are mixed: one report concerning a nine year clinical trial suggests that autologous EC lining improves the patency of small-diameter vascular grafts (6mm ePTFE grafts) (Deutsch, Meinhart, *et al.*, 1999), while other reports of similar trials give disheartening results (Herring, Smith, *et al.*, 1994). Expressive of the failure in these clinical trials is the low rate of survival of EC *in vivo* shortly after implantation (with up to 95% of the cells getting lost within 24 hours) (Rosenman, Kempczinski, *et al.*, 1985). There have also been studies suggesting that some improvement made to the cell seedling/culturing procedure is responsible for increased rate of cell survival, thus making clinical results less disheartening (Bordenave, Fernandez, *et al.*, 2005).

There have also been trials where other types of cells are seeded onto the synthetic vascular grafts, including smooth muscle cells (SMC) and fibroblasts, because they were reported to promote formation of endothelial tissues (Weinberg and Bell, 1986).

Recently, stem cells have become increasingly popular in the research and development of bioengineered vascular grafts, because of their high capacity for proliferation and ability to differentiate into various types of cells, e.g., EC (Bell, Owens, *et al.*, 2008) and SMC (DiMuzio, Harris, *et al.*, 2011).

10.2.2. Scaffolds

A scaffold for a bioengineered vascular graft is expected to provide a temporary support for cells to attach to, and to grow on. The cells will secrete a new extracellular matrix that will eventually replace the temporary scaffold. It should have appropriate biomechanical properties so as to maintain the strength and shape of the graft. It serves as a substrate for the regulators that guide/promote the growth of cells. More importantly, it should be biocompatible so that it does not to cause host response.

A variety of biomaterials have been used in scaffolds for bioengineered vascular grafts, including natural and synthetic polymers. Early development of bioengineered vascular grafts involved seeding ECs onto a non-absorbable graft (e.g., Dacron) (Pasic, Muller-Glauser, *et al.*, 1996), ePTFE (Meinhart, Deutsch, *et al.*, 1997), resulting in improved patency in the graft. However, such an approach has its limitations, including (1) difficulties in the long-term survival and proliferation of ECs on the synthetic material; and (2) the likelihood for the non-absorbable scaffold to impede the normal remodeling process of the vascular system so as to cause the synthetic material to become a physical barrier to long-term adaptation of the vessel (Nerem and Seliktar, 2001).

Due to these limitations, recent efforts on bioengineered vascular grafts have been concentrated on bio-absorbable polymers. Collagen is a frequently used natural polymer for vascular tissue engineering, since it is an important component in the native vessels. Although collagen (usually in the form of a gel matrix) provides an ideal scaffold for cell attachment and proliferation, it has inherent physical weakness, which makes it difficult for the bioengineered graft to sustain cyclic load imposed by the hemodynamic environment. As a result, the early collagen-based bioengineered vascular graft had to adopt supporting sleeves made from Dacron (Weinberg and Bell, 1986).

Since then, extensive research has been devoted to the development of scaffolding materials/structures with both adequate biocompatibility and mechanical properties to be used in a hemodynamic environment. As a result of such efforts, electrospun bio-absorbable nanofibers have attracted keen attention, largely because of the versatility of the electrospinning technique, a technique for the production of nanofibers from a variety of polymers. Electrospun nanofibrous mats provide scaffolds with good mechanical properties. Other textile structures (e.g., woven, filament winding) have also been explored. They include the many bio-absorbable polymers, as explained in the following.

PGA (polyglycolic acid) and PLA (polylactic acid) are usually used in combination for the construction of scaffolds for bioengineered vascular grafts. Nonwoven meshes of PGA fibers is a good choice for scaffolds that support cell growth and tissue development, but may be deficient in stability to resist compressive forces *in vivo*. PLA can serve as a good external support to stabilize the structure (Mooney, Mazzoni, *et al.*, 1996). For this purpose, PGA and PLA can be combined with other bio-polymers via mixing, coating or copolymerization. A clinical trial using bioengineered vascular grafts composed of PGA/PLA or PGA/PCL (Polycaprolactone) on young patients (range 1–24 years) with an average of 5.8-year follow-up indicates no graft-related mortality or major problems (e.g., graft aneurysm [abnormal widening], graft rupture and graft infection), although the major mode of graft failure and graft stenosis (abnormal narrowing) needs further follow-up and monitoring (Hibino, McGillicuddy, *et al.*, 2010). Other scaffolding structures constructed from PGA and/or PLA include electrospun nanofibrous tubes (Wang, Zhang, *et al.*, 2009) and stacked sheets wrapped into a tubular shape (Iwasaki, Kojima, *et al.*, 2008).

PCL is another biocompatible and bio-absorbable polymer used for bioengineered vascular grafts. It provides good mechanical properties, including high strength and excellent compliance (McClure, Wolfe, *et al.*, 2011). PCL has been fabricated into films (via hot press (Serrano, Portoles, *et al.*, 2005) or casting from its solution (Zhu, Gao, *et al.*, 2002). PCL has also been electrospun into nanofiber mesh for bioengineered vascular grafts. PCL scaffolds usually need surface treatments to improve their hydrophilicity and cell attachment. Alkali (e.g., NaOH) treatment can be used to induce surface hydrolysis, which produces hydrophilic groups (i.e., carboxyl and hydroxyl groups) (Serrano, Portoles, *et al.*, 2005). Grafting of biocompatible and hydrophilic polymers (e.g., gelatin) onto a PCL surface is another route to achieving the same goal (Ma, He, *et al.*, 2005). There are also studies about the combination of PCL with other polymers via bi-layered electrospinning (Vaz, van Tuijl, *et al.*, 2005), or copolymerization with PLA (Hanson, Jamshidi *et al.*, 1988) for better scaffolding materials. To date, related results are obtained only from animal models involving PCL-based bioengineered vascular grafts, indicating the potential usefulness of such scaffolding materials for vascular tissue engineering (Watanabe, Shin'Oka, *et al.*, 2001).

Collagen is a good material for tissue engineering applications because of its natural abundance in the human body, although its mechanical weakness limits its application. Extensive work, therefore, has been devoted to the improvement in the mechanical properties of collagen scaffolds. Crosslinking is the most frequently used method to enhance the mechanical strength of collagen scaffolds which are usually in the form of gels. Crosslinking can be achieved by using chemical agents (e.g., glutaraldehyde, carbodiimide), UV irradiation, or dehydrother-mal treatment (Berglund, Mohseni, *et al.*, 2003; Madaghiele, Piccin-no, *et al.*, 2009). The crosslinking agent glutaraldehyde is possibly to blame for the resulting toxicity that may adversely affect tissues *in vivo* (Friess, 1998). Other optional crosslinking methods are therefore pre-ferred. Electrospinning is an approach to the production of scaffolds containing collagen fibers and having better mechanical properties (Matthews, Wnek, *et al.*, 2002). Collagen can also be combined with other biocompatible polymers in the fabrication of tissue-engineered scaffolds to provide better mechanical strength. Various constructs for such a combination include the blending of different polymers in elec-trospun nanofibrous structures. These include collagen and a copolymer of PLLA-PCL (He, Yong, *et al.*, 2005), a freeze-dried collagen sponge reinforced by an electrospun PLGA nanofibrous layer (Jeong, Kim, *et al.*, 2007), and a multi-layered tube containing collagen and elastin fibrils extracted from animal tissues (Koens, Faraj, *et al.*, 2010). Elastin is a natural protein existing in human/animal native tissues, inlucing vessels.

An alternative choice for bioengineered vascular scaffolds is the de-cellularized vessel. Such a construct has been processed from blood vessels from humans (e.g., umbilical arteries) (Gui, Muto, *et al.*, 2009), canines (Zhou, Liu, *et al.*, 2009), sheep (Zhao, Zhang, *et al.*, 2011) and bovines (Grandi, Baiguera, *et al.*, 2011) by removing the cells from their ECM. Encouraging results from such an approach include only slightly decreased but not significantly altered average burst pressure (840 mmHg), as compared to that of the original vessels (970 mmHg) (Gui, Muto, *et al.*, 2009), and the construction of patent grafts that were still exhibiting a high degree of re-endothelialization 6 months after the implantation (Zhou, Liu, *et al.*, 2009). Another advantage of such de-cellularized grafts is the likelihood that a larger number of off-the-shelf grafts can be provided when needed. However, their drawbacks include the limitations in tailoring contents of the matrix and designing of struc-tures (McClure, Wolfe, *et al.*, 2011). Their reported long-term stability and performance also need further investigation and verification.

10.2.3. Regulators

A vital part of the application of tissue engineering is the delivery of various drugs or regulators from the scaffold to the cells/tissues. Useful drugs such as anti-coagulants (e.g., heparin) and regulators (especially growth factors) can be covalently bound into scaffolding materials to increase the patency of vascular grafts (Zhou, Liu, *et al.*, 2009; Koens, Faraj, *et al.*, 2010).

A naturally occurring substance (usually a protein or a steroid hor-

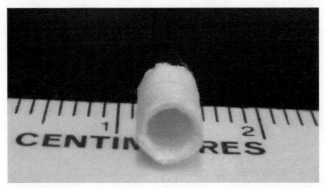

FIGURE 10.1. *An electrospun nanofibrous tubular scaffold for bioengineering vascular graft.*

mone) capable of stimulating cellular growth, proliferation and cellular differentiation, the *growth factor* is important for regulating a variety of cellular processes. Frequently applied in vascular tissue engineering are VEGF (vascular endothelial growth factor) (Zhou, Liu, *et al.*, 2009), bFGF (basic fibroblast growth factor) (Polykandriotis, Arkudas, *et al.*,

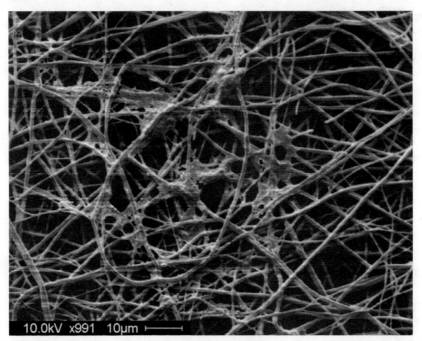

FIGURE 10.2. *Smooth muscle cells seeded on a PCL/gelatin nanofibrous scaffold for vascular tissue engineering.*

2011), PDGF (platelet-derived growth factor) (Mooney, Richardson, *et al.*, 2001) and SDF (stromal cell-derived factor) (Tang, Thevenot, *et al.*, 2010), well known for their ability to promote cell proliferation and tissue development. Specifically, VEGF plays an important role in promoting endothelial cell proliferation and neovascularization (i.e., development of new blood vessels); bFGF stimulates angiogenesis (i.e., formation and development of blood vessels) (Iwasaki, Kuwahara, *et al.*, 2004); PDGF recruits smooth muscle cells and promotes ECM deposition to stabilize new blood vessels; and SDF assists in angiogenesis by recruiting endothelial progenitor cells from the bone marrow (McClure, Wolfe, *et al.*, 2011). These regulators or their genes can usually be incorporated into the scaffolds in a variety of ways: (1) the regulator(s) is(are) mixed with the scaffolding polymer(s) before the fabrication of a scaffold, so that the regulator(s) will be physically embedded into the scaffolding structure and rapidly released from the scaffold during the application (Mooney, Shea, *et al.*, 1999); (2) the regulator(s) is(are) encapsulated into microspheres or nanoparticles before they are mixed into the polymer scaffolding structure, so that the regulator(s) will be released from the scaffold in a sustained manner (Mooney, Richardson, *et al.*, 2001); or (3) the regulator(s) can be immobilized onto/into a scaffold via conjugation with the scaffolding polymer (Feng, Ye, *et al.*, 2011).

Despite extensive research and development work in the last few decades, bioengineered vascular grafts are still in the stage of experimentation or, at most, undergoing clinical trials. One important reason is that, by using man-made materials/structures, it is difficult to simulate the complex and heterogeneous structure and functions of a natural vessel. The wall of a native artery is of three different types of structure with different mechanical properties: the tunica intima (inside), the tunica media (middle) and the tunica adventitia (outside). Tunica adventitia is composed mainly of a longitudinally-arranged collagen fibrous matrix. In the tunica media, smooth muscle cells (SMC) produce elastin, collagen and proteoglycans, which impart excellent mechanical elasticity and recovery to the vessel. Tunica intima is composed of endothelial cells (EC) and loose connective tissues. There is a gradient of mechanical stiffness and strength along the radial direction of the native artery vessel—that is, the loose connective tissue and endothelial cell layers of the tunica intima (inside) have low stiffness and strength, while the smooth muscle cells, elastin and collagen of the tunica media (middle) have a higher stiffness and strength, and the tunica adventitia (outside) has the highest strength to help prevent the vessel from rupturing at a very high pressure (Wagenseil and Mecham, 2009). Although there have already been pilot research and development of bioengineered vascular grafts with multiple layers containing different materials, structures and/or cell types (McClure, Sell, *et al.*, 2011), their long-term stability and performance need further investigation and monitoring.

10.3. BIOENGINEERED EXTRACORPOREAL DEVICES

As contrasted to traditional extracorporeal devices, bioengineered (bioartificial) extracorporeal devices are some of the products resulting from recent research and development endeavors in the field of tissue engineering. Those that have attained a degree of maturity are described as follows.

As discussed in Section 9.5, the artificial kidney or hemodialyzer has been used to take over some of the functions normally performed by the natural human kidney, including hemodialysis and ultrafiltration. The so-called *bioengineered extracorporeal kidney* is supposed to perform, in addition to the usual dialysis and ultrafiltration, more complicated tasks, termed as metabolic, endocrine, and immune. Namely, it will do much more than the mere task of filtration, all in order to increase the chances of survival for patients with acute or chronic renal failure (Fissell, Kimball, *et al.*, 2001). Such a bioartificial kidney is similar to the conventional hemodialyzer, except that viable cells are incorporated into the extracapillary or intracapillary spaces so as to get attached to the outer surfaces of hollow fibers. Alternatively, these cells can be entrapped in gels or immobilized onto polymeric microcarriers so that they will not block the pores or frustrate mass exchange across the membrane. These viable cells have been extracted from such sources as human kidneys unsuitable for cadaver transplant and porcine kidney cells. After harvesting, culturing and seeding them onto the hollow fibrous bioreactors, it is possible that they will perform some of the metabolic functions on behalf of a kidney (Fissell, Kimball, *et al.*, 2001; Saito 2003). In an initial clinical trial treatment using bioartificial kidneys, human renal cells were grown to confluence along the inner surface of the hollow fibers in a commercial hemodialyzer, and the resulting bioartificial kidney demonstrated functional and metabolic performance for up to 24 hours of use in 10 patients, showing encouraging promise of applicability of this new approach (Humes, Weitzel, *et al.*, 2004). Further clinical studies on its long-term performance and safety are yet to be conducted.

The liver is a major metabolic and synthetic organ that performs multiple functions critical to human life. Hepatic failure can lead to life crisis. The therapy of liver transplantation is always limited by the availability of suitable donors. Blood purification is therefore an alternative treatment for patients who suffer from hepatic failure. Different from the human kidney that removes water soluble wastes from the body, the liver is responsible for removing protein-bound toxins. To achieve such a function, mechanical liver support has been developed to remove toxins from the patient's blood or plasma via adsorption devices (Naruse, Tang, *et al.*, 2007). However, such a device is unable to perform, on behalf of the natural liver, the other important functions, including metabolism and protein synthesis. This has led to the development of the *bioartificial liver* (BAL) based on tissue engineering approaches.

Hollow fiber-based bioartificial liver devices can also be developed by culturing living hepatocytes (from animals or the human) inside the hollow fibers and causing the blood of the patient to circulate in the extracapillary space. Toxic components in the blood that generally diffuse through the hollow fiber membrane into the luminal space are metabolized by the entrapped hepatocytes, and will then either diffuse back into the bloodstream or be washed out by way of the intraluminal stream. Alternatively, such cells can be cultured outside the hollow fiber and the blood goes through the luminal space (Tzanakakis, Hess, *et al.*, 2000). It is crucial and challenging in the development of bioartificial liver devices to ensure that hepatocytes will function in such an *in vitro* environment.

Polymers used for hemo-dialyzers, including polysulfone and cellulose acetate, have also been used for bioartificial liver devices. They worked positively in a clinical trial treatment for up to 5 days (Lanza, Langer, *et al.*, 2007), but long-term performance of these BAL devices for clinical uses needs further investigation.

In addition, special polymers or polymers with special structures/treatments have been studied. Various types of carbohydrate-immobilized phosphorylcholine (MPC) polymers can be used for both flat and hollow fiber membranes as interfaces with living cells (Iwasaki, Takami, *et al.*, 2008). Cells adhering to the carbohydrate-immobilized MPC polymer surface function more efficiently than cells adhering to the poly(n-butyl methacrylate) (PBMA) surface. The polymer is therefore believed to be able to provide a suitable surface for the cultivation of hepatocytes, manifesting its potential use in the construction of reliable BAL devices. In the design of a cross hollow fiber bioreactor intended to support the long-term maintenance and differentiation of human hepatocytes, two types of hollow fiber membranes that are alternatively cross-assembled can be used: one is the modified polyetheretherketone (PEEK-WC) that provides the cells with an oxygenated medium containing nutrients and metabolites, and the other is polyethersulfone that removes metabolites and cell-specific products from the cell compartment (De Bartolo, Salerno, *et al.*, 2009). In this way, the two types of membranes mimic the *in vivo* arterial and venous blood vessels. According to the report, the human hepatocytes will maintain their metabolic function for up to 18 days in such a system. In another design (Chu, Shi, *et al.*, 2009), a multi-layer, radial-flow bioreactor based on a galactosylated chitosan nanofiber scaffold is made of 65 layers of stacked polycarbonate plates, onto which electrospun chitosan nanofibers will be deposited to support the hepatocytes. These galactosylated chitosan nanofiber membranes will function more efficiently due to improved cell adhesion. In addition, the use of pig red blood cells in the culture medium is recommended because they provide oxygen for the hepatocytes. Research results suggest that this type of pre-bioreactor may provide short-term support for patients with hepatic failure.

Since similar polymer materials are generally used in the construction of bioartificial kidneys and bioartificial liver, it is proposed that a well-designed hollow fiber filter system can be applied in an advanced total hemopurification system of bioartificial kidney and liver assist devices (Ye, Watanabe, *et al.*, 2005; 2006). In such a system, blood taken from a patient suffering from both renal and hepatic failure is pumped into a plasmapheresis device to separate blood cells from plasma. Plasma thus separated enters a biohybrid liver assist reactor for detoxification. The detoxified plasma is then passed first through a hemofilter that performs the traditional function of hemofiltration and then through a biohybrid renal tubule, where re-absorption is carried out.

Fiber bioreactors have also been used in the development of the *bioartificial pancreas* for treating diabetes (Velez, Stephens, *et al.*, 1997; Boyd, Lopez, *et al.*, 1998; Morita, 1998; Chae, Kim, *et al.*, 2001). Related research work is focused on the integration of islets of Langerhans into flat sheet or hollow fiber membranes. These membranes separate the cells from the blood and are permeable for glucose and insulin but impermeable to immunoglobulins and lymphocytes (Beck, Angus, *et al.*, 2007). Related research work has only been carried out in laboratories, however.

10.4. SUMMARY

The ultimate goal of tissue engineering is, theoretically and ideally, to custom-build every vital organ of the human body—the skin, kidney, liver, bladder, heart, bone, cartilage, ligament, etc.—when the original organs start to fail to perform their functions. The diseased or failing organs are not rebuilt piece by piece, however, but kind of "tissue by tissue"; namely, they have to be repaired or restored by causing the related "tissues" to *regain* the ability to live normally (hence the term "tissue regeneration") as a result of healing diseased or damaged tissues and/or making and using substitutes for those that have failed to work. Since the regeneration of tissues is directed by the physical presence and/or chemical activities of *biomaterials* (many of which are textiles, as discussed in Chapter 9), this chapter for "tissue engineering" must be biomaterials-oriented.

The success of a tissue engineering approach depends upon the combined performance of cells, scaffold and regulator(s), kind of a "tripod". Of these three components, *scaffold* is entirely a matter of biomaterials (including textile materials), and is therefore what we hope our readers will pay utmost attention to.

Thus, besides emphasizing scaffolding in the related texts, we have constantly drawn attention to the benefits and use of materials for the purpose of tissue engineering. That is why, for instance, we name PCL as a "biocompatible and bio-absorbable" polymer for bioengineered vascular grafts, due to its mechanical performance, such as high strength and excellent compliance. In addition, even when we talk about "cells", which is not a matter of materials, we make it clear that their function can be materials-related; for example, cells arranged to adhere to the carbohydrate-immobilized MPC polymer surface function more efficiently than cells adhering to the poly(n-butyl methacrylate) (PBMA) surface.

While we have only mentioned some of the efforts in this chapter, tissue engineering has the ambition to heal or restore every human organ. This is an exciting field of research which will undoubtedly develop extensively in the future.

10.5. REFERENCES

Beck, J., R. Angus, *et al.* (2007). Islet encapsulation: strategies to enhance islet cell functions. *Tissue Engineering* **13**(3): 589–599.

Bell, E., A.W. Owens, *et al.* (2008). Differentiating dermal stem cells into vascular endothelial cells for use in tissue engineering vascular grafts. *Journal of Molecular and Cellular Cardiology* **44**(4): 801–801.

Berglund, J.D., M.M. Mohseni, *et al.* (2003). A biological hybrid model for collagen-based tissue engineered vascular constructs. *Biomaterials* **24**(7): 1241–1254.

Bordenave, L., P. Fernandez, *et al.* (2005). In vitro endothelialized ePTFE prostheses: clinical update 20 years after the first realization. *Clinical Hemorheology and Microcirculation* **33**(3): 227–234.

Boyd, R.F., M. Lopez, *et al.* (1998). Solute washout experiments for characterizing mass transport in hollow fiber immunoisolation membranes. *Annals of Biomedical Engineering* **26**(4): 618–626.

Caldwell, F.T., Jr., B.H. Wallace, *et al.* (1996). Sequential excision and grafting of the burn injuries of 1,507 patients treated between 1967 and 1986: end results and the determinants of death. *Journal of Burn Care and Rehabilitation* **17**(2): 137–146.

Chae, S.Y., S.W. Kim, *et al.* (2001). Bioactive polymers for biohybrid artificial pancreas. *Journal of Drug Targeting* **9**(6): 473–484.

Chu, X.H., X.L. Shi, *et al.* (2009). In vitro evaluation of a multi-layer radial-flow bioreactor based on galactosylated chitosan nanofiber scaffolds. *Biomaterials* **30**(27): 4533–4538.

Clark, R.A.F., K. Ghosh, *et al.* (2007). Tissue engineering for cutaneous wounds. *Journal of Investigative Dermatology* **127**(5): 1018–1029.

Curran, M.P. and G.L. Plosker (2002). Bilayered bioengineered skin substitute (Apligraf®)—A review of its use in the treatment of venous leg ulcers and diabetic foot ulcers. Biodrugs **16**(6): 439–455.

De Bartolo, L., S. Salerno, *et al.* (2009). Human hepatocyte functions in a crossed hollow fiber membrane bioreactor. *Biomaterials* **30**(13): 2531–2543.

Deutsch, M., J. Meinhart, *et al.* (1999). Clinical autologous in vitro endothelialization of infrainguinal ePTFE grafts in 100 patients: a 9-year experience. *Surgery* **126**(5): 847–855.

DiMuzio, P.J., L.J. Harris, *et al.* (2011). Differentiation of adult stem cells into smooth muscle for vascular tissue engineering. *Journal of Surgical Research* **168**(2): 306–314.

Eaglstein, W.H. and V. Falanga. (1997). Tissue engineering and the development of Apligraf®, a human skin equivalent. *Clinical Therapeutics* **19**(5): 894–905.

Edmonds, M.E., A.V. Foster, *et al.* (1997). 'Dermagraft': a new treatment for diabetic foot ulcers. *Diabetic Medicine* **14**(12): 1010–1011.

Ehrenreich, M. and Z. Ruszczak. (2006). Update on tissue-engineered biological dressings. *Tissue Engineering* **12**(9): 2407–2424.

Feng, Z.G., L. Ye, *et al.* (2011). Heparin-conjugated PCL scaffolds fabricated by electrospinning and loaded with Fibroblast Growth Factor 2. *Journal of Biomaterials Science-Polymer Edition* **22**(1-3): 389–406.

Fette, A. (2005). Integra artificial skin in use for full-thickness burn surgery: benefits or harms on patient outcome. *Technology and Health Care: Official Journal of the European Society for Engineering and Medicine* **13**(6): 463–8.

Fissell, W.H., J. Kimball, *et al.* (2001). The role of a bioengineered artificial kidney in renal failure. *Bioartificial Organs III: Tissue Sourcing, Immunoisolation, and Clinical Trials* **944**: 284–295.

Friess, W. (1998). Collagen—biomaterial for drug delivery. *European Journal of Pharmaceutics and Biopharmaceutics* **45**(2): 113–136.

Grandi, C., S. Baiguera, *et al.* (2011). Decellularized bovine reinforced vessels for small-diameter tissue-engineered vascular grafts. *International Journal of Molecular Medicine* **28**(3): 315–325.

Green, H., O. Kehinde, *et al.* (1979). Growth of cultured human epidermal-cells into multiple epithelia suitable for grafting. *Proceedings of the National Academy of Sciences of the United States of America* **76**(11): 5665–5668.

Gui, L.Q., A. Muto, *et al.* (2009). Development of decellularized human umbilical arteries as small-diameter vascular grafts. *Tissue Engineering Part A* **15**(9): 2665–2676.

Hanson, S.J., K. Jamshidi, *et al.* (1988). Mechanical evaluation of resorbable copolymers for end use as vascular grafts. *ASAIO transactions/American Society for Artificial Internal Organs* **34**(3): 789–93.

He, W., T. Yong, *et al.* (2005). Fabrication and endothelialization of collagen-blended biodegradable polymer nanofibers: potential vascular graft for blood vessel tissue engineering. *Tissue Engineering* **11**(9-10): 1574–1588.

Herring, M., A. Gardner, *et al.* (1978). Single-staged technique for seeding vascular grafts with autogenous endothelium. *Surgery* **84**(4): 498–504.

Herring, M., J. Smith, *et al.* (1994). Endothelial seeding of polytetrafluoroethylene femoral popliteal bypasses—the failure of low-density seeding to improve patency. *Journal of Vascular Surgery* **20**(4): 650–655.

Hibino, N., E. McGillicuddy, *et al.* (2010). Late-term results of tissue-engineered vascular grafts in humans. *Journal of Thoracic and Cardiovascular Surgery* **139**(2): 431–U233.

Humes, H.D., W.F. Weitzel, *et al.* (2004). Initial clinical results of the bioartificial kidney containing human cells in ICU patients with acute renal failure. *Kidney International* **66**(4): 1578–1588.

Iwasaki, A., M. Kuwahara, *et al.* (2004). Basic fibroblast growth factor (bFGF) and vascular endothelial growth factor (VEGF) levels, as prognostic indicators in NSCLC. *European Journal of Cardio-Thoracic Surgery* **25**(3): 443–448.

Iwasaki, K., K. Kojima, *et al.* (2008). Bioengineered three-layered robust and elastic artery using hemodynamically-equivalent pulsatile bioreactor. *Circulation* **118**(14): S52–S57.

Iwasaki, Y., U. Takami, *et al.* (2008). Interfacing biomembrane mimetic polymer surfaces with living cells: surface modification for reliable bioartificial liver. *Applied Surface Science* **255**(2): 523–528.

Jeong, S.I., S.Y. Kim, *et al.* (2007). Tissue-engineered vascular grafts composed of marine collagen and PLGA fibers using pulsatile perfusion bioreactors. *Biomaterials* **28**(6): 1115–1122.

Kamolz, L.P., W. Haslik, *et al.* (2007). First experiences with the collagen-elastin matrix Matriderm® as a dermal substitute in severe burn injuries of the hand. *Burns* **33**(3): 364–368.

Kamolz, L.P., D.B. Lumenta, *et al.* (2008). Tissue engineering for cutaneous wounds: an overview of current standards and possibilities. *European Surgery-Acta Chirurgica Austriaca* **40**(1): 19–26.

Koens, M.J.W., K.A. Faraj, *et al.* (2010). Controlled fabrication of triple layered and molecularly defined collagen/elastin vascular grafts resembling the native blood vessel. *Acta Biomaterialia* **6**(12): 4666–4674.

Langer, R. and J.P. Vacanti (1993). Tissue engineering. *Science* **260**(5110): 920–926.

Lanza, R.P., R.S. Langer, *et al.* (2007). Principles of tissue engineering. San Diego, CA: Academic Press.

Ma, Z.W., W. He, *et al.* (2005). Grafting of gelatin on electrospun poly(caprolactone) nanofibers to improve endothelial cell spreading and proliferation and to control cell orientation. *Tissue Engineering* **11**(7-8): 1149–1158.

Madaghiele, M., A. Piccinno, *et al.* (2009). Collagen- and gelatine-based films sealing vascular prostheses: evaluation of the degree of crosslinking for optimal blood impermeability. *Journal of Materials Science-Materials in Medicine* **20**(10): 1979–1989.

Matthews, J.A., G.E. Wnek, *et al.* (2002). Electrospinning of collagen nanofibers. *Biomacromolecules* **3**(2): 232–238.

McClure, M.J., S.A. Sell, *et al.* (2011). Tri-layered electrospinning to mimic native arterial architecture using polycaprolactone, elastin, and collagen: a preliminary study. *Journal of Visualized Experiments* **47**: e2084.

McClure, M.J., P.S. Wolfe, *et al.* (2011). Bioengineered vascular grafts: improving vascular tissue engineering through scaffold design. *Journal of Drug Delivery Science and Technology* **21**(3): 211–227.

Meinhart, J., M. Deutsch, *et al.* (1997). Eight years of clinical endothelial cell transplantation - Closing the gap between prosthetic grafts and vein grafts. *ASAIO Journal* **43**(5): M515–M521.

Mooney, D.J., T.P. Richardson, *et al.* (2001). Polymeric system for dual growth factor delivery. *Nature Biotechnology* **19**(11): 1029–1034.

Mooney, D.J., L.D. Shea, *et al.* (1999). DNA delivery from polymer matrices for tissue engineering. *Nature Biotechnology* **17**(6): 551–554.

Mooney, D.T., C.L. Mazzoni, *et al.* (1996). Stabilized polyglycolic acid fibre based tubes for tissue engineering. *Biomaterials* **17**(2): 115–124.

Morita, S. (1998). An experimental study on the bioartificial pancreas using polysulfone hollow fibers. *Japanese Journal of Transplantation* **33**(3): 169–180.

Naruse, K., W. Tang, *et al.* (2007). Artificial and bioartificial liver support: A review of perfusion treatment for hepatic failure patients. *World Journal of Gastroenterology* **13**(10): 1516–1521.

Nerem, R.M. and D. Seliktar (2001). Vascular tissue engineering. *Annual Review of Biomedical Engineering*. **3**: 225–243.

Pasic, M., W. Muller-Glauser, *et al.* (1996). Endothelial cell seeding improves patency of synthetic vascular grafts: manual versus automatized method. *European Journal of Cardio-Thoracic Surgery* **10**(5): 372–379.

Polykandriotis, E., A. Arkudas, *et al.* (2011). The impact of VEGF and bFGF on vascular stereomorphology in the context of angiogenic neo-arborisation after vascular induction. *J. Electron Microsc. (Tokyo)* **60**(4): 267–74.

Rosenman, J.E., R.F. Kempczinski, *et al.* (1985). Kinetics of endothelial-cell seeding. *Journal of Vascular Surgery* **2**(6): 778–784.

Saito, A. (2003). Development of bioartificial kidneys. *Nephrology* **8**: S10–S15.

Serrano, M.C., M.T. Portoles, *et al.* (2005). Vascular endothelial and smooth muscle cell culture on NaOH-treated poly (epsilon-caprolactone) films: a preliminary study for vascular graft development. *Macromolecular Bioscience* **5**(5): 415–423.

Sheridan, R.L. and R.G. Tompkins (1995). Cultured autologous epithelium in patients with burns of 90-percent or more of the body-surface. *Journal of Trauma-Injury Infection and Critical Care* **38**(1): 48–50.

Tang, L.P., P.T. Thevenot, *et al.* (2010). The effect of incorporation of SDF-1 alpha into

PLGA scaffolds on stem cell recruitment and the inflammatory response. *Biomaterials* **31**(14): 3997–4008.

Tzanakakis, E.S., D.J. Hess, *et al.* (2000). Extracorporeal tissue engineered liver-assist devices. *Annual Review of Biomedical Engineering* **2**: 607–632.

Vaz, C.M., S. van Tuijl, *et al.* (2005). Design of scaffolds for blood vessel tissue engineering using a multi-layering electrospinning technique. *Acta Biomaterialia* **1**(5): 575–582.

Velez, G.M., C.L. Stephens, *et al.* (1997). Mass transfer in hollow fiber-type artificial pancreas devices. *FASEB Journal* **11**(3): 1676–1676.

Wagenseil, J.E. and R.P. Mecham (2009). Vascular extracellular matrix and arterial mechanics. *Physiological Reviews* **89**(3): 957–989.

Wainwright, D.J. (1995). Use of an acellular allograft dermal matrix (alloderm) in the management of full-thickness burns. *Burns* **21**(4): 243–248.

Walles, T., H. Gorler, *et al.* (2004). Functional neointima characterization of vascular prostheses in human. *Annals of Thoracic Surgery* **77**(3): 864–868.

Wang, S.D., Y.Z. Zhang, *et al.* (2009). Fabrication and properties of the electrospun polylactide/silk fibroin-gelatin composite tubular scaffold. *Biomacromolecules* **10**(8): 2240–2244.

Watanabe, M., T. Shin'Oka, *et al.* (2001). Tissue-engineered vascular autograft: inferior vena cava replacement in a dog model. *Tissue Engineering* **7**(4): 429–439.

Weinberg, C.B. and E. Bell (1986). A blood-vessel model constructed from collagen and cultured vascular cells. *Science* **231**(4736): 397–400.

Ye, S.H., J. Watanabe, *et al.* (2005). Design of functional hollow fiber membranes modified with phospholipid polymers for application in total hemopurification system. *Biomaterials* **26**(24): 5032–5041.

Ye, S.H., J. Watanabe, *et al.* (2006). High functional hollow fiber membrane modified with phospholipid polymers for a liver assist bioreactor. *Biomaterials* **27**(9): 1955–1962.

Yim, H., Y.S. Cho, *et al.* (2010). The use of AlloDerm on major burn patients: AlloDerm prevents post-burn joint contracture. *Burns* **36**(3): 322–328.

Zhao, Y.L., Z G. Zhang, *et al.* (2011). Preparation of decellularized and crosslinked artery patch for vascular tissue-engineering application. *Journal of Materials Science-Materials in Medicine* **22**(6): 1407–1417.

Zhou, M., Z. Liu, *et al.* (2009). Development and validation of small-diameter vascular tissue from a decellularized scaffold coated with heparin and vascular endothelial growth factor. *Artificial Organs* **33**(3): 230–239.

Zhu, Y.B., C.Y. Gao, *et al.* (2002). Surface modification of polycaprolactone with poly(methacrylic acid) and gelatin covalent immobilization for promoting its cytocompatibility. *Biomaterials* **23**(24): 4889–4895.

CHAPTER 11

Intelligent Medical and Healthcare Textiles

INTELLIGENCE is a capacity of human beings and some living creatures. The most admirable of such intelligence is man's ability to
"sort of know" something simply according to some "feeling", without
resorting to any extra, material means (a tool, for example), and to respond to that something (regarded as a "stimulus") by modifying one's
behavior to effect positive outcomes. People have for centuries been
dreaming of, and busying themselves with, making tools that also possess that remarkable capacity to know, react and adapt to stimuli.

An even bolder dream is the incorporation of intelligence into materials (metals, textiles, etc.). This dream may have been prompted by
the great multiplicity of stimuli (e.g., mechanical, thermal, chemical,
electrical and magnetic) that stand in the way (or "the environment", to
use a modern phrase) as inconveniences, obstacles, hazards, etc. This is
the classical dream of having an extra "sense" (i.e., one in addition to
the corporal "five senses"), a dream for making man abler and stronger.

A word of comfort is that such materials no longer exist only in our
dreams. Over the decades, as is the concern of this book, a variety of
intelligent textiles and smart products have been used to promote health
and quality of life. This chapter will address such textiles and their applications in the medical and healthcare sectors.

11.1. INTELLIGENT MATERIALS

Textiles are the traditional (and the most common) material able to
protect us from cold, heat, or other environmental hazards. In order to
improve and add to such protective functions, innovations and development implemented in material science and technology have brought
about new textile materials and products capable of playing more active

251

roles towards man's better quality of life and increased health and well-being. Related to a rather new field of research and development, *intelligent textiles,* interchangeably termed as *smart* or *active* textiles, refer to textile materials and/or structures that are potentially able to sense, react and/or adapt to environmental stimuli, and therefore can be used in products for performing these functions, as discussed in Section 11.2.

11.1.1. Chromic (Color Changing) Materials

Chromism refers to the phenomenon of color change. Materials that exhibit reversible color change upon the change of external conditions are known as chromic (color changing) materials. They are usually incorporated into textile products in the form of chromic dyes, pigments, or coatings. Chromic textiles that act upon such color change are also known as chameleon textiles. Different kinds of chromism are named after the stimuli that cause color changes (Bamfield, 2001; Langenhove, 2007). They include the photo-, thermo-, electro-, and halochromic materials.

Photochromism is brought about by sunlight or UV light. The chemical structure of a photochromic material can be changed temporarily as a result of UV irradiation. This change in chemical structure leads to a shift in its absorption of electromagnetic waves to the visible part of the spectrum, upon which the color changes from colorless to colored. A reverse change in its chemical structure, and consequently in its electromagnetic waves absorption spectrum, can take place in the absence of UV rays. As a result, the material returns to its original colorless state.

Many photochromic compounds have been identified or developed for different applications. For example, they can be coated on spectacle lenses to have the lenses darken when exposed to strong sunlight while reverse to colorless in dim light. However, most of the inorganic photochromic substances, which are usually based on metals, are not suitable for treating textile materials. Some organic photochromic dyes, therefore, are often used to produce chromic textiles. Photochromic textiles have mostly been used for fashion and decoration purposes since they were commercialized in the 1980s. They are also used for military purposes to provide protection by camouflage.

Thermochromism is brought about by heat. Thermochromic materials change their molecular or supramolecular structure and absorption spectrum as a result of the variation in environmental temperature.

Application of inorganic thermochromic materials in textiles is limited due to the fact that a high temperature and/or a solvent are usually required to induce a change of color. This explains why organic thermochromic compounds are preferable for treating textiles, because their color changing temperatures are often between the ambient and body temperatures. The structural changes of organic thermochromic compounds may include rearrangement of molecules (e.g., cleavage of covalent bonds or changes in spatial configuration of a molecule) and changes in crystalline structures. Thermochromic dyes can be used for decoration and fashion. They are also used as an indicator of temperature or in thermometers (e.g., thermodiagnostics and skin thermometers).

Electrochromism is induced by electrical current. Electrochromic materials may experience a reversible change of color as a result of the gain or loss of electrons, which is an indication of redox reactions (i.e., oxidation and reduction). This process usually involves the passage of a weak electric current or potential at a voltage no more than a few volts. Electrochromic substances include some inorganic metal-based compounds and conductive polymers (e.g., polypyrrole, polyaniline, etc.).

The first commercialized electrochromic devices are self-dimming, anti-glare, rear-view car mirrors. Electrochromic materials have also been used to produce "smart windows" that automatically darken when the sunlight reaches a certain level so as to reduce the heat, and become clear again when the sunlight dims so as to allow more light in.

Halochromism is a color-changing phenomena caused by pH value. Halochromic dyes have been developed and used for textiles, and the resulting halochromic fibers or textiles can be applied in the making of pH sensors. For example, for burn patients, their skin pH values vary during the healing process; incorporation of halochromic molecules into a wound dressing allows the monitoring of the wound recovery process without causing disturbance to the wound bed (Osti, 2008). Halochromic textiles can also be used in geotextiles or protective clothing that provides real time indication of changes in environmental pH values.

Other types of chromism include piezochromism (mechanical pressure), tribochromism (mechanical friction), ionochromism (ions), solvatochromism (solvent polarity) and hygrochromism (moisture).

11.1.2. Phase Changing Materials

Phase (or structure) changing materials are a group of intelligent materials that change their morphology (e.g., shape, porosity, solubility, state, molecular structure) upon predetermined stimuli (e.g., thermal, chemical). Discussed in the following are materials in this group that are used more often: thermal regulation phase changing materials, intelligent hydrogels, and the various shape memory materials.

Typically, phase changing materials (PCM) are remarkable for their capacity to store or release heat upon changes of their states over a narrow range of temperature, and can therefore be used for the purpose of thermal regulation. Specifically, *thermal regulation phase changing materials* absorb latent heat as a result of phase change (e.g., changing from a solid state into a liquid one) during the heating process, a process during which temperature of PCM and their surroundings remains almost constant. Conversely, the materials release the stored latent heat into the environment due to a reverse phase change (e.g., changing from a liquid state into a solid one) during the cooling process, again a process during which the materials and their surroundings undergo almost negligible changes in temperature. Namely, PCM's thermal regulation capacity depends on their ability to absorb or release a large amount of heat with little temperature change.

A good example of natural PCM with high latent heat storage capacity is water, which absorbs a latent heat of about 335J/g upon being heated (i.e., melting) from ice to liquid water, but it will absorb only about 4J/g when it is further heated as a liquid. For that reason, ice can be a theoretically good thermal regulation material when the purpose is to reduce heat (i.e., to have a lot of heat absorbed).

Some PCMs may differ in their phase change temperature ranges and heat storage capacities. The most commonly used PCM are paraffins, which are linear long chain hydrocarbons and a by-product of oil refining with the general formula C_nH_{2n+2}. For instance, hexadecane ($C_{16}H_{34}$) melts at 18.5°C and crystallizes at 16.2°C, with a latent heat storage capacity of 237 J/g, and eicosane ($C_{20}H_{42}$) melts at 36.1°C and crystallizes at 30.6°C, with a heat storage capacity of 247 J/g. The paraffins can be mixed for a desirable phase changing temperature range. In order to prevent loss of PCM during their liquid stage, they are usually encapsulated into microspheres with diameters ranging from 1–20 μm. These PCM-encapsulated microspheres can be further incorporated into textiles via a number of ways: (1) The micro-capsules are embedded into the fibers by mixing the micro-capsules with the spinning solution before spinning; (2) the micro-capsules are mixed into a coating compound which is then applied topically onto a textile substrate; (3) the micro-capsules are mixed into a foaming compound which is then applied topically onto or laminated with a textile substrate; or (4) the micro-capsules are dispersed into the porous structures of a fibrous substrate (e.g., nonwoven) (Langenhove, 2007). Other PCMs include hydrated inorganic salts (e.g., $Na_2SO_4 \cdot 10H_2O$), PEG (polyethylene glycol) and fatty acids (Mondal, 2008).

The incorporation of PCM into textile materials and products was first investigated in the early 1980s by the US National Aeronautics and Space Administration (NASA) as part of the efforts to improve the thermal performance of space suits, which were expected to provide protection against the extreme temperature variations in outer space. A recent trend is the development of PCM-incorporated textiles for consumer apparel products, to meet the demand of those who wish that their clothes would be so smart as to be able to thermally regulate as the environment requires.

Currently, PCM-incorporated textiles have already been used in the healthcare and medical sectors in such products as heating and cooling pads/blankets. Heating and cooling pads are made of a PCM-incorporated polymer matrix embedded in a textile cover. A heating pad can be used for thermal therapy: it can be heated to a desirable temperature in a microwave or oven and, when it is brought into contact with the diseased part of the body, it functions by having the heat stored in the PCM slowly released to help heal that part. On the other hand, a cooling pad can be applied to a body part that is suffering inflammation: the pad absorbs the heat and provides cooling that is gentler than an ice pack, and it does not require refrigeration to regenerate. PCM can also be incorporated into bedding products or surgical protective gowns to enhance their thermal comfort (Langenhove, 2007).

As mentioned in Chapters 6 and 8, hydrogels are made of a water-swollen, three-dimensional network, composed of physically or chemically cross-linked hydrophilic polymers. Environmental stimuli-responsive, *intelligent hydrogels* are usually designed to undergo reversible volume transformation (e.g., expansion or contraction) due to changes of environmental conditions, such as temperature, pH, electrical field, solvent composition, and concentration of certain chemical compounds.

A wide variety of polymers have been developed as intelligent hydrogels capable of responding to different stimuli. Alginate, for example, is a natural, ion-sensitive hydrogel that is responsive to Ca^{2+} or other divalent ions. Cellulose-based electrolyte hydrogel containing NaCMC (sodium carboxymethyl cellulose) is pH sensitive.

A major application of intelligent hydrogels is in controlled drug delivery. For such hydrogels, environmental stimuli (e.g., pH, temperature) trigger the swelling-shrinking transition, which in turn changes the molecular mesh size. A drug or other bioactive molecule can therefore be designed to be either entrapped in (when the hydrogel shrinks) or released from (when the hydrogel swells) its hydrogel matrix (Peppas, 1997).

Shape memory materials have the capacity to "remember" their original shape; for example, they can return to their previous shape upon exposure to a stimulus, such as deformation due to external stress. The most frequently used are thermally-induced, shape memory materials, which are discussed in this section. Certain metal alloys and polymers demonstrate such a smart capacity. A reversible change in the shape of a shape memory material results from a phase transition during the heating process at a certain temperature: for a shape memory alloy (e.g., the Nickel-Titanium alloy), reversible crystal transformation is involved; for a shape memory polymer (SMP), there usually occurs a reversible transformation from a glassy state to a rubbery state (Langenhove, 2007).

SMPs are usually block-copolymers containing both hard and soft segments. The hard segments (e.g., polyurethane) form a crystalline region and determine the permanent shape. The soft segments (e.g., polyether or polyester diol), on the other hand, construct an amorphous region that is responsible for the deformation, retaining the temporary shape, and returning to the original shape upon exposure to the predetermined stimulus.

SMPs have been used for a variety of biomedical applications, including stents, sutures, and surgical gowns, as detailed below.

Introduced in the 1980s, the metallic *vascular stent* is an expandable device to support and prevent the narrowing of a blood vessel. Polymer coatings were later developed to provide drug-eluting stents (DESs), in which the polymer coatings improve biocompatibility and serve as carriers for drugs that reduce thrombosis (O'Brien and Carroll, 2009). Recently, SMPs have found potential applications in vascular stents because of their enhanced biocompatibility, biodegradability, drug loading capacity, compliance and strain recovery capacity as compared to polymer-coated metal. SMP stents are usually programmed to have an activation temperature closely proximate to the body temperature. As a result, such an "intelligent" stent can be inserted into the human body through a small delivery instrumentation so as to ensure minimal invasion, and will then deploy to fit the vessels (Yakacki and Gall, 2010), as shown in Figure 11.1. Both thermoplastic (e.g., polyurethane) (Wache, Tartakowska, *et al.*, 2003) and thermoset (e.g., acrylates) (Gall, Yakacki, *et al.*, 2005) polymers have been developed for this purpose. Research and development work for vascular stents made from SMPs is, however, still in the stage of *in vitro* tests in labs, and performance of such devices have to be justified through further characterization and *in vivo* experiments.

Biocompatible and biodegradable SMPs were first introduced as a potential material for *intelligent sutures,* and as a solution to the well-known challenge in endoscopic surgery: it is very difficult to use normal instruments to form a knot to close an incision with an appropriate stress. That is, if the knot is formed with a force that is too strong, it may cause damage to the surrounding tissue; if the force is too weak, there may be the danger of hernia due to scar tissue that is lower in mechanical strength than healthy tissue. As a result, it is desirable that

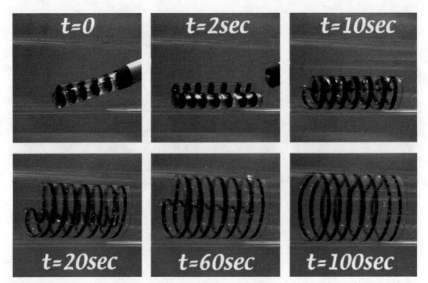

FIGURE 11.1. *The sequence of an SMP stent being deployed: it was delivered via an 18 Fr. catheter and expanded into a 22 mm ID glass tube containing body temperature water at 37°C. [Reprinted with permission from Yakacki, Shandas et al., 2007. Copyright (2007) Elsevier].*

the suture is so smart that it can be temporarily elongated and applied loosely into the surgical position so that the temperature can be raised above the traditional point, and then the suture will duly shrink and tighten the knot to provide an optimum force. A suitable polymer material for this application can also be made to consist of a hard and a soft segment. For example, a degradable multi-block polymer is reported to contain a hard segment of oligo(*p*-dioxanone)diol and a soft segment of oligo(e-caprolactone)diol, the two segments being coupled with 2,2(4),4-trimethylhexanediisocyanate. *In vitro* and animal model tests have validated its status as an "intelligent" suture, as shown in Figures 11.2 and 11.3 (Lendlein and Langer, 2002).

Piezoelectric materials have a unique property in that they generate an electric voltage when mechanically deformed, and conversely, with the application of an external electric field, it becomes mechanically deformed again. A well-known piezoelectric material in our everyday life is quartz (silica dioxide or SiO_2), its piezoelectric properties allowing it to be used as a frequency standard (quartz clocks or watches). Other piezoelectric materials include crystals, ceramics and polymers. Piezoelectric polymers include polyvinylidene fluoride (PVDF), polyacrilonitrile (PAN) and odd-numbered nylons like nylon-11 and nylon-7.

Piezoresistive materials have characteristics similar to those of piezoelectric materials, but are different in that they change their conductivity/resistivity (instead of producing an electric voltage) upon

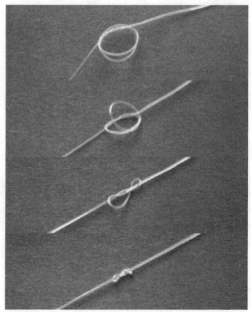

FIGURE 11.2. *A suture of thermoplastic shape-memory polymer, which can be pre-stretched for about 200% before forming a loose knot, with its two ends fixed (the photo series showing, from top to bottom, how the knot tightened in 20 seconds when heated to 40°C. [Reprinted with permission from Lendlein and Langer, 2002. Copyright ©2002, American Association for the Advancement of Science].*

applied mechanical stress. Polymeric piezoresistive materials include conducting polymers (e.g., polypyrrole, polyaniline) and carbon-loaded elastomers (Schwarz, 2010).

Piezoelectric and piezoresistive materials have been used in sensors (e.g., for the measurement of mechanical strength and pressure), resonators, actuators, and so on (Tichý, Erhart, *et al.*, 2010). In the medical or healthcare sectors, they have been studied for their applications in intelligent clothing for healthcare and disease management.

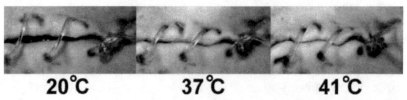

FIGURE 11.3. *A degradable shape-memory suture for wound closure, the photo series from an animal experiment showing (left to right) shrinkage of the suture with increased temperature. [Reprinted with permission from Lendlein and Langer, 2002. Copyright © 2002, American Association for the Advancement of Science].*

11.2. INTELLIGENT TEXTILE PRODUCTS

There is currently a need for intelligent or smart products due to increased recognition of the importance for the elderly and people with chronic diseases or disabilities to live "independently", obviously a matter of higher life quality for them. To that end, extensive efforts have been made, for example, to promote "active aging". A major goal of such efforts is to give the elderly the ability to perform activities and functions required in daily life with no or little help from others (WHO, 2002). A promising approach to achieving this goal has been to use intelligent textiles in healthcare products (articles, devices, units, etc.) and therapeutic treatments, often by way of health monitoring and disease management, so that these people may not have to be confined to hospitals for healthcare or treatment.

Smart devices made from intelligent textiles are expected to provide remote monitoring of a patient's physiological and physical data and signs via non-invasive sensors embedded in clothing materials. These data or signs can be used to support diagnosis and personalized management of chronic diseases like diabetes, arthritis, lung and heart disease, and hypertension. Such technologies allow patients to be treated at home instead of hospitals; they also allow early detection of diseases and timely treatment (Cho and Lee, 2007).

To perform their functions, these smart textile products are often combined into a system, which typically contains the following components: (1) sensors; (2) signal/data processing devices; (3) actuation devices; (4) telecommunication devices; (5) data management devices; and (6) decision support units. Among these, components 1–4 can be integrated on a wearable textile/clothing platform; components 5 and 6 are usually located in the central mentoring unit, in which local healthcare professionals can analyze the data and monitor the health status of the patient, make decisions or be dispatched to offer help in the shortest amount of time. Such a system can be applied in home healthcare for the elderly, people with chronic diseases, or individuals in rehabilitation.

Depending on the functions and behaviors of intelligent textile systems, they can be divided into three categories: (1) a textile system with only a sensing function, referred to as *passive smart textile;* (2) a textile system with both sensing and actuating functions, or an *active smart textile;* and (3) a textile system with an adaptive function (i.e., able to adapt its behavior to the environment), known as a very smart textile system (Tao and Textile Institute, Manchester, England, 2001).

A system of intelligent textile products mimics living creatures (mostly the human being) in the way in which they sense and respond to stimuli, as shown in Figure 11.3: the sensors in the system mimic the nervous system in a human body to detect signals from the outer environment; the signals are analyzed or evaluated by a processor (simulating part of the human brain's function); then the actuators will, upon input of the processor in a pre-determined manner or as guided by the central control unit, act properly in response to the stimuli.

Smart functions of such a system are endowed by the intelligent materials, which are often embedded or incorporated in the fiber, yarn or fabric structures. These materials can be classified according to the types of stimuli, such as the mechanical, light, thermal, chemical, electrical and magnetic. They can also be categorized by the way they respond to these stimuli, such as color change, structural change and shape change (deformation), as discussed in section 11.1.

Application of smart devices made from intelligent textiles can be conveniently discussed under two subtitles: the sensor (a typical, central smart device), and the smart clothing system, which is a typical smart textile system.

11.2.1. The Sensor

Although a wide variety of intelligent functions have been developed for textile products, sensing remains to be the most progressive area for intelligent textiles. A number of healthcare parameters can now be measured by fiber- or textile-based sensors. These parameters include: body temperature, biopotentials (e.g., cardiogram), acoustics (e.g., heart and lung), ultrasound (blood flow), motion (e.g., respiration and motion), pressure (e.g., blood), and mechanical and electric parameters of the skin.

Temperature sensors can be integrated into clothing systems to help monitor body temperature, a basic health parameter. It is important that

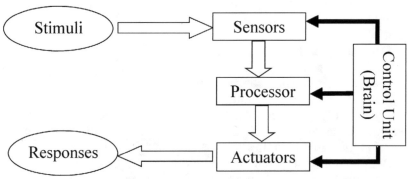

FIGURE 11.4. *A smart textile system.*

these sensors be designed in such a way as to cause minimum disturbance to the wearer. Currently, resistance temperature detectors (RTDs) or resistance temperature sensors are the most popular sensors used for this purpose. Their working mechanism is that the resistance (R) of a conductor increases with the increase in temperature (T):

$$(R - R_0)/R_0 = \alpha(T - T_0) \tag{11.1}$$

where α is the temperature coefficient of resistance, and R_0 the resistance of the material at reference temperature T_0.

Platinum (Pt) thin film is a frequently used material for RTDs. These RTDs, usually in the form of micro temperature-sensing arrays, can be integrated onto a flexible platform via the micro-electronic-mechanical system (MEMS) technology (Xiao, Che, *et al.*, 2007; Kinkeldei, Zysset, *et al.*, 2009). Figure 11.5 shows an example of such a MEMS fabrication process in these steps: (1) as shown in Figure 11.5(a), a flexible polyimide film, Kapton, is pre-treated to achieve a clean surface; (2) a layer of sensing material (usually a metal, e.g., Pt) is then deposited onto the substrate, as demonstrated in Figure 11.5(b); (3) the coated substrate is then attached to a clean glass side with drops of de-ionized water to keep the substrate flat during procedures, as shown in Figure 11.5(c); (4) a thin layer of pre-patterned resist is thereafter deposited on top of the sensing material layer to temporarily shield the selected areas of the sensing material during subsequent procedures, as shown in Figure 11.5(d); (5) the sensing material layer goes through an etching procedure to remove the areas that have not been protected by the resist layer, leaving behind the protected areas with a pre-designed pattern, as shown in Figure 11.5(e); (6) the final product (i.e., a flexible substrate integrated with sensing arrays, is obtained by removing the temporary resist layer and the underlying glass slide, as shown in Figure 11.5(f). Subsequently, the sensor-incorporated substrate is cut into single strips, which can be further inserted into a fabric during the weaving or knitting process (Kinkeldei, Zysset, *et al.*, 2009).

A number of chronic or acute diseases affect the respiration of patients. Respiratory sensors are therefore useful for home care of patients who need long-term respiratory monitoring, as well as athletes who need long-term performance monitoring. A respiratory sensor is usually embedded in a wearable system and placed next to the thorax to detect its expansion during respiration.

Figure 11.6 illustrates one of the designs for a respiratory sensor system, a system based on a capacitive pressure sensor made of multiple layers of fabric with different structures and functions. The core of this

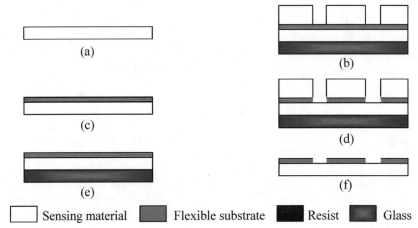

FIGURE 11.5. *A process of fabrication of RTDs on a flexible platform (adapted from Kinkeldei, Zysset, et al., 2009).*

symmetric structure is a 3D spacer fabric that determines the sensitivity of the system to applied force. The 3D spacer fabric is sandwiched between conductive fabrics which serve as the electrode of the plate capacitor. The fabric is endowed with conductivity by the incorporation of silver. Outside each of the conductive fabric layers, a layer of waterproof fabric is added to protect the sensor from being penetrated and affected by moisture. Furthermore, a layer of grounded conductive fabric is mounted on each side to shield the sensor from the external field. Finally, the multilayered sensor is protected by an extra layer of waterproof fabrics on each side. Such a sensor is thus based on the principle of a plate capacitor that is formed by two conductive textiles with a separating distance equal to the thickness of the spacer fabric. An external force (i.e., expansion of the human thorax) can change the thickness (d) of the spacer fabric and consequently the capacitance (C)

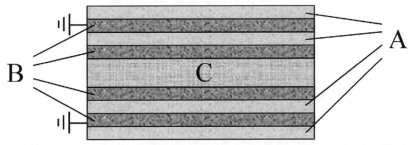

FIGURE 11.6. *A textile capacitive sensor composed of multiple layers at a cross section (A: waterproof fabrics, B: conductive fabrics, C: a 3D spacer fabric) (Hoffmann, Eilebrecht, et al., 2011).*

of the sensor, according to Equation (11.2). A continuous monitoring of the capacitance of the sensor allows detection of the wearer's respiratory pattern (Hoffmann, Eilebrecht, *et al.*, 2011).

$$C = \varepsilon_0 \varepsilon_r A / d \qquad (11.2)$$

where ε_0 is the permeability in vacuum, ε_r the relative permittivity and A the area of the capacitor.

Strain sensors, when integrated into a wearable system, are useful for physical therapists, rehabilitation and sports care professionals to monitor the motion and posture of the human body or joints. Different types of strain sensors are available for such purposes. Piezoresistive materials are good choices for strain sensors. For instance, a commercially available strain sensor is composed of a thermoplastic elastomer thread (0.3 mm in diameter) filled with 50% w/w carbon black powder. Able to change its resistivity with length, such a sensor can be incorporated in a clothing system during fabrication of the fabrics, and placed in regions of the clothing that will deform with parts of the body (Mattmann, Amft, *et al.*, 2007). Textile fabrics printed with silver in a predetermined pattern have also been developed as piezoresistive textiles for strain sensing (Calvert, Patra, *et al.*, 2007). Alternatively, piezoelectric film strips can be incorporated into a clothing system to sense the angle of a joint or a force resulting from a motion, as piezoelectric materials generate a voltage in response to the deformation or applied force (Martin, Jones, *et al.*, 2004). Micro-fabrication technology has also been applied in the fabrication of strain sensors on a flexible platform (Lichtenwalner, Hydrick, *et al.*, 2007).

Electrochemical sensors provide a faster, simpler and cheaper means to obtain a variety of healthcare-related analytical information than traditional laboratory-based assays. For example, hand-held glucose meters have been widely used for personal diabetes monitoring. Most of the currently available glucose meters involve the use of single-use sensor strips. A patient has to prick his/her finger, place a small drop of blood onto the sensor strip, and obtain a blood-glucose concentration reading. More recently, non-invasive approaches are developed for continuous glucose monitoring as an option to replace the inconvenient finger-pricking sampling (Wang, 2002), utilizing electroosmosis of glucose across intact skin (Tierney, Kim, *et al.*, 2000). Electroosmosis refers to the transport of a liquid under the influence of an applied electric field across a porous material.

Integration of electrochemical sensors onto a wearable system obviously benefits people who have chronic conditions (e.g., diabetics) and

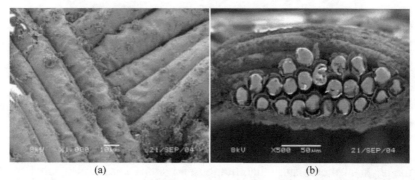

(a)   (b)

FIGURE 11.7. *A nylon fabric printed with silver in a predetermined pattern: potentially useful for strain sensors. [Reprinted with permission from Calvert, Patra et al., 2007. Copyright (2007) SPIE].*

need such arrays on a regular basis. It is important for such designs and development that performance of the integrated sensors should not be affected by the constant deformation of the clothing system. Micro-fabrication technology (e.g., screen printing) is a widely used approach to forming thick-film electrochemical sensors onto clothing structures. In a screen printing process, carbon-based ink can be printed through a patterned stencil to form a carbon electrode array onto a textile fabric substrate, followed by curing for stabilization (Wang, Yang *et al.*, 2010).

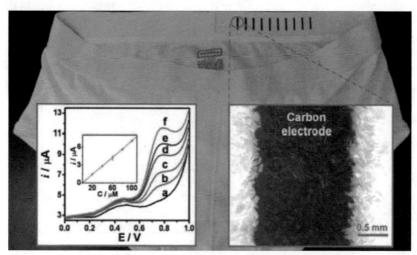

FIGURE 11.8. *Image of the screen-printed carbon electrodes on underwear along with the morphology of a single electrode (right inset) and linear-scan voltammetric response for increasing NADH concentrations over the 0–100 mM range (left inset). (Wang, Yang, et al., 2010)—Reproduced by permission of The Royal Society of Chemistry.*

In addition to the sensors discussed above, there are similar devices available to detect other important health parameters of the human body. They are usually integrated into a clothing system via one or more of the methods discussed above. For example, textile-based pressure sensors can be fabricated in a way similar to the capacitive sensor for respiratory monitoring (Holleczek, Ruegg, *et al.*, 2010); fiber-shaped sensors (including yarns/fibers coated with conductive materials, and yarns spun with a blend of normal textile fibers and conductive fibers) can be directly woven or knitted into fabrics for the monitoring of such vital signs as ECG (electrocardiographic activity) (Silva, Catarino, *et al.*, 2009); microfabrication (or MEMS) technology is another popular approach to the integration of various sensors onto a wearable system (Guler and Ertugrul, 2007; Meng, Xu, *et al.*, 2007). Readers who are interested in or need more detailed data will find them in the above references, although they represent but a portion of the extensive studies and publications available in this area.

11.2.2. The Smart Clothing System

To date, of the many devices that constitute a *smart clothing system,* the signal or data processing devices made of textile materials have not been achieved; electronic devices are still needed to provide these functions.

The *actuator* in a smart clothing system reacts to the signal released from a sensor or data processing unit. For example, an actuator may provide mechanical support to a patient with disabilities by compensating his/her lost motor functions or assisting him/her in physiotherapeutic restoration; it may also support sports training or rehabilitation by preventing risks related to abnormal stress distributions and overloading. However, the research and development of actuator-integrated textiles are still in their initial stages. A variety of smart materials, including conducting polymers, been investigated for their potential applications in wearable actuators, but there have been few reports on the effective integration of actuating functions into textiles (Carpi and De Rossi, 2005).

A *telecommunication unit* is essential for a smart system to be connected to both its wearer and the data management devices or/and decision support unit. Wireless technology is usually used for this purpose. Conductive fibers and fabrics have aided the development of textile-based antennas, which are now available in different shapes and sizes. Among these, micro-strip patch antennas are most suitable for a clothing system. Such an antenna can be composed of a metallic patch on top of a dielectric substrate (insulator), which is mounted onto a conducting ground plane. In a design of wearable antennas, the conductive components of a micro-strip patch antenna can be replaced by metal (e.g., copper and tin)-plated textile fabrics (e.g., woven nylon fabrics), and the dielectric substrate be replaced by a fleece substrate, thus making the antenna more flexible and allowing easier handling and integration into a clothing system (Hertleer, Tronquo, *et al.*, 2008), as shown in Figure 11.9. On the other hand, the communication between a smart garment and its wearer can be achieved by a flexible display, which may consist of plastic optical fibers that form a screen with a number of pixels or arrays of LED (light-emitting diode) pixels mounted on a flexible substrate (Schwarz, 2010).

Although there have been numerous research and development reports on individual components (e.g., sensors, actuators, communication devices) of a smart system, prototyping or production of an integrated intelligent clothing system remains challenging. This is because it is important that the incorporation of the smart components should cause minimum disturbance to the wearer and should not decrease the aesthetic appeal and comfort of the clothing system. Also, the smart components must work properly even when the materials are subjected to deformation caused by temperature and humidity changes, the act of wearing and cleaning, and so on. A couple of such intelligent clothing systems are cited below as instances.

WEALTHY is a wearable health care system developed in Italy. In this system, integrated on a knitted fabric platform are a number of smart sensors (in fiber and yarn forms), signal processing devices and the telecommunication unit. Specifically, the smart system has been designed to provide measurements of various parameters, such as respiration (measured by electrodes placed on the thoracic position of the clothing system for impedance pneumography), core and skin temperature (by two non-textile microelectronic sensors, one being placed under the arm for core temperature and the other near the shoulder for skin temperature), joint movement (by piezoresistive sensors next to joint locations), and electrocardiogram (ECG), as shown in Figure 11.10 (http://www.wealthy-ist.com/). Among the sensors, the piezoresistive ones are composed of a Lycra® fabric coated with carbon-loaded rub-

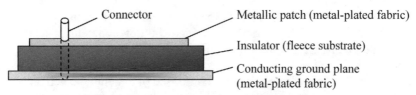

FIGURE 11.9. *Cross section of a microchip patch antenna.*

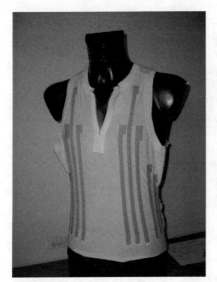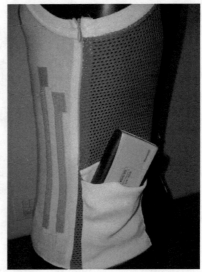

FIGURE 11.10. The WEALTHY system (with the permission from Smartex laboratories, Italy).

ber and a commercial conductive yarn. The fabric electrodes are made of two stainless steel fibers twisted around a viscose rayon textile yarn, and these connections are made from textiles using the circular knitting technique (Schwarz, 2010).

In addition, a small portable electronic device, known as the portable patient unit (PPU), is developed to collect signals from the sensor, pre-process the data and transfer the signals to such data management devices as computers, PDA (personal digital assistant) or mobile phones via wireless technology (bluetooth/GPRS[General packet radio service]). The size of the PPU is small enough to be fit into the pocket of a garment. Finally, a WEALTHY central monitoring software is designed to interpret data received from PPU for the reference of healthcare personnel to respond to (e.g., to alert the patients or provide medical assistance) when necessary.

An initial clinical trial of the WEALTHY system with ECG monitoring capacity in cardiac patients suggested that such a smart system is capable of providing real time monitoring and transmitting ECG with a comparable quality to a commonly used telemetry system, and is reasonably comfortable to wear (Coli, Grassi, *et al.*, 2006).

The *MYHEART* project was aimed at developing intelligent biomedical clothing for monitoring, diagnosing and treating cardiovascular disease (CVD) (http://www.hitech-projects.com/euprojects/myheart/). The resultant intelligent clothing system is based on a woven fabric with thin insulated copper fibers. As the building block for the fabric, the copper fibers allow the measurement of body temperature (a function based on the fact that the electrical resistance of the copper has a linear relationship with temperature). Movement of the wearer can be detected by a capacitive pressure sensor based on a spacer fabric sandwiched between two conductive patches on both sides (Schwarz, 2010). In addition, an automatic chewing sound analysis system is developed for dietary monitoring, as part of the project is to promote healthy lifestyle and increase prevention of CVD. It has been demonstrated that the sound from the users' mouth can be used to recognize the types of food being consumed (Amft, Stager, *et al.*, 2005). So far, the sounds are acquired with a microphone located inside the ear and, therefore, further efforts may have to be made so that the system can be integrated into the clothing platform.

A number of other intelligent clothing systems have been or are being developed for the purpose of health monitoring and disease control. They usually share concepts of design with systems introduced above. These intelligent clothing systems can also be applied in other areas, functioning as sports and recreational devices, protective devices, and uniforms for military and firefighting personnel. As such they may provide new solutions to traditional problems or hazards and enhance welfare and safety for people with medical conditions or in a life-threatening environment. Research and development work in this area remain pretty elementary to date, and few intelligent systems have been commercialized to benefit end users so far.

11.3. SUMMARY

Intelligent materials are important for those who are weak or disabled, have diseases, and those in high-risk occupations, because they enable these people to depend more on things and less on other people (doctors, nurses, etc.). These materials make it more likely that they will be able to live "independently", which means to them a much improved quality of life; intelligent textiles and smart products are valued largely for that remarkable benefit.

Materials are "intelligent" or "smart" because they *work* or *think* on their own, as it were, so that they are able to detect a stimulus (which more often than not stands for a danger) and react to it. This chapter introduces a series of intelligent textile materials classified according to the types of stimuli and how they react to them. Various chromic (color changing) materials are intelligent because they are able to react to the various stimuli by changing their colors. Chromic materials can be subjected to subdivision because different stimuli cause color changes in different materials; for example, electro-chromic materials are able to change their colors upon gaining or losing electrons. Similarly, phase changing materials will change their phases (shape, structure, etc.) when they react to external stimuli. Again, since there are a variety of stimuli to cause such phase changes, there are many different phase changing materials, especially the various shape changing (shape memory) materials.

A discussion of such materials necessitates a discussion of their application in relevant products, often integrated into a smart system in specific applications. This chapter discusses a typical product (the *sensor*, a smart textile-based device) and a system of such products, i.e., the *smart clothing system* as an instance or illustration of these smart systems.

Intelligent textiles and smart products for healthcare and medical applications have been the result of highly interdisciplinary research and development endeavors made in many fields: material science, telecommunication technology, engineering, and biomedicine, to name a few. Only decades ago, talk of such materials and products would sound like fairy tales or happenings in wonderlands, which justifies the fact that this book reports achievements that seem so elementary, and that the true success stories have to be found in many future books of this nature.

11.4. REFERENCES

Amft, O., M. Stager, *et al.* (2005). Analysis of chewing sounds for dietary monitoring. *Ubicomp 2005: Ubiquitous Computing, Proceedings* **3660**: 56–72.

Bamfield, P. (2001). Chromic phenomena technological applications of colour chemistry. Cambridge, UK: Royal Society of Chemistry.

Calvert, P., P. Patra, *et al.* (2007). Piezoresistive sensors for smart textiles. *Electroactive Polymer Actuators and Devices (EAPAD)* 2007 6524.

Carpi, F. and D. De Rossi (2005). Electroactive polymer-based devices for e-textiles in biomedicine. *IEEE Transactions on Information Technology in Biomedicine* **9**(3): 295–318.

Cho, H.Y. and J. Lee (2007). A development of design prototype of smart healthcare clothing for silver generation based on bio-medical sensor technology. *Human-Computer Interaction, Pt 2, Proceedings* **4551**: 1070–1077.

Coli, S., F. Grassi, *et al.* (2006). Successful real time ECG recording and transmission in cardiac patients with a wearable system based on smart textiles: first clinical experience of the WEALTHY project. *European Heart Journal* **27**: 871–871.

Gall, K., C.M. Yakacki, *et al.* (2005). Thermomechanics of the shape memory effect in polymers for biomedical applications. *Journal of Biomedical Materials Research Part A* **73A**(3): 339–348.

Guler, M. and S. Ertugrul (2007). Measuring and transmitting vital body signs using MEMS sensors. Istanbul: Istanbul Technical Univ.

Hertleer, C., A. Tronquo, *et al.* (2008). The use of textile materials to design wearable microstrip patch antennas. *Textile Research Journal* **78**(8): 651–658.

Hoffmann, T., B. Eilebrecht, *et al.* (2011). Respiratory monitoring system on the basis of capacitive textile force sensors. *IEEE Sensors Journal* **11**(5): 1112–1119.

Holleczek, T., A. Ruegg, *et al.* (2010). Textile pressure sensors for sports applications. *2010 IEEE Sensors*: 732–737.

Kinkeldei, T., C. Zysset, *et al.* (2009). Development and evaluation of temperature sensors for textile integration. *2009 IEEE Sensors,* Vols 1–3: 1502–1505.

Langenhove, L.V. (ed.) (2007). Smart textiles for medicine and healthcare : materials, systems and applications. Cambridge, England: Woodhead Pub.

Lendlein, A. and R. Langer (2002). Biodegradable, elastic shape-memory polymers for potential biomedical applications. *Science* **296**(5573): 1673–1676.

Lichtenwalner, D.J., A.E. Hydrick, *et al.* (2007). Flexible thin film temperature and strain sensor array utilizing a novel sensing concept. *Sensors and Actuators A-Physical* **135**(2): 593–597.

Martin, T., M. Jones, *et al.* (2004). Modeling and simulating electronic textile applications. *ACM Sigplan Notices* **39**(7): 10–19.

Mattmann, C., O. Amft, *et al.* (2007). Recognizing upper body postures using textile strain sensors. *Eleventh IEEE International Symposium on Wearable Computers, Proceedings* 29–36.

Meng, M., Y. Xu, *et al.* (2007). Intelligent textiles based on MEMS technology. *57th Electronic Components & Technology Conference, 2007 Proceedings.* IEEE: 2030–2034.

Mondal, S. (2008). Phase change materials for smart textiles—an overview. *Applied Thermal Engineering* **28**(11–12): 1536–1550.

"MyHeart Project." http://www.hitech-projects.com/euprojects/myheart/. Retrieved Oct 13, 2011.

O'Brien, B. and W. Carroll (2009). The evolution of cardiovascular stent materials and surfaces in response to clinical drivers: A review. *Acta Biomaterialia* **5**(4): 945–958.

Osti, E. (2008). Skin pH variations from the acute phase to re-epithelialization in burn patients treated with new materials (Burnshield®, Semipermeable Adhesive Film, Dermasilk®, and Hyalomatrix®). Non-invasive preliminary experimental clinical trial. *Annals of Burns and Fire Disasters* **11**(2): 73–77.

Peppas, N.A. (1997). Hydrogels and drug delivery. *Current Opinion in Colloid & Interface Science* **2**(5): 531–537.

Schwarz, A. (2010). A roadmap on smart textiles. Oxford, UK: Taylor & Francis.

Silva, M., A. Catarino, *et al.* (2009). Study of vital sign monitoring with textile sensors in swimming pool environment. *IECON: 2009 35th Annual Conference of IEEE Industrial Electronics, Vols 1–6*: 4202–4207.

Tao, X. and Textile Institute (Manchester, England) (2001). Smart fibres, fabrics and clothing. Boca Raton, FL: CRC Press.

Tichý, J., J. Erhart, *et al.* (2010). Fundamentals of piezoelectric sensorics: mechanical, dielectric, and thermodynamical properties of piezoelectric materials. Berlin: Springer.

Tierney, M.J., H.L. Kim, *et al.* (2000). Electroanalysis of glucose in transcutaneously extracted samples. *Electroanalysis* **12**(9): 666–671.

Wache, H.M., D.J. Tartakowska, *et al.* (2003). Development of a polymer stent with shape memory effect as a drug delivery system. *Journal of Materials Science-Materials in Medicine* **14**(2): 109–112.

Wang, J. (2002). Portable electrochemical systems. *Trac-Trends in Analytical Chemistry* **21**(4): 226–232.

Wang, J., Y.L. Yang, *et al.* (2010). Thick-film textile-based amperometric sensors and biosensors. *Analyst* **135**(6): 1230–1234.

"WEALTHY—Wearable Health Care System." http://www.wealthy-ist.com/. Retrieved Oct 13, 2011.

WHO. (2002). Active aging: a policy framework. Retrieved November 9, 2010, from http://whqlibdoc.who.int/hq/2002/who_nmh_nph_02.8.pdf.

Xiao, S.Y., L.F. Che, *et al.* (2007). A cost-effective flexible MEMS technique for temperature sensing. *Microelectronics Journal* **38**(3): 360–364.

Yakacki, C.M. and K. Gall. (2010). Shape-memory polymers for biomedical applications. *Shape-Memory Polymers* **226**: 147–175.

Yakacki, C.M., R. Shandas, *et al.* (2007). Unconstrained recovery characterization of shape-memory polymer networks for cardiovascular applications. *Biomaterials* **28**(14): 2255–2263.

Glossary

Allograft "a graft from an allogeneic donor of the same species as the recipient" (Dirckx, 2001).

Amphiphile a molecule with both hydrophilic and hydrophobic blocks and properties.

Aortofemoral bypass a bypass joining the abdominal aorta and the femoral arteries.

Atherosclerosis a condition in which fatty materials accumulate along the artery walls, thickening, hardening, and eventually blocking the arteries.

Autograft "tissue or an organ transferred by grafting into a new position in the body of the same individual" (Dirckx, 2001).

Biocompatibility (1) "The ability of a material to perform with an appropriate host response in a specific application." (Williams, 1987). (2) "Acceptance of an artificial implant by the surrounding tissues and by the body as a whole. The biomaterial must not be degraded by the body environment, and its presence must not harm tissues, organs, or systems. If the biomaterial is designed to be degraded, then the products of degradation should not harm the tissues and organs." (Park and Lakes, 2007).

Biodegradation A chemical process in which a long-chain polymer is cleaved in a biological environment, resulting in molecules with smaller sizes (Ratner, Hoffman, *et al.*, 2004).

Bioinert   "The capacity of a material to maintain a stable material/ tissue interface, that is, the constituent of the tissue and material neither react chemically with each other nor dissolve into each other." (Wise, 2000).

Biomaterial   (1) "A nonviable material used in the fabrication of a medical device and intended to react with biological system." (Williams, 1987). (2) "Any material used to make devices to replace a part or a function of the body in a safe, reliable, economic, and physiologically acceptable manner." (Park and Lakes, 2007).

Bioresorption (bioabsorption)   The process of a polymer and/or its degradation products being removed by the cellular activity (e.g. phagocytosis) in a physiological condition. (Ratner, Hoffman, *et al.*, 2004).

Biostability   "Ability of a biomaterial to maintain its original dimensions, and its mechanical and chemical properties during long-term implantation or exposure to a hostile biological environment." (Williams, 1987)

Biotextile   "a structure composed of textile fibers and designed for use in a specific biological environment, where its performance depends on its interactions with cells and biological fluids as measured in terms of "biocompatibility" and "biostability" (Martin and Burg, 2003).

Blood compatibility   "the property of a material or device that permits it to function in contact with blood without inducing adverse reactions." (Ratner, Hoffman, *et al.*, 2004).

Chromic (color changing) materials   materials that exhibit reversible color change upon the change of external conditions.

Chromism   the phenomenon of color change.

Chronic wound (or chronic cutaneous ulcer)   a wound that has failed to heal within a reasonable length of time (e.g. 3–4 months) (Shai and Maibach, 2005).

Coated fabric   "a flexible material composed of a fabric and any adherent polymeric material applied to one or both surfaces" (ASTM, 2008).

Coaxial electrospinning   an electrospinning process in which a special coaxial spinneret is used to fabricate bi-component nanofibers with a core/sheath structure.

Combustion or ignition temperature (T_c) the temperature at which a combustible polymer ignites when heated.

Comfort "a pleasant state of physiological, psychological and physical harmony between a human being and the environment" (Slater, 1985).

Composite material a material that is composed of two or more physical distinct components, one of which (i.e. the reinforcement) can be dispersed into the other(s) to achieve optimum properties; The final material may have superior properties to the properties of the individual components (Hull, 1981; Swanson, 1997).

Contact urticaria or the contact urticaria syndrome (CUS) the immediate inflammatory reactions that appear, usually within minutes, after contact with the eliciting substance (Marzulli, Zhai, *et al.*, 2008).

Dialysate bath for hemodialysis, a water solution of electrolytes, the concentration of which is approximately the level normal for the human blood serum.

Diaper rash (or diaper dermatitis) a term used to describe any inflammatory eruption of the skin occurring in the diaper area as a consequence of disruption of the barrier function of the fragile skin through prolonged contact with feces and urine (Atherton, 2004; Scheinfeld, 2005).

Dilation the enlargement of the grafted vessel diameter after implantation.

Disposable capable of being disposed of easily; especially designed to be thrown away after use with only negligible loss.

Edema an accumulation of an excessive amount of watery fluid in cells, tissues, or body cavities.

Electret fibers filter-forming fibers that carry an electric charge, produced by corona charging.

Electrospinning a method to produce ultra-fine (in nanometers) fibers by charging and ejecting a polymer melt or solution through a spinneret under a high-voltage electric field and to solidify or coagulate it to form a filament.

Emulation a mixture of two immiscible liquids, one of which is an aqueous solution and dispersed as microscopic or ultramicroscopic droplets throughout the other oily solution.

Emulsion electrospinning an electrospinning process in which a water-in-oil emulsion is electrospun to produce bi-component nano-fibers with a core/sheath structure.

Fabric   "a planar structure consisting of yarns or fibers" (ASTM, 2008).

Fiber   "in textiles, a generic term for any one of the various types of matter that form the basic elements of a textile and that is characterized by having a length at least 100 times its diameter" (ASTM, 2008).

Flame resistant (or flame retardant)   "the property of a material whereby flaming combustion is prevented, terminated, or inhibited following application of a flaming or nonflaming source of ignition, with or without subsequent removal of the ignition source" (ASTM, 2008).

Friction blistering   a skin problem that results from frictional forces that mechanically separate epidermal cells at the level of the stratum spinosum. The area of separation is filled with a fluid that is similar in composition to plasma but has a lower protein level (Knapik, Reynolds, *et al.*, 1995).

Glass transition temperature (T_g)   the temperature at which a polymer changes from a glassy state to a rubbery state when heated.

Granulation tissues   a tissue containing a large number of pink tiny granules, which are actually newly formed young blood vessels.

Growth factor   a naturally occurring substance (usually a protein or a steroid hormone) capable of stimulating cellular growth, proliferation and cellular differentiation.

Hemodialysis   "dialysis of soluble substances and water from the blood by diffusion through a semi-permeable membrane; separation of cellular elements and colloids from soluble substances is achieved by pore size in the membrane and rates of diffusion" (Dirckx, 2001).

Hernia   the protrusion of a structure, or a part of a structure, through the tissues normally containing it (Dirckx, 2001).

Hydrogel   a water-swollen three-dimensional network composed of physically or chemically cross-linked hydrophilic polymers (Peppas, Huang, *et al.*, 2000).

Hydrolysis   a chemical decomposition due to which a compound (e.g. polymer) is split into other compounds by reacting with water.

Immune system   in an organism, a system of cells, tissues and their products (e.g., signal molecules) that recognizes, attacks and destroys what is foreign to the body (Mak and Saunders, 2006).

Inflammation   "the reaction of vascularized living tissue to local injury" (Ratner, Hoffman, *et al.*, 2004).

Intelligent hydrogel   an intelligent material that undergoes reversible volume transformation (e.g. expansion or contraction) due to changes of environmental conditions (e.g. temperature, pH, electrical field, solvent composition, or concentration of certain chemical compounds).

Intelligent (or smart, active) textiles   textile materials and/or structures that are potentially able to sense, react and/or adapt to environmental stimuli.

In vitro   a process or reaction occurring in an artificial environment, such as in a test tube or culture medium (Dirckx, 2001).

In vivo   a process or reaction occurring in a living body (Dirckx, 2001).

Knitted fabric   "a structure produced by interlooping one or more ends of yarn or comparable materials" (ASTM, 2008).

Laminated fabric   a structure composed of at least one layer of fabric and another component like film(s), fabric(s) or foam(s). The different layers are bonded together by adhesives or the adhesive properties of one or more of the components.

Ligaments   strong and highly elastic strips of tissue that connect one bone to another.

Limiting oxygen index (LOI)   the minimum oxygen concentration that supports the combustion of a fiber material.

Manufactured fiber   any fiber that is "derived by a process of manufacture from any substance which, at any point in the manufacturing process, is not a fiber" (FTC, 1958).

Melting temperature (T_m)   when a thermoplastic polymer is heated, the temperature at which it changes from a solid to a liquid.

Microclimate   a general term that describes the temperature, humidity and micro-space air-stream between the skin and clothing (Li and Layton, 2001).

N95 respirators   a protective respirator that filters at least 95% of airborne particles but is NOT resistant to oil, according to "Respiratory Protective Devices" (42 CFR Part 84) issued by NIOSH.

Nanofiber   a fiber with a diameter less than 1 micrometer. It can be produced by different approaches including electrospinning, drawing, phase separation or self-assembly.

Natural fiber   "any fiber that exists as such in the natural state" (FTC, 1958).

Nonwoven fabric   "a textile structure produced by bonding or interlocking of fibers, or both, accomplished by mechanical, chemical, or solvent means and combinations thereof" (ASTM, 2008).

Nosocomial infection   infection acquired in healthcare facilities.

Nylon fibers   "manufactured fibers in which the fiber forming substance is any long chain synthetic polyamide in which less than 85% of the amide linkages are attached to two aromatic rings" (FTC, 1958).

Patency   the condition of being open and unobstructed, such as in blood vessels.

Phase changing material (PCM)   an intelligent material that changes its morphology (e.g., shape, porosity, solubility, state or molecular structure) upon predetermined stimuli (e.g., thermal or chemical).

Piezoelectric material   an intelligent material that generates an electric voltage when it is mechanically deformed, and conversely, with the application of an external electric field, it becomes mechanically deformed again.

Piezoresistive material   an intelligent material that changes its conductivity/resistivity upon applied mechanical stress.

Polyelectrolyte   a charged macromolecule formed in an aqueous solution by dissociation of its charged units.

Polyester fibers   "manufactured fibers in which the fiber forming substance is any long-chain polymers composed of at least 85% by weight of an ester of a substituted aromatic carboxylic acid" (FTC, 1958).

Polymer   "a macromolecular material formed by the chemical combination of monomers having either the same or different compositions" (ASTM, 2008).

Pressure garments   tightly fit garments, or gloves, masks, sleeves, orstockings that can be worn to cover part of the human body and exert pressure on a compromised skin that has healed from a burn injury (i.e., the wound is closed and able to sustain pressure).

Pressure ulcer (or bedsore, decubitus ulcer, or pressure sore)   "localized injury to the skin and/or underlying tissue usually over a bony prominence, as a result of pressure, or pressure in combination with shear" (EPUAP and NPUAP, 2009).

Proteolysis the degradation or digestion of proteins by enzymes (Bennett, 1988; Moy, Waldman, *et al.*, 1992).

Re-epithelialization in wound healing, a process of resurfacing injured tissue via the migration and proliferation of keratinocytes from the free edges of the wound.

Regulator a type of biomolecules that may promote the growth and/ or guide the differentiation of the cells in tissue engineering.

Scaffold a 3-dimensional, porous, solid biomaterial that has been developed to perform some or all of the following functions in tissue engineering to (1) provide an environment that is suitable for the cells to live and will promote cell adhesion and proliferation; (2) allow transport of gas, nutrients and regulators that are necessary for the cells to perform their functions and to proliferate; (3) biodegrade at a controllable manner; and (4) cause minimal host responses.

Secondary infection infection due to the re-suspension of entrapped pathogens from a protective mask as a result of human sneezing/ coughing and mechanical handling (Reponen, Wang, *et al.*, 1999).

Sensorial comfort the elicitation of various neural sensations when a textile comes into contact with skin. These sensations are free from pain, prickle and itch (Li and Layton, 2001).

Shape memory material an intelligent material that has the capacity to "remember" its original shape; for example, it can return to its previous shape upon exposure to a stimulus (e.g., deformation due to external stress).

Stem cells biological cells that have the capacity for proliferation and differentiation into one or more types of specialized cells, including embryonic and adult tissue stem cells.

Stratum corneum (SC) the most superficial layer of the skin that is in direct contact with the fabric. It consists of multiple layers of keratinized cells (corneocytes), which are dead cell layers originating from the underlying basal layer.

Superabsorbent polymers (SAPs) a group of cross-linked hydrophilic polymers able to absorb large volumes of water and aqueous solutions (up to hundreds of times of their original weight) in a short period of time and to retain them under a slight mechanical pressure.

Surface tension a measure of the amount of energy required to increase the surface area of a liquid by one unit.

Synthetic fiber a fiber that is composed of a polymer originating from small organic molecules via the process of polymerization to form long linear chains.

Tendon a fibrous cord or band that connects a muscle with its bony attachment (Dirckx, 2001).

Textile "a general term for fibers, yarn intermediates, yarns, fabrics, and products that retain all the strength, flexibility, and other typical properties of the original fiber or filaments" (ASTM, 2008).

Textured yarn a yarn that is endowed with significantly enhanced apparent volume, by the introduction of coils or loops into the fibers, via physical, chemical and/or heat treatments.

Thermoneutral zone the range of ambient temperature within which the basal metabolic rate of a human being is minimal and constant.

Thermophysiological comfort the attainment of a comfortable thermal and wetness state. It involves transport of heat and moisture through a fabric (Li and Layton, 2001).

Thrombosis the formation of thrombus, a fibrin clot that forms in a blood vessel or chamber of the heart.

Tissue engineering "an interdisciplinary field that applies the principles of engineering and the life sciences toward the development of biological substitutes that restore, maintain, or improve tissue function" (Langer and Vacanti, 1993).

Top-sheet (or cover, coverstock, coversheet or facing) a layer in a modern diaper (sanitary napkin, or similar disposable products) that is placed next to the skin.

Transepidermal water loss (TEWL) an insensible loss of water from the human body through the skin—specifically, a passive flux of water that takes place towards the more superficial stratum corneum layers from the deeper, highly hydrated layers of the epidermis and dermis (Agache and Humbert, 2004).

Twist "the helical or spiral configurations induced by turning a strand about its longitudinal axis" (ASTM, 2008).

Waterproof and breathable textiles textile fabrics that prevent penetration of liquid water but allow the transmission of water vapor.

Wetting the displacement of a solid-air interface with a solid-liquid interface.

Wicking   the spontaneous flow of a liquid in a porous substrate, driven by capillary forces.

Wound   "a disruption in the normal continuity of a body structure" (Shai and Maibach, 2005).

Wound care   prevention of wound complications and promotion of wound healing.

Woven fabric   "a structure produced when at least two sets of strands are interlaced, usually at right angles to each other, according to a predetermined pattern of interlacing, and such that at least one set is parallel to the axis along the lengthwise direction of the fabric" (ASTM, 2008).

Yarn   "a generic term for a continuous strand of textile fibers, filaments, or material in a form suitable for knitting, weaving, or otherwise intertwining to form a textile fabric" (ASTM, 2008).

REFERENCES

Agache, P. G. and P. Humbert (2004). *Measuring the skin: non-invasive investigations, physiology, normal constants.* Berlin; New York, Springer.

ASTM (2008). D123-07 Standard Terminology Relating to Textiles. West Conshohocken, PA, American Society for Testing and Materials.

Atherton, D. J. (2004). "A review of the pathophysiology, prevention and treatment of irritant diaper dermatitis." *Curr Med Res Opin* **20**(5): 645–9.

Bennett, R. G. (1988). "Continuing Medical-Education—Selection of Wound Closure Materials." *Journal of the American Academy of Dermatology* **18**(4): 619–640.

Dirckx, J. H. (2001). Stedman's Concise Medical Dictionary for the Health Professions: Illustrated, 4th Edition. Baltimore, Lippincott Williams & Wilkins.

EPUAP and NPUAP (2009). Treatment of pressure ulcers: Quick Reference Guide. Washington DC, European Pressure Ulcer Advisory Panel and National Pressure Ulcer Advisory Panel

FTC (1958). The Textile Fiber Products Identification Act: 15 U.S.C. § 70, Federal Trade Commission

Hull, D. (1981). *An Introduction to composite materials.* Cambridge, Cambridge University Press.

Knapik, J. J., K. L. Reynolds, *et al.* (1995). "Friction blisters. Pathophysiology, prevention and treatment." *Sports Med* **20**(3): 136–47.

Langer, R. and J. P. Vacanti (1993). "Tissue Engineering." *Science* **260**(5110): 920–926.

Li, Y. and J. M. Layton (2001). *The science of clothing comfort: a critical appreciation of recent developments.* Manchester, Textile Institute International.

Mak, T. W. and M. E. Saunders (2006). *The immune response: basic and clinical principles.* Amsterdam; Boston, Elsevier/Academic.

Martin, J. and K. J. L. Burg (2003). "Textiles and biomedical devices." *Aatcc Review* **3**(11): 41–44.

Marzulli, F. N., H. Zhai, *et al.* (2008). *Marzulli and Maibach's dermatotoxicology.* Boca Raton, CRC Press.

Moy, R. L., B. Waldman, et al. (1992). "A Review of Sutures and Suturing Techniques." *Journal of Dermatologic Surgery and Oncology* **18**(9): 785–795.

Park, J. B. and R. S. Lakes (2007). Biomaterials an introduction. New York, NY, Springer: xi, 561 p.

Peppas, N. A., Y. Huang, et al. (2000). "Physicochemical, foundations and structural design of hydrogels in medicine and biology." *Annual Review of Biomedical Engineering* **2**: 9–29.

Ratner, B. D., A. S. Hoffman, et al. (2004). Biomaterials science. *An introduction to materials in medicine.* Amsterdam; Boston, Elsevier Academic Press: xii, 851 p.

Reponen, T. A., Z. Wang, *et al.* (1999). "Survival of mycobacteria on N95 personal respirators." *Infection Control and Hospital Epidemiology* **20**(4): 237–241.

Scheinfeld, N. (2005). "Diaper dermatitis: a review and brief survey of eruptions of the diaper area." *Am J Clin Dermatol* 6(5): 273–81.

Shai, A. and H. I. Maibach (2005). *Wound Healing and Ulcers of the Skin.* Berlin, Springer.

Slater, K. (1985). *Human comfort.* Springfield, Ill., U.S.A., C.C. Thomas.

Swanson, S. R. (1997). *Introduction to design and analysis with advanced composite materials.* Upper Saddle River, N.J., Prentice Hall.

Williams, D. F. (1987). *Blood compatibility.* Boca Raton, Fla., CRC Press.

Williams, D. F. (1987). *Definitions in Biomaterials.* Proceedings of a Consensus Conference of the European Society for Biomaterials, Chester, England, Elsevier, New York.

Wise, D. L. (2000). *Biomaterials and bioengineering handbook.* New York, Marcel Dekker.

Appendix

Textile (polymeric) Materials and their Applications in the Healthcare Sector

Fiber Type		Features	Applications	Chapters
Natural fibers	Cotton	Soft, hydrophilic	Next-to-skin clothing, wound dressings	4, 8
	Wool	Highly absorbent, highly elastic, may be itchy	Clothing for cold weather	4
	Silk	Tough, biocompatible	Sutures	9
Natural regenerated/ modified fibers	Viscose rayon	Soft, highly absorbent	Wound dressings	3, 8
	Cellulose acetate/ Cuprophane	Less absorbent than other natural fibers, blood compatible	Hollow fiber bioreactors for extracorporeal devices	3, 9
	Silk fibroin	Biocompatible and bioabsorbable	Scaffolds for tissue engineering	3, 10
	Carboxymethyl cellulose (CMC)	Superabsorbent polymer	Absorbent core for disposable hygiene products, wound dressings	6, 8
Special natural fibers for medical uses	Catgut	Derived from the small intestines of sheep or cattle, collagen as the major component, low biocompatibility, bioabsorbable	Sutures	9
	Alginate	Derived from seaweed, biocompatible and bioabsorbable	Wound dressings	8
	Collagen	Biocompatible and bioabsorbable	Wound dressings, scaffolds for tissue engineering	3, 8, 10
	Gelatin	Biocompatible and bioabsorbable	Wound dressings, scaffolds for tissue engineering	3, 8, 10
	Chitin/Chitosan	Derived from crab and shrimp shells, biocompatible and bioabsorbable, antibacterial	Wound dressings, scaffolds for tissue engineering	3, 8, 10

(continued)

283

Textile (polymeric) Materials and their Applications in the Healthcare Sector (continued).

Fiber Type		Features	Applications	Chapters
Synthetic fibers	Polyester	High mechanical strength, toughness, abrasion resistance and elasticity, hydrophobic and inert	Sutures, vascular grafts, ligament prosthesis	9
	Polypropylene	Zero absorbency, inert, high wicking capacity, low static buidup	Disposable hygiene products (e.g. diapers), carpets (antistatic), sutures	6, 7, 9
	Nylon	High mechanical strength and elasticity, hydrophobic, inert	Pressure garments, sutures	9
	Acrylic	Allow modification by copolymerization	(Modacrylic) antibacterial, flame retardant products	7
	PTFE	Most inert polymer	Protective clothing (waterproof and breathable fabrics), sutures, vascular grafts, ligament prosthesis	9
	Lycra (elastic)	Highly elastic	Blended with other fibers for pressure garment, dressing retentions	8
Special synthetic fibers for medical uses	Polysulfone	Blood compatible	Hollow fiber bioreactors for extracorporeal devices	9
	Polyglycolic acid (PGA)	Biocompatible and bioabsorbable	Absorbable sutures, scaffolds for tissue engineering	3, 9, 10
	Polylactic acid (PLA)	Biocompatible and bioabsorbable	Scaffolds for tissue engineering	3, 10
	PLGA	Biocompatible and bioabsorbable	Absorbable sutures, scaffolds for tissue engineering	3, 9, 10
	PCL	Biocompatible and bioabsorbable	Scaffolds for tissue engineering	3, 10
	Polydioxanone	Biocompatible and bioabsorbable	Absorbable sutures	9

Index